USMLE S~~tep~~

1st Edition

USMLE Step 2 Review

1st Edition

975
Questions & Answers

Samuel L. Jacobs, MD
Assistant Professor
Department of Obstetrics and Gynecology
Medical College of Pennsylvania and
Hahnemann University
Philadelphia, Pennsylvania
Associate Director
Women's Fertility Institute, PC
Voorhees, New Jersey

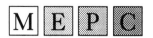

APPLETON & LANGE
Stamford, Connecticut

Copyright © 1996 by Appleton & Lange
A Simon & Schuster Company

96 97 98 99 00 / 10 9 8 7 6 5 4 3 2 1

Prentice Hall International (UK) Limited, *London*
Prentice Hall of Australia Pty. Limited, *Sydney*
Prentice Hall Canada, Inc., *Toronto*
Prentice Hall Hispanoamericana, S.A., *Mexico*
Prentice Hall of India Private Limited, *New Delhi*
Prentice Hall of Japan, Inc., *Tokyo*
Simon & Schuster Asia Pte. Ltd., *Singapore*
Editora Prentice Hall do Brasil Ltda., *Rio de Janeiro*
Prentice Hall, *Upper Saddle River, New Jersey*

ISBN 0-8385-6270-1

9 780838 562703

90000

ISSN: 1086-0959
Acquisitions Editor: Marinita Timban
Production Service: Inkwell Publishing Services
Designer: Mary Skudlarek

PRINTED IN THE UNITED STATES OF AMERICA

CONTENTS

CONTRIBUTORS

Samuel L. Jacobs, MD, FACOG
  Assistant Professor
  Department of Obstetrics and Gynecology
  Medical College of Pennsylvania and
    Hahnemann University
  Philadelphia, Pennsylvania

Carlyle Chan, MD
  Department of Psychiatry and Behavioral Medicine
  Medical College of Wisconsin
  Milwaukee, Wisconsin

Esther K. Chung, MD, MPH
  General Pediatric Fellow
  Children's Hospital of Pennsylvania
  Philadelphia, Pennsylvania

Susan V. Donelan, MD
  Assistant Professor of Clinical Medicine
  Division of Infectious Diseases
  SUNY at Stony Brook
  Stony Brook, New York

Stephan R. Glicken, MD
  Assistant Professor
  Department of Pediatrics
  New England Medical Center
  Boston, Massachusetts

William H. Greene, MD
  Associate Chief
  Division of Infectious Diseases and
    Associate Professor of Clinical Medicine
  SUNY at Stony Brook
  Stony Brook, New York

Richard H. Hart, MD, DrPh
Dean, School of Public Health
Loma Linda University
Loma Linda, California

Michael Metzler, MD
Associate Professor of Surgery
Chief, Division of General Surgery and Surgical Critical Care
University of Missouri Hospitals and Clinics
Columbia, Missouri

William Schwartz, MD
Associate Chair–Clinical Activities
Children's Hospital of Pennsylvania
Philadelphia, Pennsylvania

PREFACE

To be a competent practitioner, the modern physician has the increasing responsibility to know the most recent developments in the field of medicine. Even at the medical student level, the size of this body of knowledge is growing by leaps and bounds. In conjunction with the Federation of State Medical Boards of the United States, the National Board of Medical Examiners administers the United States Medical Licensing Examination Step 2 (USMLE Step 2) as an objective measure of these clinical sciences covered in the third and fourth years of medical education.

Formerly known as the NBME Part II, the relatively new USMLE Step 2 has been redesigned and reformatted to reflect this ever expanding knowledge base and growing emphasis on primary health care. Our intention has been to produce a comprehensive boards review textbook with the most up-to-date information and the most recent references available.

As a director of medical student education in the department of obstetrics and gynecology at Hahnemann University School of Medicine, I have had extensive exposure to the students' feelings and criticisms of the review literature available to them. Almost unanimously, they have asked for a boards text with a comprehensive "answers" section at the end of each chapter.

We have responded to their request in this review book. Each answer has been presented in a detailed, concise, and readable manner, with key words and extensive up-to-date references. All references are from only the top literature of the field and the most respected peer review journals. In addition, detailed photographs, figures, tables, and graphs have been included in the text to help clarify the material for the reader.

The scope of this review book is comprehensive and current, based on the outline of the USMLE Step 2 bulletin. This is to ensure that all topics are covered adequately and completely. A total of over 975 questions are covered in this edition. Approximately 150 questions are covered in each of the major clinical disciplines: Obstetrics and Gynecology/Women's Health Care, Pediatrics, Internal Medicine, Surgery, Psychiatry, Public Health/Preventive Medicine, and Normal Growth and Development/General Principles of Care.

We hope that medical students, as well as educators, will find this review book a welcome addition to their regular clinical textbook in the preparation for the USMLE Step 2 exam.

SAMUEL L. JACOBS, MD

1

Normal Growth and Development

Stephan R. Glicken, MD

DIRECTIONS: Each of the questions or incomplete statements below is followed by a list of suggested answers or completions. Select the **one** that is best in each case.

1. The stage of adolescent development classified as "midadolescence" is characterized by all of the following **EXCEPT**
   A. strong peer group alliance
   B. Tanner stage IV development
   C. egocentrism
   D. full physical maturity
   E. dating behavior

2. A 16-year-old young woman comes to you because she is worried about pregnancy. She does not want you to share this information with her parents who have been physically abusive in the past. You should
   A. refuse to perform a pregnancy test without parental consent because she is not emancipated
   B. agree to examine and counsel her because you feel she is an emancipated minor
   C. explain that your only option is to inform her parents because she is covered by their insurance
   D. suggest she buy and use a home pregnancy test
   E. refer her directly to an obstetrician

3. The highest incidence of completed suicide among 15- to 19-year-old Americans occurs among
   A. Asian males
   B. white males
   C. white females
   D. African-American males
   E. African-American females

4. Risk factors for completed adolescent suicide involve all the following **EXCEPT**
   A. depression
   B. prior attempt
   C. family history of suicide
   D. substance abuse
   E. exposure to music with suggestive lyrics

5. Which of the following public health measures would **MOST LIKELY** reduce the rate of adolescent suicide?
   A. Gun control laws
   B. Suicide hot lines for teenagers
   C. Reduced toxicity of sedative drugs
   D. Screening questionnaires in high school
   E. Limiting sensational publicity

6. Which of the following DSM-III R diagnostic criteria is **NOT** essential for the diagnosis of bulimia nervosa?
   A. Recurrent episodes of binge eating
   B. Minimum average of 2 binges per week for at least 3 months

    C. Feeling of lack of control over eating behavior
    D. Self-induced vomiting
    E. Persistent overconcern with body weight and shape

7. Newly published AMA Guidelines for Adolescent Preventive Services (GAPS) recommend that all adolescents have
    A. clinician visits at 12–15 and 16–18 years of age
    B. annual physical examinations
    C. annual preventive health care visits
    D. HIV testing at least once in late adolescence
    E. routine urine drug screening

8. Treatment of attention deficit (ADD) might reasonably include any of the following **EXCEPT**
    A. methylphenidate (Ritalin)
    B. environmental manipulation
    C. pemoline
    D. hypoallergenic diet
    E. amphetamines

9. Which is **TRUE** about ADD?
    A. Treatment is indicated only when it causes significant problems for the child or peers
    B. It clearly involves cerebral dysfunction
    C. Its characteristic behaviors are clearly different from normal
    D. Methylphenidate (Ritalin) acts specifically on ADD children in a way different from normal peers
    E. It is rarely seen after 9 years of age

10. In annual surveys, about what percentage of male high school seniors report drinking five or more alcoholic beverages in a row during the preceding two weeks?
    A. 10%
    B. 25%
    C. 45%
    D. 65%
    E. 90%

11. Routine indications for pelvic examination in an adolescent include all the following **EXCEPT**
    A. menstrual cramps
    B. sexual activity
    C. pregnancy
    D. vaginal discharge
    E. lower abdominal pain

12. Primary amenorrhea refers to the absence of menstruation by age
    A. 11.0 years
    B. 12.5 years
    C. 13.0 years
    D. 16.0 years
    E. 18.0 years

13. The first sign of puberty in males is **USUALLY**
    A. lengthening of the phallus
    B. appearance of pubic hair
    C. growth spurt
    D. deepening of the voice
    E. enlargement of the testes

14. A very short child with an elevated weight-to-height ratio has a bone age (epiphyseal maturation) 4 standard deviations below the chronologic age. You are **MOST** concerned about
    A. chronic malabsorption
    B. endocrine abnormalities
    C. familial microsomia
    D. hyperthyroidism
    E. wasting

15. Approximately what percentage of teenage girls who become pregnant carry their pregnancies to term?
    A. 10%
    B. 20%
    C. 30%
    D. 40%
    E. 50%

16. In familial short stature
   A. height and weight fall off simultaneously around 9 months of age
   B. head circumference is proportional to height
   C. final height can be predicted at the time of birth
   D. triceps skin folds will be greater than normal
   E. bone age is usually depressed

17. Failure to thrive may be seen in situations where a parent does not perceive the hunger of the child and respond appropriately. Which of the following does **NOT** illustrate this?
   A. Parental retardation
   B. Parental psychopathy
   C. Parental depression
   D. Parental poverty
   E. Parental psychosis

18. A child starved in a third-world country over a prolonged period stops his linear growth. Upon refeeding, he regains a normal weight-to-height ratio but has a low height for his age and a depressed bone age. This represents
   A. stunting
   B. malabsorption
   C. depression
   D. wasting
   E. retardation

19. The standard measure of overall intelligence in a 4-year-old child is achieved with the
   A. Revised Denver Developmental Screening Test
   B. Wide Range Aptitude Test (WRAT)
   C. Wechsler Preschool and Primary Scale of Intelligence (WPPSI)
   D. Wechsler Intelligence Scale for Children (WISC)
   E. Kaufmann Assessment Battery for Children

20. Which of the following is **NOT** an effective safety measure for homes with small children?
   A. Fencing in a backyard that has a swimming pool in it
   B. Safety proof caps on all medications
   C. Reducing the hot water temperature to 125°
   D. Placing bars in stairway windows to prevent young children from climbing out
   E. Removing all handguns from the home

21. Which of the following conditions is the leading cause of death for American children over the age of one year?
   A. Bacterial infection
   B. Motor vehicle accidents
   C. Suicide
   D. AIDS
   E. Leukemia

22. When can children safely graduate from specially designed car seats to adult lap/shoulder belts with a booster seat?
   A. At 1 year of age
   B. At 25 lb
   C. At 40 lb
   D. At 3 years old
   E. At 55 lb

23. Typical injuries for children during ages 5 to 9 include all of the following **EXCEPT**
   A. bicycle accidents
   B. drowning
   C. car accidents
   D. choking
   E. burns

24. Which of the following is **TRUE** about the racial breakdown of adolescent (15- to 19-year-old) mortality statistics?
   A. Suicide is the most common cause of death among white teenagers
   B. The suicide rate for African-American teenagers is twice as common as for white teenagers
   C. White teenagers are twice as likely as African-American teenagers to die from accidents

    D. Homicides occur equally among African-American and white teenagers

    E. Alcohol is uncommonly associated with accidental deaths in either group

25. Overall, the age group with the highest risk of death from injury is
   A. less than 1 year old
   B. 1 to 4 years old
   C. 5 to 9 years old
   D. 10 to 14 years old
   E. 15 to 24 years old

26. At 4 months of age, most children play with their hands and learn to grasp objects. This is an example of
   A. separation from the mother
   B. discovery of the relation between sight and touch
   C. use of recall memory
   D. initial ability to comprehend reality on a symbolic basis
   E. "clumsiness" seen as new muscles are coordinated in the acquisition of new skills

27. At 8 months of age, drooling is an example of
   A. separation anxiety
   B. discovery of the relation between sight and touch
   C. use of recognition memory
   D. initial ability to comprehend reality on a symbolic basis
   E. "clumsiness" seen as new muscles are coordinated in the acquisition of the new skill of syllable repetition

28. When children first begin to attach meaning to their utterance of repeated syllables, this indicates
   A. separation from the mother
   B. discovery of the relation between sight and touch
   C. use of recognition memory
   D. initial ability to comprehend reality on a symbolic basis
   E. "clumsiness" seen as new muscles are coordinated in the acquisition of new skills

29. When a child cries because her mother has left the room, this illustrates which stage?
    A. Fear of punishment
    B. Discovery of the relation between sight and touch
    C. Use of recall memory
    D. Inability to comprehend reality on a symbolic basis
    E. "Clumsiness" seen as new muscles are coordinated in the acquisition of new skills

30. When a child is born, visually s/he will show preference for all the following **EXCEPT**
    A. round objects
    B. slowly moving objects
    C. faces
    D. near objects
    E. brown objects

31. The tendency of a 2-month-old child to show calming at the presence of a particular person indicates the presence of
    A. bonding
    B. stranger anxiety
    C. poor discipline
    D. object permanence
    E. recall memory

32. The average American newborn male is what size?
    A. Weight 2 kg, height 50 cm, head circumference 35 cm
    B. Weight 2.5 kg, height 55 cm, head circumference 40 cm
    C. Weight 3.5 kg, height 60 cm, head circumference 35 cm
    D. Weight 3.5 kg, height 50 cm, head circumference 35 cm
    E. Weight 4 kg, height 45 cm, head circumference 35 cm

Questions 33–37 all refer to developmental milestones. Pick the age that **BEST** fits the descriptive phrase.

    A. 3–6 months
    B. 8–12 months
    C. 12–16 months
    D. 18–24 months
    E. 24–30 months

33. The Babinski response, normally present at birth, disappears

34. The Moro response disappears

35. The first few intelligible words appear

36. Separation anxiety becomes marked

37. Walking normally begins

Questions 38–46 all refer to developmental milestones. Pick the age that **BEST** fits the descriptive phrase.

    A. 0–18 months
    B. 18–36 months
    C. 3–6 years
    D. 6–11 years
    E. 12–17 years
    F. 17–30 years
    G. 30–60 years
    H. 60+ years

38. Eriksonian period of generativity vs. stagnation

39. Freudian anal period

40. Piagetian sensorimotor period

41. Upper limit for normal menarche

42. Most common appearance of schizophrenia

43. Piagetian formal operational period begins

44. Full command of English grammar

45. Understanding of first words

46. Magical thinking

47. The pubertal height growth spurt occurs at approximately what ages?
    A. Female 11, male 13
    B. Female 10, male 14.5
    C. Female 12, male 13
    D. Female 11.5, male 11
    E. Female 10, male 12.5

48. Peak growth rate in males during puberty occurs at what age?
    A. 11 years
    B. 12 years
    C. 13 years
    D. 14 years
    E. 15 years

49. Peak growth rate in females during puberty occurs at what age?
    A. 11 years
    B. 12 years
    C. 13 years
    D. 14 years
    E. 15 years

50. The first event in male puberty is
    A. testicular enlargement
    B. growth spurt
    C. gynecomastia
    D. nocturnal emission
    E. loss of body fat

Questions 51–55 all refer to stages of adolescent development. Match the phrases with the **MOST APPROPRIATE** stage.

    A. Early adolescence
    B. Midadolescence
    C. Late adolescence
    D. None of the above

51. Most rapid rate of growth

52. Dating intimacy

53. Bonding with same sex peers

54. Rise of abstract thinking

55. Career planning

56. Gender identity is generally solidified by what age?
  A. 2 years
  B. 5 years
  C. 9 years
  D. 13 years
  E. 17 years

57. In working with teenagers it is common for young, recently trained physicians to
  A. be seen as someone who can't understand teenagers' problems
  B. carry their own parenting conflicts into a countertransference
  C. foster dependency
  D. make parents defensive about their authority roles
  E. overidentify with the parents in family conflicts

58. Which of the following is **TRUE** of developmental dyslexia?
  A. It is a rare form of isolated learning disorder
  B. The boy-to-girl ratio is approximately equal
  C. There is a strong family history in about one-third of cases
  D. Delays in speech and language development are seen in 80% of cases
  E. Neurologic investigations frequently reveal associated deficits

59. Which of the following is **TRUE** of attention deficit hyperactivity disorder (ADHD)?
  A. The diagnosis is often made in conjunction with a diagnosis of childhood psychosis
  B. Associated learning problems are generally extremely rare
  C. Children with ADHD, while abnormal at home, may exhibit totally normal behavior in the closed environment of the school
  D. 25% of affected children will respond positively to a regimen of stimulant medication
  E. Many parents of these children will report distractibility and hyperactivity in the preschool years

Questions 60–64: Match the age group with the typical developmental anxiety associated with that period of life.

    A. Early infancy
    B. 1 year
    C. 2–6 years
    D. School age
    E. Adolescent to adult

60. Fear of loss of loved one

61. Fear of sudden loud noises or unpredictable stimuli

62. Fear of failure and concern about social acceptance

63. Fear of dark and imaginary creatures

64. Separation distress

65. Which of the following is **TRUE** of autistic individuals?
    A. One of the best prognostic factors will be the development of significant symbolic language skills by age 5 years
    B. Autism has not convincingly been linked to other significant neurologic dysfunctions
    C. Most have normal intelligence despite bizarre behaviors
    D. Most affected individuals will eventually outgrow their disorder and become relatively functional adults
    E. The onset may not be recognized until a child enters the school years

66. What percentage of people over age 85 reside in nursing homes?
    A. 10%
    B. 20%
    C. 30%
    D. 40%
    E. 50%

67. Which of the following is **NOT** an age-related physiologic change in the central nervous system?
    A. Brain atrophy leading to senescent forgetfulness
    B. Decreased brain dopamine synthesis leading to stiff gait

C. Decreased righting reflex leading to body sway
D. Decreased catecholamine synthesis leading to frank depression
E. Drop in stage IV sleep leading to insomnia

68. The normal changes in body systems associated with aging may result in what effects?
A. The decrease in body fat results in decreased volume of distribution for fat-soluble drugs and increased toxicity
B. Increased colonic motility results in diarrhea
C. Urethral mucosal atrophy leads to bacteriuria
D. The increase in total body water results in increased volume of distribution for water-soluble drugs and need for increased dosage
E. Increased vitamin D absorption may lead to hypercalcemia

69. Which of the following is **TRUE** of dementia?
A. It affects 25% of people over 65 years old
B. 60–70% of the cases are due to Alzheimer disease
C. Benign senescent forgetfulness often leads to Alzheimer disease
D. Alzheimer disease may be slowed by treatment with aspirin
E. Multiinfarct dementia is associated with hypotensive episodes that cause ischemia

70. Which of the following is **NOT TRUE** regarding the appearance of pathologic symptoms in elderly patients?
A. The organ system most commonly associated with a given symptom is less likely statistically to be the cause of that symptom in an elderly patient
B. Because of changes in compensatory systems, disease in elderly patients often presents later in the course than with younger patients
C. Because many homeostatic mechanisms are compromised, there is usually a single abnormality amenable to treatment
D. Because elderly people are more likely than the young to suffer disease, they are less likely to benefit from therapy
E. Findings that are abnormal in younger patients, when they occur in the elderly, should be assumed to be the cause of presenting symptoms

Questions 71–74: Match the following stages in the accommodation of people to their deaths with the appropriate statements.

    A. Denial
    B. Anger
    C. Bargaining
    D. Depression
    E. Acceptance

71. A 73-year-old patient goes to her fifth alternative medical care practitioner for advice on controlling her metastatic breast cancer, sure that an alternative diagnosis can be found

72. A 17-year-old boy with end-stage inoperable astrocytoma requests visits from favorite friends and relatives and begins calmly giving away his favorite possessions to them

73. A 47-year-old man whose wife has malignant melanoma unpredictably tries to fire her family practitioner whom he blames for her rapidly downhill course

74. A 21-year-old college senior begs his physician to find a treatment that will allow him to graduate college, so that he can die with a sense of achievement

75. Various muscle training and other exercises in the elderly
    A. are dangerous and can lead to serious injury
    B. may cause osteopenia
    C. are useful in preventing falls
    D. may worsen postural hypotension
    E. aggravate their common vestibular dysfunction

Questions 76–83: Match the appropriate approximate age in children with the correct milestone of language development.

    A. 4 months
    B. 10 months
    C. 1 year
    D. 18–24 months
    E. 2 years

76. Understandable two word phrases

77. Use of pronouns

78. First consonantal sounds

79. All vowels correct

80. Repetitive syllables (e.g., baba, lala, dada)

81. Begins use of personal "jargon"

82. First word other than "Mama, Dada"

83. Two-word phrases

Questions 84–90: Match the appropriate approximate age in children with the correct milestone of visual-motor development.

    A. 1–2 months
    B. 3–5 months
    C. 6–8 months
    D. 9–11 months
    E. 12 months
    F. 18 months
    G. 24 months
    H. 3 years

84. Can throw a ball

85. Grasps and brings objects to mouth

86. Copies a circle in imitation

87. Sits alone briefly

88. Puts a garment on

89. Follows objects through visual field

90. Imitates patty cake

91. Which of the following is **TRUE** about growth?
   A. Newborns lose up to 20% of their birth weight in the first few days of life
   B. Fetal weight growth slows down during the last two months of intrauterine life
   C. By 1 year of age children should weigh twice their birth weight
   D. Energy requirements for growth rise during the second year of life
   E. Genetic factors influencing height manifest after 6 months of age

92. Physical development of the nervous system shows what characteristics?
   A. At birth, head circumference is half the adult size
   B. Myelinization of the brain precedes that of the spinal cord *in utero*
   C. Cranial nerves 3–12 are well myelinated at birth
   D. The autonomic system is poorly matured at birth
   E. The cerebellum is the earliest part of the gray matter to develop

93. Which of the following is **TRUE** about child abuse?
   A. Prolonged separation from the mother due to neonatal illness is associated with increased incidence of abuse
   B. A large proportion of perpetrators of child abuse are strangers to the child
   C. Less than 1% of American children are estimated to have been abused annually
   D. Physical neglect is often directly attributable to inadequate family income
   E. The most common manifestation of significant emotional neglect in infancy is endogenous depression

94. Which of the following radiologic findings is **NOT** typical of child abuse?
   A. Metaphysial or "bucket handle" fractures
   B. Posterior rib fractures
   C. Spiral fractures of long bones in toddlers
   D. Subdural hematomas
   E. Fractures of two different ages

95. Drug use is common among children and teenagers. Which of the following statements is correct regarding drug usage?
  A. Many more eighth graders are smoking alcohol than using marijuana
  B. The use of cocaine is steadily rising among high school seniors
  C. The use of alcohol in high school seniors is occasional—less than 20% report using it during the past month
  D. Less than 20% of high school seniors smoke cigarettes daily
  E. Substance abuse is always caused by, but never is the cause of, family dysfunction

96. Which of the following statements about sexual activity and contraception among teenagers is **NOT TRUE**?
  A. Sexually active adolescent females wait about one year before seeking contraception
  B. Half of teenage pregnancies in the United States occur within six months of initiation of sexual activity
  C. Homosexual teenagers often "act out" by engaging in excessive heterosexual activity
  D. The polyurethane vaginal pouch or "female condom" is no more effective than regular condoms in preventing pregnancy and STDs
  E. The regulation of menses into predictable cycles makes subdermal contraceptive implants particularly attractive for teenagers

97. Criteria for diagnosis of anorexia nervosa include all the following **EXCEPT**
  A. weight at least 15% below that expected for age and height
  B. fear of weight gain or obesity
  C. female sex
  D. interruption of menses for at least 3 months
  E. delusion of being obese despite inanition

98. Children at about 6 months of age exhibit the mental milestone of "object permanence." This represents
   A. a belief by the child that the mother is always present
   B. the ability to hold a mental image of an object in the mind after its disappearance, and the ability to anticipate its reappearance
   C. the beginnings of separation and individuation in which the child is able to protest, or object to, unwanted stimuli
   D. children's ability to control their physical grasp of objects and alternately flex and release muscles of finger flexion
   E. visible signs of fear in a child of new faces or environments

99. In Piaget's period of concrete mental operations
   A. children become more cognizant of rules and cause and effect in general
   B. boys are more advanced than girls in academic pursuits
   C. children welcome differences in their peers and expand their social groups
   D. children are usually fraught with anxiety over their abilities
   E. thought processes are not yet logical and coherent

100. Primary caregiver dysfunction refers to situations where proper parenting is not provided due to parental vulnerability or disability. Signs and symptoms suggestive of this include all the following **EXCEPT**
   A. sleep disorders
   B. physical neglect
   C. frequent, nonspecific medical visits
   D. feeding problems
   E. abnormally rapid development

Normal Growth and Development

Answer Key

1. D	26. B	51. A	76. D
2. B	27. E	52. C	77. E
3. A	28. D	53. A	78. A
4. E	29. C	54. B	79. E
5. A	30. E	55. C	80. B
6. D	31. A	56. A	81. C
7. A	32. D	57. D	82. C
8. D	33. C	58. C	83. D
9. A	34. A	59. E	84. F
10. C	35. D	60. D	85. B
11. A	36. B	61. A	86. H
12. D	37. C	62. E	87. C
13. E	38. G	63. C	88. G
14. B	39. B	64. B	89. A
15. E	40. A	65. A	90. D
16. A	41. E	66. B	91. E
17. D	42. F	67. D	92. C
18. A	43. E	68. C	93. A
19. C	44. C	69. B	94. C
20. A	45. A	70. A	95. D
21. B	46. C	71. A	96. E
22. C	47. A	72. E	97. C
23. D	48. D	73. B	98. B
24. C	49. B	74. C	99. A
25. E	50. A	75. C	100. E

Normal Growth and Development

Answers and Comments

1. **(D)** Midadolescents strongly identify and use as a reference the feelings and current concerns of their peer group. They often feel invincible as they reflect on their own existence as individuals. Dating generally begins in this period, but full maturity is achieved in late adolescence. (**Ref. 2**, pp. 96–98)

2. **(B)** In general, a contract for confidentiality must be set up with the family prior to the adolescent's seeing the doctor alone. In many states, issues regarding sexually transmitted disease and pregnancy are confidential issues by statute, or may remain so in cases of mature minors when revelation may put the adolescent at risk of physical or emotional injury. This varies by locale. (**Ref. 2**, pp. 87–94)

3. **(A)** Asian and Native Americans have a higher rate of suicide than the general population. Males have three to four times the risk of females of completed suicide, while female attempts are much more common. (**Ref. 1**, p. 526)

4. **(E)** Suicide risk is greatest in older adolescent boys with the histories noted. There is little if any evidence to suggest that exposure to popular entertainment has any effect on suicidal behavior. (**Ref. 2**, pp. 183–185)

5. **(A)** Most successfully completed adolescent suicides involve firearms, generally obtained in the home. Poisonings are common, yet gestures outnumber completed suicides by as much as 200:1. Questionnaires are of dubious value, and publicity is probably associated with transient rises in suicidal gestures. (**Ref. 1**, p. 526)

6. **(D)** Self-induced vomiting, while common, is *not* essential for the diagnosis of bulimia. What is essential is the presence of an eating disorder characterized by uncontrollable bouts of binging as described. (**Ref. 4**, pp. 67–68)

7. **(A)** Current AMA recommendations are for physical assessments twice during the adolescent years. HIV testing is recommended on an as-needed basis and drug screening only in cases involving legal or psychiatric problems where the adolescent consents to the procedure. (**Ref. 5**, pp. 1–11)

8. **(D)** All stimulant medications have been shown to be effective in alleviating symptoms in up to 70% of children with ADD. Environmental manipulation in the classroom is useful. More questionable is behavior modification. Dietary management has been a recurrent fad, but has proven effective only in extremely rare situations. (**Ref. 2**, pp. 150–152)

9. **(A)** ADD has effects that persist through adulthood. The etiology is still debated, and all its characteristics may be seen in normal people some of the time. There is no evidence that the effect of methylphenidate is specific for any group. (**Ref. 2**, pp. 150–152, 188–189)

10. **(C)** Reports of research conducted by the University of Michigan Institute for Social Research have shown that 43.5% of male and 30.4% of female high school students report heavy drinking during the previous month. Overall, 44% of seniors report this behavior. Even more depressing, 50% of ninth graders have used alcohol in the past month and 27.7% report drinking heavily. (**Ref. 6**, September 18, 1992, pp. 698–703; November 15, 1991, pp. 776–777, 783–789)

11. **(A)** Generally, dysmenorrhea can be managed by the use of NSAIDs such as ibuprofen or naproxen sodium. If these fail or if

pain is severe, pelvic examination may be indicated. Screening for STDs, evaluation of lower abdominal pain, evaluation of pathological discharges, and evaluation of extent of pregnancy are also reasonable indications. Some advocate routine pelvic exam at 16 years for Papanicolau smear if one has never been performed. (**Ref. 2,** pp. 117–119)

12. (**D**)   In the presence of normal secondary sexual characteristics, primary amenorrhea is the absence of any menses by age sixteen. Causes include anatomic abnormalities, endocrine deficiencies, and enzyme defects. (**Ref. 2,** 113–117)

13. (**E**)   Under the influence of LH and FSH, the testes are the first target organs to visibly respond. Early pubic hair development follows, with growth spurt occuring relatively later in boys, followed by voice changes and shaft lengthening. (**Ref. 2,** pp. 94–96)

14. (**B**)   While severe nutritional deficiency can result in delays in the bone age, these are all characterized by markedly low weight-to-height ratios. Hyperthyroidism results in advances in the bone age. Familial microsomia may cause a slightly delayed bone age, but weight-to-height ratio is normal. Endocrine deficiencies, especially growth hormone (HGH), cause the most severe distortions. (**Ref. 2,** pp. 881–885)

15. (**E**)   More than 1 million teenage pregnancies occur yearly in the United States. Of these, 40% result in abortion, 13% in miscarriage, and 47% in live births. Almost half of 15- to 19-year-old girls are sexually active and over one-third will become pregnant within two years of onset of sexual activity. (**Ref. 2,** pp. 125–126)

16. (**A**)   Familial or constitutional short stature is characterized by slower than normal rate of growth in the first year of life. Body proportions are normal and at least one parent is usually short. They usually have normal body fat and bone age. (**Ref. 2,** pp. 881–885)

17. (**D**)   Poverty does not affect the ability of a parent to care for a child adequately in any but the most severe circumstances. Mental health problems, especially depression may prevent proper responses to a child's needs, as can psychopathy, retardation, or psychosis. (**Ref. 2,** pp. 881–885)

18. **(A)** Prolonged starvation results in inhibition of epiphyseal growth. With adequate refeeding, the loss of fat and muscle tissue reverses, but bone growth will continue to lag. Wasting refers to the primary loss of fat and muscle tissue with undernutrition, and causes the drop in weight-to-height ratio. Depression and retardation may lead to undernutrition, but have no distinct effect on bone age. **(Ref. 2,** pp. 881–885)

19. **(C)** The Denver Test is a crude screening tool used to help decide whether further evaluation is necessary. The WRAT and WISC are appropriate tools for reading, school-age children. The Kaufman Battery measures specific, narrowly defined skills. **(Ref. 2,** pp. 136–139)

20. **(A)** Most pool drownings and accidental handgun fatalities occur on the child's own home property. Safety caps have reduced poisonings by 75–90%. Lowering water heater temperatures will prevent full-thickness scalds. Window bars effectively prevent falls. **(Ref. 7,** pp. 697–712)

21. **(B)** Accidents in general and motor vehicle accidents specifically far outnumber all other causes of death after the first year of life. In teenagers as a special subgroup, suicide and homicide together are about as common as motor vehicle accidents. **(Ref. 7,** pp. 697–712)

22. **(C)** The general guidelines depend mainly on weight. At 20 lb, children may sit facing the front of a car. Above 60 lb, they may use an adult lap-belt alone. At 60 lb and a height over 48 in., they use a lap/shoulder belt on the normal seat of the car. **(Ref. 2,** pp. 284–286)

23. **(D)** All those listed are typical except that choking rarely occurs after 4 years of age. It is the most common cause of accidental death in the home for children approximately 2 years of age. **(Ref. 2,** pp. 284–286)

24. **(C)** Unintentional injury is the most common cause of death for white teenagers. Suicide and motor vehicle accidents are much more common for white than African-American adolescents. All mortality due to trauma is strongly correlated with alcohol use;

about one-third of teenage drivers involved in fatal accidents have been drinking. (**Ref. 2,** pp. 85–87)

25. (**E**)   Above 1 year of age, accidents are the leading cause of death in all age groups. There are two peaks, in the 1- to 4-year-old group and in the 15- to 24-year-old group. But the older group has a mortality rate over twice as high. (**Ref. 1,** pp. 148–149)

26. (**B**)   At 4 months of age, myelinization has progressed to the point that conscious control of the hands is achieved easily. Infants spend considerable time studying their hands and learning relationships between proprioception, vision, and touch. Recall memory later allows them to recognize what is real and present in the environment but not to refine early motor skills. They are clumsy at this stage, but this is not relevant to the question. (**Ref. 2,** pp. 65–75)

27. (**E**)   At 8 months, babies have a high state of separation anxiety, but this is reflected in their responses to environment. Recognition memory is present probably from birth and represents the ability to respond to familiar stimuli. Symbolic thinking is important to language development: the motor correlate is the learning of fine control of the anterior structures of the mouth. (**Ref. 2,** pp. 65–78)

28. (**D**)   With the advent of recall memory, infants can use signifiers of a mental reality as tools to manipulate mental images and later to influence the behavior of others. "Baby talk" is connected with the ability to control the vocal apparatus in repeating syllables containing consonant sounds, then applying meaning to them through symbolic thinking and recall. (**Ref. 2,** pp. 65–78)

29. (**C**)   With recall memory, a child can create or bring up a mental image of an environment, then realize how that image compares with a current situation. Anxiety is produced when a desired object is perceived to be missing from the real environment. It is connected with symbolic thinking. (**Ref. 2,** pp. 65–78)

30. (**E**)   Infants are born with vision in approximately the 20/400 range, possibly due to lack of compliance of their lenses. They see best objects about 16 in. from their faces. They prefer patterns, faces, red or brightly colored objects and those in motion. (**Ref. 2,** pp. 65–66)

31. (A) Children quickly learn the sound, smell, and sight of their parents. With a good, normal relationship, their positive associations with the parents' presence leads to positive responses to their presence, or "bonding." Object permanence occurs with recall memory, when children will retain a mental image of an object that has temporarily left their field of perception. Stranger anxiety appears much later than bonding. (**Ref. 2,** pp. 17–18, 65–75)

32. (D) A useful mnemonic is that head circumference (HC) and length (L) are related by HC = L/2 + 10 cm. Average weight for white children is 3.5 kg. African-American children are smaller. Birth size generally has little relationship to parental size. (**Ref. 2,** pp. 9–14, 68–74)

33. (C) (**Ref. 2,** pp. 69–74)

34. (A) (**Ref. 2,** pp. 69–74)

35. (D) (**Ref. 2,** pp. 76–78)

36. (B) (**Ref. 2,** pp. 67–68, 154–155)

37. (C) (**Ref. 2,** pp. 80–82)

38. (G) (**Ref. 2,** p. 67)

39. (B) (**Ref. 2,** pp. 66–68)

40. (A) (**Ref. 2,** pp. 66–68)

41. (E) (**Ref. 2,** pp. 82–83, 112–117)

42. (F) (**Ref. 2,** pp. 67, 169–170)

43. (E) (**Ref. 2,** p. 67)

44. (C) (**Ref. 2,** pp. 76–79)

45. (A) (**Ref. 2,** pp. 76–79)

46. (C) (**Ref. 2,** pp. 76–79)

47. (A) Girls begin their growth spurts about two years earlier than boys. Their growth spurt is also shorter, lasting about three years for girls, as opposed to four years for boys. (**Ref. 2,** pp. 94–96)

48. (D) Boys' peak growth rate occurs around 14 years of age. At that age they are growing at approximately 4 in./year (9.5 cm/year ± 1.5 cm). (**Ref. 2,** pp. 94–96)

49. (B) Girls' growth peaks around 12 years of age, when they are growing at about 3 in./year (8.3 cm/year ± 1.2 cm). (**Ref. 2,** pp. 94–96)

50. (A) The normal order for male puberty, with some variation is testicular enlargement, pubarche, growth spurt, penile enlargement, loss of body fat, and nocturnal emission. Gynecomastia may occur at any time and is not considered a pubertal milestone. (**Ref. 2,** pp. 94–96)

51. (A) (**Ref. 2,** pp. 96–98)

52. (C) (**Ref. 2,** pp. 96–98)

53. (A) (**Ref. 2,** pp. 96–98)

54. (B) (**Ref. 2,** pp. 96–98)

55. (C) (**Ref. 2,** pp. 96–98)

56. (A) By age 5 or 6, a definite sense of personal masculinity or femininity is established. In latency, most children are aware of feelings of "crushes" but generally don't act on them sexually until the teen years. But the sense of oneself as male or female antedates all the other sexual identity milestones. Sexual preference and orientation are not defined until later, probably after the teenager reaches the formal operational stage and can think of him- or herself abstractly within the larger social context. (**Ref. 2,** pp. 97–98)

57. (D) Teenagers are notorious for their ability to sense the vulnerabilities of authority figures. Older physicians who themselves have teenagers may overidentify with parents' perspectives in family conflicts and thereby lose credibility in the eyes of adolescent patients. Because of the realities of the adolescent years, fostering dependency is rarely achieved. Young physicians often go to extremes in seeing the teenager's perspective and thereby make the parents uncomfortable with their roles. (**Ref. 2,** pp. 87–94)

58. **(C)** Dyslexia is the most common specific learning disorder. It is much more common in boys (3:1) and in 34% of cases there is a strong family history, especially among male relatives. Specific neurologic problems are found only occasionally. Speech and language delays are seen in one-third of cases. (**Ref. 2,** pp. 141–145)

59. **(E)** With an onset before 7 years of age, ADHD is found in children with at least a 6-month history of distractibility, short attention span, hyperactivity, and impulsivity, which often can be traced back to the preschool years. It may be associated with aggressive behavior, but psychosis effectively eliminates the diagnosis. Associated learning problems are common, and normal behavior at school, where attention is critical, rules out the diagnosis. Fifty to eighty percent of affected children respond well to medical management, though counseling is almost always recommended for the associated behavioral and emotional problems. (**Ref. 2,** pp. 150–152, 172–174)

60. **(D)** (**Ref. 2,** pp. 154–166)

61. **(A)** (**Ref. 2,** pp. 154–166)

62. **(E)** (**Ref. 2,** pp. 154–166)

63. **(C)** (**Ref. 2,** pp. 154–166)

64. **(B)** (**Ref. 2,** pp. 154–166)

65. **(A)** Autism is a pervasive developmental disorder usually evident in infancy or very early childhood. About three-quarters of these children are measurably retarded. The disorder is lifelong, though one-sixth may become independent adults and another sixth can function in sheltered environments. About 25% develop seizure disorders, and there are frequently other inherited or perinatally acquired disorders affecting brain development. (**Ref. 2,** pp. 168–169)

66. (B) The majority of the extreme elderly in the United States live without any significant impairment. Only one-third have a serious problem with any particular activity of daily living. Life expectancy for persons 85 years of age is currently six years, and 80% live on their own without need for extended nursing care. (**Ref. 3,** pp. 30–32, 47–48)

67. (D) Depression is always considered pathological and is not a consequence of normal aging. Changes in the cerebellum can lead to body sway, but falls usually are the result of several problems acting in concert, such as body sway with weakness and poor vision. Similarly, movements may stiffen, but Parkinsonism is always considered pathological. (**Ref. 3,** pp. 36–40)

68. (C) Mucosal atrophy can also lead to dyspareunia. Older people develop increased body fat and decreased total body water, causing the opposite effects from those noted above. They have decreased vitamin D absorption and metabolism, which contributes to osteopenia. Constipation is commonly seen which results from diminution in colonic and anorectal function. (**Ref. 3,** pp. 30–35)

69. (B) Dementia is an acquired persistent and progressive impairment of intellectual function with compromise in at least two areas among the following: language, memory, visual-spatial skills, emotional behavior, and cognition. It affects 5–10% of people over 65, but the prevalence rises as people age to perhaps 47% for those over 85. Fifteen to twenty percent are vascular and another 15–20% are mixed Alzheimer-vascular. Multiinfarct dementia may be slowed by use of antihypertensives, smoking cessation, aspirin, and treatment of arrhythmias. (**Ref. 3,** pp. 36–40)

70. (A) Uncommon causes of particular symptoms are more likely to be found in elderly patients, and practitioners should not be lulled into accepting common causes too quickly. Similarly, symptoms often have multiple causes, and treatment of all causes often produces appreciable results. Disease presentations are often early in the elderly because of the effects on body homeostasis of even minor abnormalities. (**Ref. 3,** pp. 30–32)

71. (A); 72. (E); 73. (B); 74. (C) Since Elizabeth Kuebler-Ross first proposed them, the "stages of death" have become part of a common medical vocabulary. Not all patients go through all five stages, nor do all experience them in the same order. Family members and loved ones go through similar progressions, but are often at different stages, which can lead to severe friction and emotional problems. Often, patients with strong moral or religious beliefs will make the best accommodations to the process. (**Ref. 3,** pp. 308, 346–347, 938–939)

75. (**C**) Carefully planned exercise programs, including range of motion, weight training, and isometrics, improve health and well-being. Falls are the most common serious injury problem for elderly people and cause significant mortality. Their frequency can be diminished with attention to environment, vision, hearing, strength, and balance, among the many contributing factors. Postural hypotension can be aided with leg exercises, and habituation training can improve unsteadiness caused by vestibular problems. Exercise is also associated by some with improvements in osteoporosis—certainly no increase in osteopenia is expected. (**Ref. 3,** pp. 40–43)

76. (**D**) (**Ref. 2,** pp. 76–78)

77. (**E**) (**Ref. 2,** pp. 76–78)

78. (**A**) (**Ref. 2,** pp. 76–78)

79. (**E**) (**Ref. 2,** pp. 76–78)

80. (**B**) (**Ref. 2,** pp. 76–78)

81. (**C**) (**Ref. 2,** pp. 76–78)

82. (**C**) (**Ref. 2,** pp. 76–78)

83. (**D**) (**Ref. 2,** pp. 76–78)

84. (**F**) (**Ref. 2,** pp. 65–82)

85. (**B**) (**Ref. 2,** pp. 65–82)

86. (**H**) (**Ref. 2,** pp. 65–82)

87. (**C**) (**Ref. 2,** pp. 65–82)

88. (G) **(Ref. 2,** pp. 65–82)

89. (A) **(Ref. 2,** pp. 65–82)

90. (D) **(Ref. 2,** pp. 65–82)

91. (E) Normal newborns should lose no more than 10% of their birth weight before fully regaining it by 7 to 10 days of age. Much of this weight loss is body water, which is relatively high at birth. Fetal weight doubles, mostly due to fat deposition during the last two months of gestation. The average 1-year-old will have tripled its birth weight. Most newborns are relatively equal in size. Only after six months will they begin to approach the familial mean height, which can mean significant percentile changes. Energy requirements at two years of age are about half those at birth. **(Ref. 2,** pp. 68–75)

92. (C) Certain parts of the nervous system are well myelinated and matured by birth, including cranial nerves 3–12 and autonomic nerves. The brain develops quickly *in utero* and by birth is three-quarters of its adult circumference. The spinal cord develops earlier than the brain, accounting for early appearance of spinal reflexes *in utero*. The cerebellum develops late in fetal life, beginning at 30 weeks gestation and continuing to one year of age, making it particularly vulnerable to trauma and insults. **(Ref. 2,** p. 69)

93. (A) The first few days of life appear to be critical for the maternal-infant relationship, though the exact implications are unclear. Most child abuse occurs within family units. Annually, at least 2–2.5% of American children are abused, resulting in over 3 million reports of abuse, of which 1.2 million are substantiated. Emotional neglect of infants most commonly presents as failure to thrive. **(Ref. 2,** pp. 205–209)

94. (C) Many typical radiologic findings are hypothesized to correlate with specific forms of physical abuse. Metaphysial fractures ("flags") are felt to be due to sudden accelerations of young children who are violently shaken. Posterior rib fractures are virtually never seen in direct, blunt trauma, but rather derive from crushing injuries to the chest wall. Fractures of two different ages are always suspicious, and subdural bleeding may be due to direct blows or shaking. Spiral fractures of long bones are rather typical "normal" fractures of toddlers, but in preambulatory children should strongly suggest abuse. (**Ref. 2,** pp. 205–209)

95. **(D)** Cigarette use is slowly declining among teenagers. About 10% of eighth graders have tried alcohol or marijuana during their lives. Cocaine use peaked in 1983, and is now declining. Alcohol remains the most commonly used drug among young people; 88% of high school seniors have used it at least once, and 51% report having had at least one alcoholic drink during the previous month. (**Ref. 2,** pp. 210–228)

96. **(E)** More than 1 million adolescent women become pregnant annually, representing an annual rate of 11%! Eighty percent of these pregnancies are unintentional, and 68% are unmarried at the time of conception. Gay youth often engages in promiscuous heterosexual activity as part of the "coming out" process. The "female condom's" main advantage is the control it offers women over condom use. The subdermal implant often results in highly irregular periods, which are often unacceptable to young women. (**Ref. 2,** pp. 125–126)

97. **(C)** Five to ten percent of anorectic patients are male. The mortality for anorexia nervosa is high, around 9%, and it affects between 4.5% and 18% of adolescent women. Depletion of body fat usually results in decreased production of endogenous estrogen and produces the typical amenorrhea of anorectics and extreme athletes. Many other characteristics are frequently seen in including laxative use, vomiting, family dysfunction, and perfectionism, but none of these is necessary to the diagnosis. (**Ref. 2,** pp. 102–105, 178–180)

98. **(B)** Children at 6 months of age begin to experience the world in a symbolic fashion. Paramount in this is the ability to hold and manipulate mental images, and to realize the difference between interior mental life and real experience. Stranger anxiety appears later and is more complex, representing the ability to recognize the foreign nature of new faces by comparing them to introjected mental images. Hand release begins earlier and has nothing to do with mental imaging. (**Ref. 2,** pp. 65–82)

99. **(A)** During this period, the senses of logic and causality take prominence in the mental lives of children. Girls often excel in this in school, doing better academically than boys. Peer groups may shrink as children are excluded as "different." Most children develop an easy sense of mastery and are comfortable with their abilities. **(Ref. 2,** p. 158)

100. **(E)** Parents who display primary caregiver dysfunction are often anxious, tense, irritable, tired, and withdrawn. They display poor control of children's behavior and inadequately reinforce positive behaviors. They may displace their anxieties onto the medical visit. Children from such families often display delays in development, possibly due to childhood depression. **(Ref. 2,** pp. 167–168)

References

1. Behrman RE (ed): *Nelson Textbook of Pediatrics.* Philadelphia, W. B. Saunders, 1992.

2. Hay WW Jr et al.: *Current Pediatric Diagnosis & Treatment,* 12th ed. Norwalk, CT, Appleton & Lange, 1995.

3. Tierney LM Jr, McPhee SJ, Papadakis MA: *Current Medical Diagnosis & Treatment,* 35th ed. Norwalk, CT, Appleton & Lange, 1995.

4. DSM-IIIR: *Diagnostic and Statistical Manual of Mental Disorders.* Washington, DC, American Psychiatric Association, 1987.

5. *Guidelines for Adolescent Preventive Services.* Department of Adolescent Health, American Medical Association, 1992.

6. *Morbidity and Mortality Weekly Report.*

7. Rudolph AM (ed): *Rudolph's Pediatrics,* 19th ed. Norwalk, CT, Appleton & Lange, 1991.

2

Internal Medicine

Susan V. Donelan, MD and
William H. Greene, MD

DIRECTIONS: Each of the questions or incomplete statements below is followed by a list of suggested answers or completions. Select the **one** that is best in each case.

Questions 1–3: A 77-year-old woman with a history of atherosclerotic cardiovascular disease and mild, compensated congestive heart failure, for which she is receiving digoxin, complains of occasional "skipped heartbeats." Cardiac auscultation and an initial EKG revealed no ectopic beats. The physician decided to monitor the patient's rhythm for 24 hours. Figure 2-1 was obtained while the patient was sleeping.

1. Which of the following procedures was used to obtain the tracing?
   A. Holter monitoring
   B. Lown monitoring
   C. Marriott monitoring
   D. Wolff monitoring
   E. Parkinson monitoring

2. The monitored strip in this patient shows which of the following?
   A. Wenckebach phenomenon
   B. Mobitz type II AV block
   C. Complete heart block
   D. Parasystole
   E. Multifocal atrial tachycardia

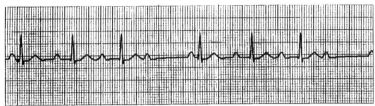

Figure 2-1

3. Which of the following would be the **MOST USEFUL** in the patient described?
   A. Starting propranolol
   B. Implanting a temporary pacemaker
   C. Implanting a permanent pacemaker
   D. Obtaining a digoxin level
   E. Starting quinidine

4. A sexually active 18-year-old man complains of a painful urethral discharge. After appropriate studies, a diagnosis of gonorrhea is made. Which of the following would **MOST LIKELY** be found on a smear of his discharge?
   A. Gram-positive rods
   B. Gram-negative rods
   C. Gram-positive cocci
   D. Gram-negative cocci
   E. Acid-fast bacilli

Questions 5-7: Figure 2-2 represents an experimental study in which groups of 20 mice were injected with propranolol alone, histamine alone, and propranolol followed by histamine.

5. Which of the following is demonstrated by this figure?
   A. Tachyphylaxis
   B. An additive effect
   C. Synergistic toxicity
   D. The effect of an alpha agonist on a vasoactive amine
   E. The effect of a beta agonist on a vasoactive amine

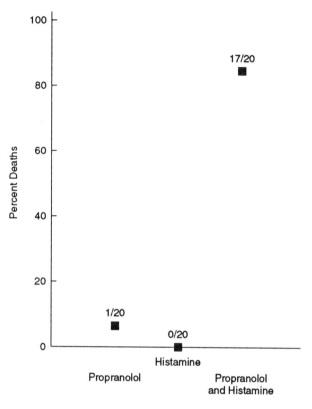

Figure 2-2

6. The sensitizing effect of propranolol is **MOST PROBABLY** mediated through
   A. blockade of alpha receptors of the autonomic nervous system
   B. blockade of beta receptors of the autonomic nervous system
   C. blockade of alpha receptors of the central nervous system
   D. blockade of beta receptors of the central nervous system
   E. blockade of delta receptors of the central nervous system

7. Because of its effects as a beta blocker, caution would also be indicated in using propranolol in subjects with all the following **EXCEPT**
   A. congestive heart failure
   B. heart block (AV node)
   C. diabetes mellitus

D. bradycardia
E. hypertension

8. According to the revised Jones Criteria for guidance in the diagnosis of rheumatic fever, all the following are considered major manifestations **EXCEPT**
   A. arthralgia
   B. subcutaneous nodules
   C. erythema marginatum
   D. carditis
   E. chorea

9. The 34-year-old man with the x-ray shown in Figure 2-3 is noted on his physical exam to have jugular venous distension, ascites, and peripheral edema. A paradoxical pulse was also noted. The **MOST LIKELY** diagnosis is
   A. aortic arch syndrome
   B. pericardial effusion
   C. nephrotic syndrome
   D. cirrhosis
   E. myocardial infarction

Figure 2-3

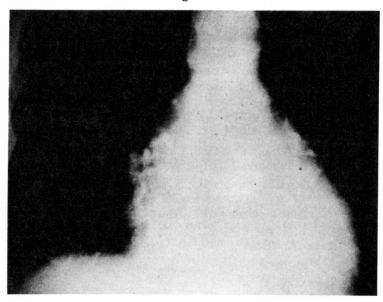

10. In patients who develop constrictive pericarditis, which of the following would **LEAST LIKELY** be found upon clinical evaluation?
   A. Wide, notched P waves on ECG
   B. A small heart on a chest x-ray
   C. T-wave inversions on ECG
   D. Atrial fibrillation
   E. Pericardial knock

11. Of the following choices, which is the **MOST COMMON** cause of constrictive pericarditis in the United States?
   A. Trauma
   B. Uremia
   C. Tuberculosis
   D. Idiopathic
   E. Connective tissue disease

12. Biopsy of a chest infiltrate in a 63-year-old man reveals the presence of blastomycosis. Which of the following medications would be **MOST LIKELY** to be indicated?
   A. Acyclovir
   B. Amphotericin B
   C. Tetracycline
   D. Tobramycin
   E. Chloramphenicol

13. During the course of therapy, the previous patient's rhythm becomes irregular. His cardiologist has been treating him with digitalis. An ECG reveals frequent PVCs. Which of the following is the **MOST LIKELY** explanation?
   A. Hypercalcemia
   B. Hypocalcemia
   C. Hyperkalemia
   D. Hypokalemia
   E. Hyperphosphatemia

14. A 48-year-old woman has had several episodes of candida vulvovaginitis. Of the following diseases, which is the patient **MOST LIKELY** to have?
   A. Diabetes mellitus
   B. Tuberculosis

C. Sarcoidosis
D. Rheumatoid arthritis
E. Lupus erythematosus

15. A 42-year-old severely depressed woman was found unconscious with an empty bottle of propoxyphene hydrochloride (Darvon) at her side. She was promptly taken to the emergency room where she was noted to be comatose. Which of the following would **LEAST LIKELY** to be found in this patient?
A. Respiratory depression
B. Apnea
C. Increase in blood pressure
D. Convulsions
E. Cardiac arrhythmias

16. After a patent airway has been ensured and artificial respiration instituted, which of the following would be **MOST HELPFUL** in treating the patient's respiratory depression?
A. Physostigmine
B. Naloxone (Narcan)
C. Atropine
D. Propranolol (Inderal)
E. None of the above

17. A 64-year-old chronic alcoholic is diagnosed as having Wernicke-Korsakoff syndrome. His main nutritional deficiency is
A. riboflavin
B. thiamine
C. pyridoxine
D. vitamin B12
E. nicotinic acid

18. Figure 2-4 was obtained in a 62-year-old man during a routine physical examination. The patient's electrical axis is approximately
A. −60°
B. −30°
C. 0°
D. +50°
E. +90°

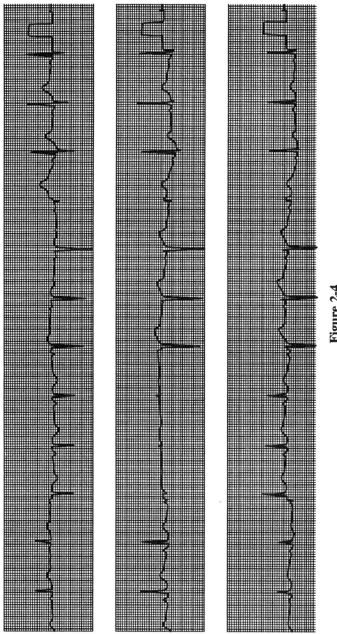

Figure 2-4

19. A 46-year-old woman with longstanding rheumatoid arthritis is started on gold therapy. Which of the following toxic reactions is the patient **MOST LIKELY** to experience?
   A. Nausea and vomiting
   B. Agranulocytosis
   C. Dermatitis and stomatitis
   D. Thrombophlebitis
   E. Alopecia

20. A 24-year-old man developed hypotension and jugular venous distension. On his chest x-ray his heart was noted to be larger than it had been on a previous chest x-ray that had been obtained because of contact with a patient with tuberculosis. Heart sounds were distant. An arterial pulsus paradoxus of 14 mm Hg was noted. The **MOST LIKELY** diagnosis is
   A. gram-negative septicemia
   B. tuberculous septicemia
   C. cardiac tamponade
   D. amyloidosis
   E. hemorrhagic pericarditis

21. It was noted during inspiration that the previous patient's neck veins became distended. This is referred to as
   A. Kussmaul's sign
   B. Jaccoud's sign
   C. Greene's sign
   D. Abraham's sign
   E. Donelan's sign

22. A 24-year-old male presents to the emergency room with myalgias, fever to 101°, and a mild headache. A careful history reveals the patient experienced a tick bite approximately one week earlier, but he cannot recall what type of tick it was. Which of the following is **NOT** a tick-borne illness?
   A. Lyme disease
   B. Ehrlichiosis
   C. Tularemia
   D. Pediculosis
   E. Babesiosis

23. A 26-year-old woman took an overdose of aspirin. Which of the following would **NOT** be considered a mild manifestation of aspirin toxicity?
    A. Nausea and vomiting
    B. Tachycardia
    C. Convulsions
    D. Tinnitus
    E. Respiratory alkalosis

24. All of the following are appropriate treatment of this patient in the emergency room **EXCEPT**
    A. control of seizures with diazepam
    B. subcutaneous administration of vitamin K
    C. parenteral fluid administration
    D. arterial blood gas analysis
    E. protection of the airway and oxygen administration

Questions 25–27: A 65-year-old man was admitted to the hospital with congestive heart failure. He responded with a rapid diuresis after receiving IV digoxin, and furosemide with potassium supplementation. His breathing improved markedly, but he complained of a pain in his left great toe. On examination his toe was slightly swollen, markedly erythematous, and exquisitely tender to touch.

25. Which of the following **MOST LIKELY** describes his condition?
    A. Septic joint
    B. Gout
    C. Janeway lesion
    D. Osteomyelitis
    E. Arterial embolism

26. Upon examination under a polarizing microscope, joint fluid from the same patient would reveal which of the following?
    A. Weakly positive birefringence
    B. Strongly positive birefringence
    C. Weakly negative birefringence
    D. Strongly negative birefringence
    E. No birefringence under polarized light but positive birefringence under light microscopy

27. Initial treatment of this patient might include all the following **EXCEPT**
   A. colchicine, oral
   B. colchicine, intravenous
   C. indomethacin
   D. allopurinol
   E. ibuprofen

Questions 28–30: A 54-year-old woman with longstanding rheumatoid arthritis developed keratoconjunctivitis sicca and xerostomia.

28. The **MOST LIKELY** diagnosis for this patient is
   A. Felty's syndrome
   B. Mikulicz's syndrome
   C. sarcoidosis
   D. Sjögren's syndrome
   E. Reiter's syndrome

29. Which of the following is **TRUE** of this syndrome?
   A. Men are more frequently affected
   B. Extraglandular involvement is rare
   C. The incidence of lymphoma is decreased
   D. Antinuclear factors occur in the majority of the patients
   E. Salivary glands are unaffected

30. In addition to biopsy, all the following have been used to help diagnose this disorder **EXCEPT**
   A. slit lamp exam
   B. rose bengal staining of the cornea
   C. Schirmer's test
   D. Ham's test
   E. salivary scintigraphy

31. The 72-year-old man whose foot is depicted in Figure 2-5 is noted to have diminished hair on his toes, dependent rubor, and nail changes. His peripheral pulses are markedly decreased. The **MOST LIKELY** explanation for these findings is
   A. acute arterial occlusive disease
   B. chronic arterial occlusive disease
   C. acute venous occlusive disease
   D. chronic venous occlusive disease
   E. thromboangitis obliterans

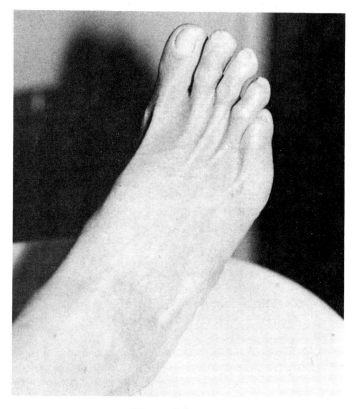

Figure 2-5

32. A 68-year-old woman was receiving a coumarin anticoagulant because of a cerebral embolism. It was noted that she was resistant to the usual therapeutic doses of the anticoagulant. Which of the following might be suspected in this patient?
    A. She is also taking a barbiturate
    B. She is on broad-spectrum antibiotics
    C. She is also taking aspirin
    D. She is also taking phenylbutazone
    E. She is also taking ibuprofen

Questions 33–35: Figure 2-6 is an EKG of a 75-year-old obese woman complaining of dizziness and weakness.

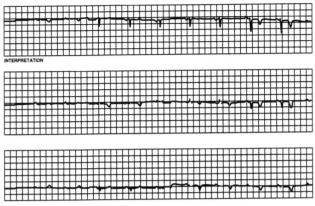

INTERPRETATION

Figure 2-6

33. Of the following which is the **MOST LIKELY** diagnosis?
    A. Inferior myocardial infarction
    B. True posterior myocardial infarction
    C. Left anterior hemiblock
    D. Right anterior hemiblock
    E. Left ventricular hypertrophy

34. All the following are consistent with the above diagnosis **EXCEPT**
    A. low voltage
    B. left axis deviation of −30° or more
    C. Q-R-S interval of 0.9 sec or more
    D. P-terminal force in V-1 of more than 0.04
    E. slow R-wave progression

35. Of the following conditions, which is this condition's **MOST COMMON** cause?
    A. Aortic insufficiency
    B. Aortic stenosis
    C. Hypertension
    D. Coarctation of the aorta
    E. Prolapsed mitral valve

36. A 65-year-old woman with a long history of congestive heart failure, for which she was taking digoxin, potassium chloride, and hydrochlorothiazide, complained of occasional skipped beats. Premature ventricular contractions were found on her EKG and another drug was added to her regimen. Digoxin levels before and after starting this additional medication are shown in Figure 2-7. Which of the following drugs was **MOST LIKELY** to have been added?
   A. Procainamide HCl
   B. Quinidine sulfate
   C. Clonidine
   D. Phenytoin
   E. Propranolol

Questions 37–38: The chemistry profile shown in Figure 2-8 was obtained in a 30-year-old man with numerous somatic complaints including diffuse aches and pains. On physical examination it was obvious that he was suffering from an endocrinological disorder.

37. Which of the following is the **MOST LIKELY** diagnosis in this patient?
   A. Addison's disease
   B. Cushing's disease

Figure 2-7

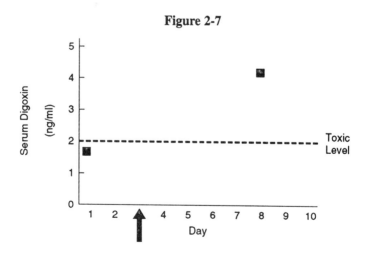

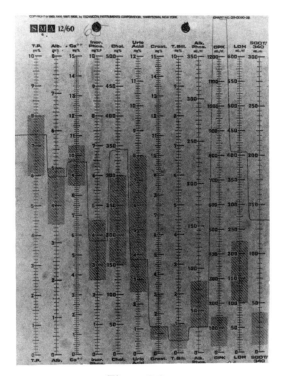

Figure 2-8

C. Primary hypothyroidism
D. Thyrotoxicosis
E. Acromegaly

38. The **MOST COMMON** cause of this disorder is
   A. drug-induced
   B. congenital
   C. autoimmune destruction
   D. iatrogenic
   E. trauma

39. A 65-year-old man is diagnosed as having carcinoma of the right colon. Which of the following would be the **MOST LIKELY** to be associated with his condition?
   A. Spiking fevers
   B. Anemia
   C. Perirectal abscess
   D. Rectal fistula
   E. Steatorrhea

40. To which of the following organs is the above patient's cancer **MOST LIKELY** to metastasize?
   A. Lung
   B. Liver
   C. Bone
   D. Stomach
   E. Skin

41. A 42-year-old woman took an intentional massive dose of acetaminophen. Which of the following is the **MOST LIKELY** organ to be severely affected in this patient?
   A. Heart
   B. Lungs
   C. Liver
   D. Kidney
   E. Brain

42. Which of the following is the **MOST EFFECTIVE** antidote for the patient above?
   A. Acetylcysteine
   B. Sodium bicarbonate
   C. Phenobarbital
   D. Sodium nitroprusside
   E. British anti-Lewisite (BAL)

Questions 43–44: Figure 2-9 was obtained in a mildly hypertensive 82-year-old woman. She was receiving no medications.

43. Which of the following is the correct interpretation of the patient's ECG?
   A. Marked left ventricular hypertrophy with strain pattern
   B. Anterior septal myocardial infarction

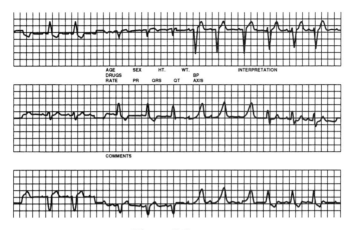

Figure 2-9

   C. Left bundle branch block
   D. Right bundle branch block
   E. Trifasicular

44. This patient's electrical axis is approximately
   A. 0°
   B. −30°
   C. −60°
   D. +30°
   E. +60°

45. A 64-year-old woman has multiple complaints, including malaise, severe unilateral headache, as well as pain and stiffness in her neck, shoulders, and back. Her appetite is poor and she has recently lost weight. Her examining physician finds that she has an oral temperature of 100.5° F, her hematocrit is 11.8%, and the sedimentation rate is 104 mm/hr. Which of the following is the **MOST LIKELY** diagnosis?
   A. Multiple sclerosis
   B. Polymyalgia rheumatica
   C. Rheumatoid arthritis
   D. Polyarteritis nodosa
   E. Gastric carcinoma

46. The **MOST FEARED** complication of giant cell arteritis (temporal arteritis) is
   A. thrombosis of the cranial artery
   B. exquisite hyperesthesia
   C. substantial fever
   D. blindness
   E. tongue pain

47. If temporal arteritis were to be demonstrated in this patient, therapy would consist of
   A. indomethacin
   B. gold thiomalate
   C. corticosteroids
   D. penicillamine
   E. aspirin

Questions 48–51: The CBC and platelet count shown in Figure 2-10 were obtained in a 69-year-old woman with a longstanding pruritus, cephalgia, and recurrent superficial phlebitis. Her spleen was markedly enlarged.

48. The **MOST LIKELY** diagnosis is
   A. acute granulocytic leukemia
   B. polycythemia vera
   C. thrombocytopenic purpura
   D. leukemoid reaction
   E. metastatic carcinoma

49. This patient's splenomegaly is **MOST PROBABLY** caused by
   A. recurrent infection
   B. increased adipose tissue
   C. myeloid metaplasia
   D. portal hypertension
   E. none of the above

50. Which of the following would be **LEAST LIKELY** in this patient?
   A. Elevated serum B12 levels
   B. Elevated leukocyte alkaline phosphatase
   C. Elevated 24-hour urinary uric acid
   D. Normal arterial blood gases
   E. Increased marrow iron stores

TECH:		
DATE REPORTED:		
TIME REPORTED:		

RESULTS	TEST	NORMAL VALUES
24.8	WBC X 10⁹/°	M 4 3-10 / F 4 3-10
7.48	RBC X 10¹²/°	M 4 4-6.0 / F 4 2-5.4
15.0	HGB g/d°	M 14-18 / F 12-16
48.5	HCT m³/d°	M 41-51 / F 37-47
65	MCV F³	80-96
20	MCH Pg	26-32
31	MCHC gm/d°	31-35

DIFFERENTIAL		RELATIVE NOR. VALUE
Seg	89	34.6-71.4
Band	1	
Lymph	7	19.6-52.7
Atypical Lymph		
MONO	2	2.4-11.8
EOSIN		0-7.8
Baso		0-1.8
Meta-Myelo		0
Myelo		0
Pro-Myelo		0

TEST	RESULT
RETIC COUNT	
PLATELET COUNT	581,000
SED RATE	
PROTH TIME	
PT CONTROL	
PTT	

RBC MORPH:
Microcytic
Normochromic
Slight Poikilocytosis
Slight Basophilia

PLATELET EST ↑

ROUTINE TODAY STAT
CBC WBC DIFF RBC HBG HCT
RETIC PLAT. CT ESR PT PTT SICKLE CELL
NAME: DATE REQUESTED: DOCTOR: CHART NO.:

Figure 2-10

51. In general, the main method of treating this patient would be
    A. $FeSO_4$
    B. phlebotomy
    C. alkylating agents
    D. total body radiation
    E. marrow transplantation

Questions 52–53: Refer to Figure 2-11.

52. The lead V1 strip shown in Figure 2-11 was obtained in an asymptomatic 81-year-old man. The patient's heart rate is approximately
    A. 82
    B. 70
    C. 54
    D. 43
    E. 30

53. The patient has which of the following?
    A. First-degree AV block
    B. Second-degree AV block
    C. Third-degree AV block
    D. Blocked PACs
    E. Slow atrial flutter

54. In which of the following conditions would digoxin be **MOST EFFECTIVE**?
    A. Heart failure secondary to anemia
    B. Heart failure secondary to arteriovenous fistula
    C. Low output heart failure
    D. Cardiac failure secondary to hyperthyroidism
    E. Infection-induced cardiac failure

55. When the patient is started on oral digoxin, what percent of the oral dose might be expected to be absorbed?
    A. 10–20%
    B. 20–35%
    C. 35–50%

Figure 2-11

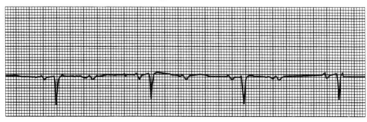

D. 55–75%
E. Over 80%

56. In young healthy subjects with normal renal function, the half-life of digoxin is approximately
   A. 12 hours
   B. 24 hours
   C. 36 hours
   D. 72 hours
   E. 96 hours

Questions 57–59: A 35-year-old man has complained of recurrent attacks of rapid heart rate and palpitations. Figure 2-12 is obtained.

57. Which of the following is **MOST LIKELY** in this patient?
   A. Anxiety reaction
   B. Floppy mitral valve
   C. Wolff-Parkinson-White syndrome
   D. Clockwise rotation of the heart
   E. Sick sinus syndrome

58. The slurring of the initial deflection of the QRS complex produces which of the following?
   A. Alpha waves
   B. Beta waves
   C. Gamma waves
   D. Delta waves
   E. Epsilon waves

59. All of the following are commonly used in the management of this entity **EXCEPT**
   A. nitroglycerin
   B. carotid sinus massage
   C. Valsalva maneuver
   D. cardioversion
   E. verapamil

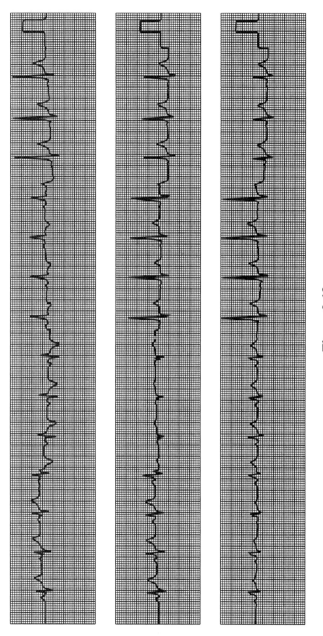

Figure 2-12

60. The woman with marked pitting edema of the lower extremities (Figure 2-13) is **MOST LIKELY** to have had during her clinical course decreased blood levels of which of the following?
A. Renin
B. Angiotensin
C. Aldosterone
D. Sodium
E. Albumin

61. Which of the following acts as a specific antagonist of aldosterone?
A. Hydrochlorothiazide
B. Spironolactone
C. Furosemide
D. Ethacrynic acid
E. Bumetamide

Figure 2-13

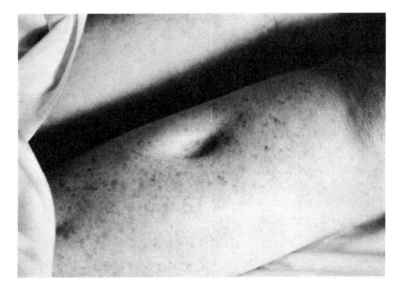

62. An 18-year-old man who has traveled to a tropical zone rapidly develops chills, recurrent fever, and severe myalgia three weeks after his return. The fevers occur in a 48-hour cycle. The **MOST LIKELY** diagnosis is
   A. varicella
   B. dengue
   C. trichinosis
   D. scarlet fever
   E. malaria

63. In congestive heart failure of beriberi heart disease, the cardiac output is
   A. variable
   B. decreased
   C. unchanged
   D. increased
   E. of no significance

64. Beriberi results from a deficiency in vitamin
   A. B1
   B. B2
   C. B3
   D. C
   E. E

65. A 24-year-old atopic man was stung by a hornet and developed a severe systemic reaction with respiratory distress and hypotension. Which of the following would be the **LEAST USEFUL** in the **IMMEDIATE** management of this patient?
   A. Oxygen
   B. Epinephrine
   C. Diphenylhydramine
   D. Intravenous corticosteroids
   E. Intravenous fluids

Questions 66–67: Figure 2-14 is that of an obese 19-year-old woman with nephrotic syndrome who recently noted increasing abdominal girth. A fluid wave and shifting dullness were noted upon physical examination of her abdomen.

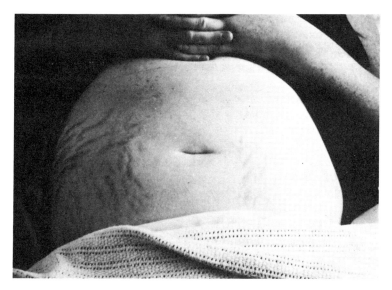

Figure 2-14

66. Which of the following would be expected if laboratory analysis of the patient's ascitic fluid were performed?
    A. A protein content of 5 g/dL
    B. 1500 WBC/mm^3
    C. Thick, cloudy ascitic fluid
    D. Bloody fluid
    E. None of the above

67. Which of the following would **LEAST LIKELY** be found in this patient?
    A. Hypoalbuminemia
    B. Marked proteinuria
    C. Hypercholesterolemia
    D. Hyperlipidemia
    E. Decreased aldosterone production

68. A young man is noted to have spider fingers, high arched palate, aortic abnormalities, and ectopic lenses. His father had a similar disease. Which syndrome does the patient have?

    A. Zollinger-Ellison syndrome
    B. Peutz-Jeghers syndrome
    C. Marfan's syndrome
    D. Reiter's syndrome
    E. Horner's syndrome

Questions 69–70: A 30-year-old African-American woman had the x-ray (Figure 2-15) done during a hospitalization for cholecystectomy. She had no pulmonary symptoms. A later x-ray was found to be normal.

69. The **MOST LIKELY** diagnosis is

    A. pulmonary embolism
    B. pneumonitis

Figure 2-15

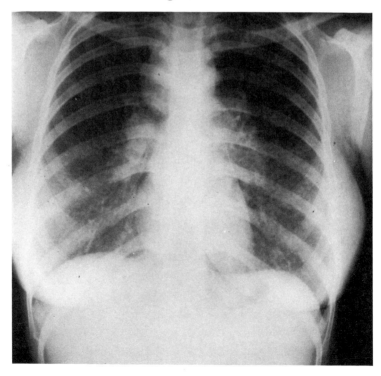

C. tuberculosis
D. sarcoidosis
E. primary pulmonary hypertension

70. Of the following skin lesions, which would have been **MORE LIKELY** to have been present in this patient?
    A. Erythema marginatum
    B. Erythema multiforme
    C. Erythema nodosum
    D. Erythema bullosum
    E. Erythema annulare centrifugum

Questions 71–73: A 22-year-old mentally retarded woman with a history of a seizure disorder is evaluated by a dermatologist because of the presence of wartlike lesions on her cheeks and forehead. The individual lesions are about 0.1 to 1.0 cm in size; they are elevated and pink-yellow. Several other family members have similar disorders.

71. This patient **MOST LIKELY** has
    A. Down's syndrome
    B. tuberous sclerosis
    C. secondary syphilis
    D. congenital rubella
    E. congenital toxoplasmosis

72. This patient's skin lesions are referred to as
    A. adenoma sebaceum
    B. neurofibromatosis
    C. condyloma acuminatum
    D. condyloma latum
    E. basal cell carcinoma

73. Which of the following is **NOT TRUE** of this condition?
    A. This disease is inherited as an autosomal dominant trait
    B. Most patients suffer from seizures
    C. Cystic lung disease is uncommon
    D. Mental retardation occurs in over 90%
    E. Brain CT may reveal calcified nodules

Questions 74–76: Refer to Figure 2-16.

74. A 28-year-old African-American man has had a persistent marked erection of his penis, which is frequently painful. Which of the following is depicted by Figure 2-16?
    A. Peyronie disease
    B. Priapism
    C. Satyriasis
    D. Balanitis
    E. Paraphimosis

75. Which of the following disorders is this patient **MOST LIKELY** to have?
    A. Pulmonary fibrosis
    B. Sickle cell anemia
    C. Nephrotic syndrome
    D. Cirrhosis
    E. Congenital heart disease

Figure 2-16

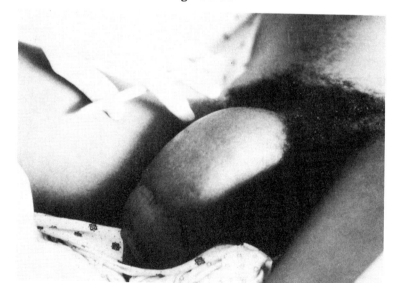

76. All the following statements concerning this patient's underlying disease are **TRUE EXCEPT**

A. his risk of developing cholelithiasis is paradoxically reduced

B. he is at risk of early stroke

C. septicemia with encapsulated organisms is common

D. Staphylococcal aureus is the most common cause of osteomyelitis in this group of patients

77. A 56-year-old woman with metastatic carcinoma of the stomach developed emboli to several organs including the brain, spleen, and kidneys. On postmortem examination, in the section of the heart shown in Figure 2-17, papillary vegetations were found on the center of each aortic valve leaflet. Which of the following did the patient **MOST LIKELY** have?

A. Amyloidosis

B. Infectious endocarditis

C. Marantic endocarditis

D. Atrial myxoma

E. Systemic lupus erythematosus

Figure 2-17

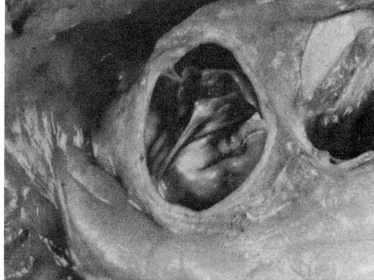

78. On routine examination, a well-developed man had an RBC of 8 million, hemoglobin of 18 g, hematocrit of 61, with normal leukocytes, thrombocytes, and O_2 saturation. There was no splenic enlargement. What test might give a clue to the probable diagnosis?
  A. Splenic aspirate
  B. Scalene node biopsy
  C. Intravenous pyelogram
  D. LE test
  E. Bronchoscopy

79. Chronic pancreatitis is **MOST FREQUENTLY** associated with
  A. duodenal ulcer
  B. alcoholism
  C. obstruction of the common duct
  D. diabetes mellitus
  E. pyogenic infection

80. Amyl nitrite is used in the treatment of cyanide poisoning because it
  A. forms methemoglobin, which competes successfully with ferricytochrome for cyanide ions
  B. improves the coronary circulation
  C. combines directly with the cyanide ions
  D. stimulates the respiratory center
  E. none of the above

81. Charcot's triad consists of all of the following **EXCEPT**
  A. fever and chills
  B. pruritus
  C. biliary pain
  D. jaundice

82. Of the following, pellagra is due to deficiency of
  A. thiamine
  B. pantothenic acid
  C. riboflavin
  D. nicotinic acid (niacin)
  E. pyridoxine

83. Inborn errors of amino acid metabolism include all the following **EXCEPT**
   A. Gaucher's disease
   B. phenylketonuria
   C. alcaptonuria
   D. maple syrup urine disease
   E. homocystinuria

84. Which of the following is **TRUE** of ascorbic acid?
   A. It is a fat-soluble vitamin
   B. It does not behave in an acidic manner
   C. It is used in the cure of pellagra
   D. It is necessary for the formation of connective tissue
   E. Its deficiency can result in beriberi

85. Lead poisoning involves all the following **EXCEPT**
   A. neuropathy with primary motor involvement
   B. blue line of fingers
   C. treatment with chelating agents
   D. seizures in the acute form
   E. urinary coproporphyrin

86. Myocarditis and pericarditis of children and adults are **MOST LIKELY** to be caused by which of the following?
   A. Coxsackie, group A
   B. Coxsackie, group B
   C. Echovirus
   D. Parainfluenza
   E. Adenovirus

87. If a Swan-Ganz catheter is passed into the pulmonary artery, which of the following should be considered a normal mean pulmonary capillary wedge pressure?
   A. −4 mm Hg
   B. 0 mm Hg
   C. 5 mm Hg
   D. 10 mm Hg
   E. 20 mm Hg

88. Cardiovascular syphilis is usually syphilis of the
  - **A.** peripheral arteries
  - **B.** coronary arteries
  - **C.** myocardium
  - **D.** aorta
  - **E.** veins

89. All the following rickettsial diseases are characterized by rash **EXCEPT**
  - **A.** Rocky Mountain spotted fever
  - **B.** primary epidemic typhus
  - **C.** Q fever
  - **D.** rickettsial pox
  - **E.** murine typhus

90. Endemic goiter is principally caused by
  - **A.** poor diet habits
  - **B.** drug toxicity
  - **C.** genetic predisposition
  - **D.** deficiency of iodine in soil and water
  - **E.** thyroid carcinoma

Questions 91–93: Each of the following options may be chosen once, more than once, or not at all.

  - **A.** Commonly presents with paranasal sinus pain, purulent nasal discharge, and lower respiratory tract symptoms
  - **B.** Commonly presents with hemoptysis, dyspnea, and hematuria
  - **C.** Commonly is associated with chronic hepatitis B antigenemia
  - **D.** Commonly presents early in the course with arthralgias of the fingers, wrists, knees, and ankles, and Raynaud's syndrome

91. Goodpasture's syndrome

92. Wegener's granulomatosis

93. Periarteritis nodosa

Questions 94–95: A 47-year-old man presents to his physician with progressive abdominal swelling. On examination, he is found to have ascites and a tender, enlarged liver.

94. If the patient describes the ascites as having been of abrupt onset and preceded by trauma, the **MOST LIKELY** diagnosis is
   A. congestive heart failure
   B. alcoholic liver disease with cirrhosis
   C. thrombosis of the hepatic vein (Budd-Chiari syndrome)
   D. portal vein thrombosis

95. If the patient describes a chronic course associated with wasting and low-grade fever, the differential diagnosis should include all the following **EXCEPT**
   A. tuberculosis
   B. cirrhosis with hepatocellular carcinoma
   C. hepatitis C
   D. chronic pancreatitis

Questions 96–98: A 67-year-old man presents to his physician with progressive dyspnea on exertion, orthopnea, paroxysmal nocturnal dyspnea, and peripheral edema. A diagnosis of hypertension and congestive heart failure is made and the patient is begun on medication. For each of the following medications, choose the subsequent effect that is **MOST LIKELY** to be associated with it. Each choice may be used once, more than once, or not at all.

   A. Digoxin
   B. Hydrochlorothiazide
   C. Coumadin
   D. Captopril
   E. Clonidine
   F. Propranolol
   G. Nifedipine

96. The patient subsequently notes the onset of swelling and tenderness of his breasts.

97. The patient begins to develop mild diarrhea as well as flushing and headache.

98. In the first month following the visit, the patient develops dysgeusia (altered taste sensation) and a nonproductive cough.

99. A 62-year-old man presents with bone pain in his legs that worsens on standing. The skin over his tibia is erythematous and warm. Laboratory studies reveal an elevated alkaline phosphatase. An x-ray taken on this patient is shown in Figure 2.18. He **MOST LIKELY** has

A. osteomalacia
B. osteoarthritis
C. calcium pyrophosphate deposition disease
D. osteomyelitis
E. Paget's disease

Figure 2-18

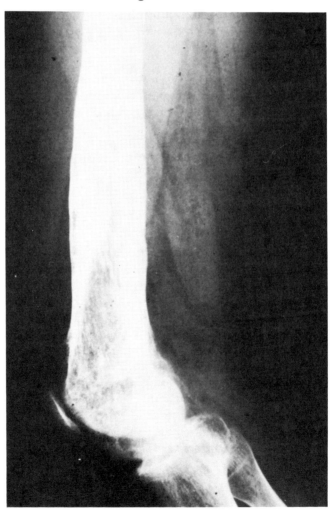

100. Use of which of the following has been found to benefit many subjects with Wegener's granulomatosis?
    A. Indomethacin
    B. Phenylbutazone
    C. Parenteral gold
    D. Cyclophosphamide
    E. Low-dose corticosteroids (<10 mg/day)

101. The organism **MOST OFTEN** causing hematogenous pyogenic vertebral osteomyelitis in patients under 65 years of age is
    A. *Escherichia coli*
    B. *Staphylococcus aureus*
    C. *Pseudomonas aeruginosa*
    D. *Mycobacterium tuberculosis*
    E. *Neisseria gonorrhea*

102. Immunosuppressive therapy is **LEAST LIKELY** to be of possible benefit in
    A. allograft rejection
    B. dermatomyositis/polymyositis
    C. Wegener's granulomatosis
    D. primary biliary cirrhosis
    E. psoriatic arthritis

103. Which of the following is **NOT** a serologic abnormality of systemic lupus erythematosis (SLE)?
    A. High titer of rheumatoid factor
    B. Positive Coomb's test
    C. Markedly increased levels of serum complement
    D. Antimitochondrial antibodies
    E. Cryoglobulinemia

104. Laboratory abnormalities found in patients with Sjogren's syndrome (SS) would **LEAST LIKELY** include
    A. rheumatoid factor
    B. hyperglobulinemia
    C. serum hyperviscosity
    D. low levels of cryoglobulin
    E. antinuclear antibodies

Questions 105–106: Figure 2-19 shows characteristic changes in the permanent upper central incisors, which present a notched appearance of the biting edges.

105. These teeth, which may be found in patients with syphilis, are referred to as
    A. Curley's teeth
    B. Clutton's teeth
    C. Hutchinson's teeth
    D. Tilton's teeth
    E. Browning's teeth

106. The patient depicted in Figure 2-19 may also have all the following **EXCEPT**
    A. cardiovascular abnormalities
    B. interstitial keratitis
    C. eighth cranial nerve deafness
    D. saddle nose
    E. arthritis of the knees

Figure 2-19

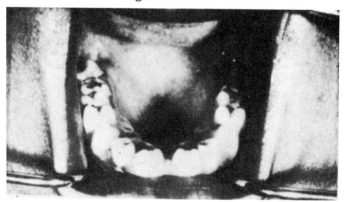

107. The hand in Figure 2-20, which is opening from a clenched position, displays atrophy and abnormal posturing of the fingers. The patient is a 42-year-old man with frontal balding, temporal muscle wasting, bilateral ptosis, and a myopathic facies. The **MOST LIKELY** diagnosis is

   A. multiple sclerosis

   B. myotonic dystrophy

   C. Duchenne's muscular dystrophy

   D. Becker's muscular dystrophy

   E. cerebral palsy

108. All the following are **TRUE** regarding *Helicobacter pylori* **EXCEPT**

   A. the organism is commonly found in histologically normal stomach tissue

   B. it may be the most common worldwide human infective agent

   C. the epidemiology of this organism is not well known

   D. it is difficult to culture

   E. it is commonly found on biopsies of patients with active antral gastritis

Figure 2-20

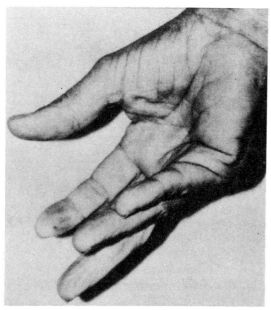

Questions 109–110: A 24-year-old patient has been in the emergency room on numerous occasions with severe abdominal pain, but no organic pathology has ever been found upon physical examination. He is thought to have a strange affect, and the resident prescribes phenobarbital. The patient returns to the emergency room a short time later with an even worse complaint of abdominal pain. He mentions that his father had undergone multiple abdominal operations without any definite diagnosis having been made. His father also exhibited several psychiatric manifestations.

109. Which of the following would be the **MOST LIKELY** diagnosis in this patient?
  A. Hypothyroidism
  B. Acute intermittent porphyria
  C. Hyperparathyroidism
  D. Addison's disease
  E. Pernicious anemia

110. The preceding disorder described results from an abnormality in the metabolism of
  A. glucose
  B. pyrrole
  C. methionine
  D. fatty acids
  E. copper

111. In a 25-year-old man weighing 150 lb, what percentage of his body weight is composed of water?
  A. 10%
  B. 20%
  C. 40%
  D. 60%
  E. 80%

Questions 112–118: The following group of questions pertains to patients with acquired immunodeficiency syndrome (AIDS). For each of the statements, select the organism or illness **MOST CLOSELY** related. Each option may be used once, more than once, or not at all.

  A. *Pneumocystis carinii*
  B. *Mycobacterium avium-intracellulare* complex (MAC)

C. Cytomegalovirus
D. Herpes simplex
E. Cryptosporidiosis
F. *Cryptococcus neoformans*
G. *Mycobacterium tuberculosis*
H. *Toxoplasma gondii*
I. Non-Hodgkin's (B cell) lymphoma
J. Kaposi's sarcoma

112. Obligate intracellular protozoan that frequently causes brain lesions

113. Most common cause of retinitis, it can also infect other organs

114. Most common cause of meningitis

115. Intractable diarrhea

116. Prophylaxis recommended when the CD4 count falls below 200

117. Wasting syndrome, fever, liver function abnormalities

118. Most frequent neoplastic manifestation of HIV infection

119. The earliest clinical manifestation of renal injury secondary to diabetes mellitus is
    A. azotemia
    B. hematuria
    C. decreased glomerular filtration rate (GFR)
    D. proteinuria

120. Which of the following organisms is thought to be responsible for one-quarter of all cases of acute urethral syndrome?
    A. *Escherichia coli*
    B. *Pseudomonas aeruginosa*
    C. *Staphylococcus aureus*
    D. *Candida albicans*
    E. *Chlamydia trachomatis*

121. All the following phrases are **TRUE** concerning multiple myeloma **EXCEPT**
    A. most patients are asymptomatic at the time of diagnosis
    B. the cause of this disease has not been definitively worked out
    C. more than half of patients are anemic at initial presentation
    D. hepatomegaly from plasma cell infiltration is uncommon

Questions 122–125: Choose the correct disease entity that **MOST CLOSELY** matches the phrase. Each choice may be used once, more than once, or not at all.

    A. Irritable bowel syndrome
    B. Crohn's disease
    C. Ulcerative colitis

122. Always involves the rectum

123. May mimic peptic ulcer disease

124. Weight loss is more common

125. Diffuse, continuous inflammation

126. Which of the following organisms is felt to be the causative agent of nearly half of the cases of nongonococcal urethritis in young men?
    A. Herpes simplex
    B. *Chlamydia trachomatis*
    C. *Candida albicans*
    D. *Trichomonas vaginalis*
    E. *Phthirus pubis*

127. All the following phrases concerning cystic fibrosis are **TRUE EXCEPT**
    A. it is inherited as an autosomal dominant disease
    B. it is the most common lethal genetic disease in the United States
    C. although up to 50% of patients have antibodies to *Aspergillus fumigatus,* only a small number develop allergic aspergillosis
    D. the median age of survival is 24 years
    E. symptomatic biliary cirrhosis occurs in 2 to 5% of patients

128. All the following statements concerning breast cancer are **TRUE EXCEPT**

    A. once a woman has had *curative* therapy for breast cancer, she can return to a routine monitoring schedule to look for future occurrences

    B. women with a positive family history and relative risk have a greater tendency to develop their cancer before age 40

    C. oral contraceptives do not appear to increase the risk of breast cancer

    D. estrogen receptor protein (ERP) is found more frequently and in higher titer in tumors from postmenopausal patients

    E. ERP-positive tumors tend to be less virulent

Questions 129–130: A 56-year-old man presents to his internist with complaints of difficulty in beginning urination, dribbling after micturition, and nocturia. He denies pain or obvious blood in his urine. The symptoms have gradually worsened over the last 6 months, but he does not feel ill. He states he would not have sought medical attention, but his wife is irritated at being awakened several times each night when he gets out of bed. There is no family history of prostate cancer, though his father died in a car accident at the age of 42. He assures you that he is monogamous.

129. All the following should be part of the initial evaluation **EXCEPT**

    A. urinalysis

    B. digital rectal examination

    C. quantitative urine culture

    D. serum prostate specific antigen determination

    E. serum VDRL

130. The patient's PSA level is 11 ng/ml (normal in the laboratory used being < 4.0 ng/ml). Which of the following statements is **INCORRECT**?

    A. This patient has a 95% likelihood of having prostate cancer

    B. This patient's symptoms are consistent with benign prostatic hypertrophy

    C. This patient's symptoms are consistent with prostate cancer

    D. Having BPH does not appear to be causally related to the development of prostate cancer

131. Which of the following is **NOT** considered a common risk factor for the development of skin cancer?
    A. The amount of exposure to electromagnetic radiation, including ultraviolet light and x-radiation
    B. The intensity of exposure to electromagnetic radiation, including UV light and x-radiation
    C. Outdoor occupation
    D. Immunosuppression
    E. Being native to an equatorial region

132. Which of the following statements concerning osteoporosis is **NOT TRUE**?
    A. The main underlying cause of fractures in osteoporosis is increased bone fragility as a result of bone loss
    B. Initial bone density is unrelated to the risk of developing osteoporosis in later years
    C. Short women of northern European extraction tend to have an increased incidence of osteoporosis
    D. Postmenopausal estrogen replacement therapy decreases the occurrence of fractures associated with osteoporosis by about one-half
    E. Smoking and high alcohol intake increase the risk of developing osteoporosis twofold

133. All the following drugs used in the treatment of osteoporosis act by decreasing bone absorption **EXCEPT**
    A. vitamin D
    B. calcium
    C. estrogen
    D. calcitonin

134. Which of the following statements concerning multiple sclerosis is **NOT TRUE**?
    A. The cause of multiple sclerosis is unknown
    B. The average age of onset is the midthirties
    C. The lesions consist of scattered areas of central nervous system myelin dissolution; however, the axon remains intact
    D. The incidence of cases rises sharply the closer you are to the equator
    E. Epidemiologic studies are suggestive of an infectious etiology

135. All the following signs and/or symptoms are **COMMON** presenting manifestations of multiple sclerosis **EXCEPT**
    A. weakness of one or more extremities
    B. unilateral vision loss
    C. incoordination
    D. paresthesias
    E. changes in intellectual function

Questions 136–138: A 19 year-old college student presents to his family physician during the Thanksgiving break with complaints of malaise, fever, a sore throat, and diminished appetite. He thought he had "the flu that is going around" since his girlfriend was similarly ill several weeks ago. He had some "leftover" ampicillin from a streptococcal throat infection back in September, which he took "to see if it worked." He has been feeling poorly for approximately two weeks, however, and his mother insisted he come to see you while he is home. He has a mild cough but denies shortness of breath, genitourinary symptoms (he is sexually active but "always" uses a condom), or change in bowel habits. He does complain of a vague "fullness" in his abdomen but denies constipation. On examination, he is febrile to 102.2° F orally; other vital signs are stable. His exam is significant for the following positive findings: tender cervical lymphadenopathy bilaterally, enlarged tonsils without exudate, mild tender hepatomegaly, splenomegaly, and a scattered macular rash. He is not jaundiced. A rapid heterophile test done in your office is highly positive.

136. The **MOST LIKELY** diagnosis, based upon the history and physical examination, is
    A. varicella viral infection
    B. recurrent streptococcal infection of the throat
    C. infectious mononucleosis
    D. acute HIV syndrome
    E. acute hepatitis B infection

137. His girlfriend comes to visit the patient and requests that you test her for evidence of recent Epstein-Barr infection. Which of the following tests would you **MOST EXPECT** to be elevated?
    A. IgG VCA (viral capsid antigen)
    B. EBNA (Epstein-Barr nuclear antigen) titer
    C. IgM VCA
    D. EA (early antigen)

138. Despite advising him to avoid contact sports, the patient is cajoled into a game of touch football on the front lawn. The game becomes somewhat rowdy, and he is tackled hard, landing under a pile of people. He does not get up. You are called to see him in the emergency room of your local hospital. His blood pressure is low, his pulse is rapid, and his abdomen is rigid. What is the **MOST LIKELY** explanation for his condition?
A. He is dehydrated from fever and exertion
B. He has ruptured his liver
C. He has ruptured his spleen
D. He had an allergic reaction to the ampicillin

139. On theoretical grounds, all the following vaccines should be avoided in pregnant women **EXCEPT**
A. measles
B. yellow fever
C. cholera
D. mumps
E. rubella

140. All the following are categories of people recommended to receive influenza vaccination **EXCEPT**
A. patients entering the hospital with an acute illness
B. patients with chronic cardiopulmonary disorders
C. residents of nursing homes or chronic care facilities
D. persons aged 65 years or older
E. children on long-term aspirin therapy

Questions 141–143: Refer to Figure 2-21.

141. The rash pictured is classic for the illness it represents. This disease is caused by
A. a fungus that lives on the keratin of the stratum corneum, nails, and hair
B. dry skin or underlying infections
C. an adverse reaction to a medication
D. a spirochetal infection passed through a tick bite

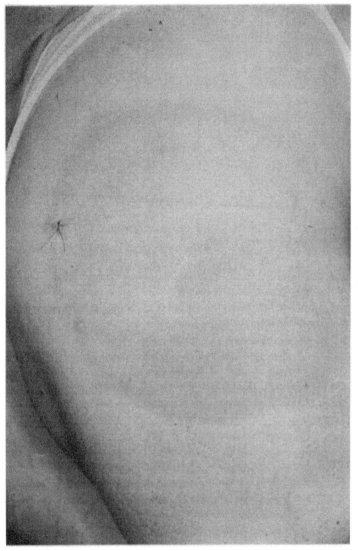

Figure 2-21

142. All the following are possible manifestations of the early form of this disease **EXCEPT**
    A. multiple annular lesions
    B. acrodermatitis chronica atrophicans
    C. fever and chills
    D. hepatomegaly
    E. generalized lymphadenopathy

143. All the following are accepted antibiotic treatment regimens for this disease **EXCEPT**
    A. trimethoprim-sulfamethoxazole
    B. amoxicillin
    C. doxycycline
    D. ceftriaxone

144. All the following statements concerning acute interstitial nephritis (AISN) are **TRUE EXCEPT**
    A. acute bacterial pyelonephritis is a rare cause
    B. methicillin is the most frequently implicated penicillin-type drug to cause AISN
    C. rifampin is the antituberculous drug most commonly causing AISN
    D. AISN may be the primary renal lesion found in some patients with systemic lupus erythematosis

Questions 145–148: You are seeing for the first time a family new to the area who wishes for their 16-year-old son to be evaluated. It appears that the child had a bout of malaise, jaundice, anorexia, and elevated liver function tests several months ago. Their pediatrician diagnosed a case of "viral hepatitis" (they do not know what types of blood tests were performed) and told them it would take awhile for their son to recover, but that he would be fine. The parents recall a similar episode a few years ago. They do not have any of the son's prior medical records besides his vaccination record, which was needed to enroll in school. Always a good student before the move, the school counselor has reported that the young man is "not living up to the potential" suggested by his old school records. He also appears to have begun to act "oddly." At first the parents attributed this to the stress of adolescence and the move to a new environment. However, they are also beginning to notice some behavioral changes, as well as deterioration of his handwriting. They want you to make sure there is nothing to worry about. While speaking to the family, you notice a slight tremor in the patient. Mental status examination suggests some organic dysfunction. His eye exam is notable for a finding of golden brown-to-greenish arcs.

145. Which of the following diseases seem **MOST LIKELY** to be causing this patient's problems?
    A. Chronic hepatitis B infection
    B. Wilson's disease
    C. Hemochromatosis
    D. Late-onset porphyria
    E. Acute intermittent porphyria

146. The lesion seen on eye examination is called a
    A. Rumpel-Leede sign
    B. Pastia's line
    C. von Willebrand ring
    D. Kaysher-Fleischer ring

147. All the following are **TRUE** regarding this disease **EXCEPT**
    A. the prevalence of disease is approximately 30 per million
    B. the metabolic mechanism of the disease has been well characterized
    C. liver copper is actually greater in presymptomatic homozygotes than in symptomatic ones
    D. The diagnosis cannot be made on the basis of histologic sections of the liver

148. Which of the following medications is the drug of choice for treatment of this disorder?
    A. Prednisone
    B. Trientine
    C. D-penicillamine
    D. Zinc

149. All the following statements regarding cigarette smoking are **TRUE EXCEPT**
   A. The use of nicotine gum has not been shown to increase the chances of smoking cessation
   B. 90% of smokers begin to smoke before the age of 20
   C. Adolescents with the least external validation of their self-worth are the ones most prone to manipulation by the advertisements of the smoking industry to improve their self-image
   D. Smoking cessation clinics have long-term success in 30 to 40% of the users who persevere in the program
   E. The use of flavorings and other additives utilized to compensate for less tobacco in some cigarettes does not need to be revealed to the public

150. All the following statements concerning gastroesophageal reflux disease (GERD) are **TRUE EXCEPT**
   A. All persons would have evidence of reflux if monitored with an intraesophageal probe over 24 hours
   B. The lower esophageal sphincter (LES) pressure is the same in persons with GERD as in normal persons
   C. Weight gain exacerbates reflux
   D. Heartburn is the most common manifestation of GERD

Internal Medicine

Answer Key

1. A	27. D	53. B	79. B
2. A	28. D	54. C	80. A
3. D	29. D	55. D	81. B
4. D	30. D	56. C	82. D
5. C	31. B	57. C	83. A
6. B	32. A	58. D	84. D
7. E	33. E	59. A	85. B
8. A	34. A	60. E	86. B
9. B	35. C	61. B	87. D
10. B	36. B	62. E	88. D
11. D	37. C	63. D	89. C
12. B	38. C	64. A	90. D
13. D	39. B	65. D	91. B
14. A	40. B	66. E	92. A
15. C	41. C	67. E	93. C
16. B	42. A	68. C	94. C
17. B	43. C	69. D	95. D
18. D	44. B	70. C	96. A
19. C	45. B	71. B	97. G
20. C	46. D	72. A	98. D
21. A	47. C	73. D	99. E
22. D	48. B	74. B	100. D
23. C	49. C	75. B	101. B
24. B	50. E	76. A	102. D
25. B	51. B	77. C	103. A
26. D	52. D	78. C	104. D

105. C	117. B	129. E	141. D
106. A	118. J	130. A	142. B
107. B	119. D	131. E	143. A
108. A	120. E	132. B	144. A
109. B	121. A	133. A	145. B
110. B	122. C	134. D	146. D
111. D	123. B	135. E	147. B
112. H	124. B	136. C	148. C
113. C	125. C	137. A	149. A
114. F	126. B	138. C	150. B
115. E	127. A	139. C	
116. A	128. A	140. A	

Internal Medicine

Answers and Comments

1. **(A)** *Key Words:* Holter monitor, congestive heart failure, arrhythmia, ECG
   The ambulatory (Holter) ECG records on magnetic tape the electrical activity of the heart, usually for a 24-hour period. The recording device is small and does not interfere with virtually any of the patient's activities except swimming and bathing. It is useful for assessing whether suspicious symptoms, such as palpitations, lightheadedness, dizziness, or syncope, in a patient with a normal resting ECG are due to an episodic arrhythmia. It can also be helpful in assessing whether episodic, but potentially life-threatening, arrhythmias are occurring in a patient with known heart disease. **(Ref. 1,** p. 737)

2. **(A)** *Key Words:* Wenckebach phenomenon, heart block
   Type 1 AV block, or the Wenckebach phenomenon, is the more benign type of second-degree AV block. The P-R interval prolongs with each cycle until a P wave fails to conduct to the ventricles. The longest R-R interval is less than twice the shortest R-R interval. **(Ref. 2,** pp. 239–240)

3. **(D)** *Key Words:* digoxin, conduction, quinidine, automaticity
   At the cellular level, exposure to excessive levels of cardiac glycosides, such as digoxin, causes increased automaticity and decreased conduction. These abnormalities are reflected in a broad array of rhythm disturbances (including but not limited to the

83

Wenckebach phenomenon) that are often difficult to distinguish from those caused by the underlying disease. Quinidine, verapamil, and amiodorone all increase steady-state serum digoxin levels, and so adding one of these agents would not be the next step in this patient's management. (**Ref. 2,** p. 204)

4. **(D)** *Key Words:* gonococcal urethritis, gram-negative diplococcus
   Gonococcal urethritis in males is characterized by a yellowish, purulent urethral discharge and dysuria. On Gram's stain it is a gram-negative diplococcus. (**Ref. 2,** p. 1756)

5. **(C)** *Key Words:* synergy, toxicity, propranolol, histamine
   Animal studies are done to help ascertain the potential toxicities of drugs used alone and in combination. The effect of some drugs can be altered markedly by the administration of other agents. Such interactions can sabotage therapeutic intent by producing excessive drug action. Two drugs may act on separate components of a common process and yield greater effects than either alone. When those effects are unwanted or dangerous, this is called synergistic toxicity, which is depicted here. The most plausible explanation for this result is that propranolol is sensitizing the animals to the subsequent administration of histamine. (**Ref. 5,** pp. 401, 403)

6. **(B)** *Key Words:* beta-receptors, propranolol, autonomic nervous system
   Propranolol is the prototypical nonselective beta-adrenergic blocking agent of the autonomic nervous system. It is considered nonselective in that it induces a competitive blockade of both beta-1 and beta-2 receptors. (**Ref. 5,** p. 424)

7. **(E)** *Key Words:* propranolol, hypertension, beta blocker
   The beta-adrenergic receptor blocking agents work to block sympathetic effects on the heart and are most effective in reducing cardiac output and in lowering arterial pressure when there is increased cardiac sympathetic nerve activity. They are most effective in controlling hypertension when used in conjunction with vascular smooth-muscle relaxants and diuretics. However, adverse effects include the precipitation of heart failure in patients in whom cardiac compensation depends on enhanced sympathetic drive. They are also contraindicated in insulin-requiring diabetics due to the predisposition of development of hypoglycemia by way

of blockade of catecholamine-mediated counterregulation and antagonism of adrenergic warning signs of hypoglycemia, as well as in patients with significant bradycardia or in patients with greater than first-degree AV block. (**Ref. 5,** pp. 424, 1125)

8. **(A)** *Key Words:* rheumatic fever, Jones criteria, erythema marginatum, carditis, chorea, arthralgia

Arthralgia is considered one of the minor clinical manifestations of rheumatic fever, along with fever and prior rheumatic fever or rheumatic heart disease. Minor laboratory manifestations of rheumatic fever include the presence of acute phase reactants (erythrocyte sedimentation rate, C-reactive protein, leukocytosis) and a prolonged P-R interval. All the other options listed are considered major manifestations; not listed is polyarthritis. The presence of two major and one minor criteria is consistent with a high probability of rheumatic fever, if also supported by evidence of a preceding streptococcal infection. (**Ref. 2,** p. 1637)

9. **(B)** *Key Words:* pericardial effusion, cardiac tamponade, jugular venous distension

Pericardial effusion from virtually any cause can progress to cardiac tamponade, which can produce all the symptoms listed. The jugular venous pressure becomes abnormally elevated; pulsus paradoxus can be detected by palpation of any arterial pulse. When extreme, the pulse disappears during inspiration; when less extreme, it diminishes but can still be palpated. (**Ref. 2,** pp. 346–347)

10. **(B)** *Key Words:* constrictive pericarditis, ECG, pericardial knock

In patients with constrictive pericarditis, ventricular filling is suddenly checked at the end of the early diastolic pressure dip; a loud third heart sound ("pericardial knock") is frequently heard. In a chest x-ray, the heart is normal in size to moderately enlarged. The ECG usually shows T-wave inversions and frequently a wide, notched P wave due to chronic elevation of left atrial pressure. In longstanding cases, atrial fibrillation often supervenes. (**Ref. 2,** p. 347)

11. **(D)** *Key Words:* constrictive pericarditis, idiopathic

In the United States and Western Europe, constrictive pericarditis is most often idiopathic, secondary to neoplasm or radiation, posttraumatic, or due to connective tissue disorders. Tuberculosis and pyogenic infections are less common causes than they used to be. (**Ref. 2,** p. 347)

12. (**B**)   *Key Words:* blastomycosis, azole, amphotericin B
    Amphotericin B has been the mainstay of therapy for the past three decades; total dosage recommendations usually range from 2.0 to 2.5 g. The azole class of compounds shows promise for further therapeutic options. (**Ref. 4,** p. 1930)

13. (**D**)   *Key Words:* digitalis, amphotericin B, arrhythmia, hypokalemia
    Amphotericin B increases the permeability of luminal membranes to potassium and therefore promotes potassium secretion. The ECG abnormalities of potassium depletion affect primarily repolarization segments, due to effects on the action potential. The common ECG manifestations of hypokalemia include sagging of the ST segment, depression of the T wave, and elevation of the U wave. In patients treated with digitalis, hypokalemia can precipitate serious arrhythmias. (**Ref. 2,** pp. 516–517)

14. (**A**)   *Key Words:* candida vulvovaginitis, diabetes mellitus, imidazole
    In a small number of patients, symptomatic vulvovaginitis infection with *Candida* species is recurrent. Therapy is with one of the imidazole compounds (clotrimazole, miconazole, butaconazole, or teraconazole). Attempts should be made to correct ancillary conditions that increase susceptibility to vaginal candidiasis: antibiotic therapy, diabetes, or oral anovulatory steroids. (**Ref. 2,** p. 1754; **Ref. 4,** p. 876)

15. (**C**)   *Key Words:* propoxyphene hydrochloride, Darvon, overdose, comatose
    The manifestations of acute overdosage with propoxyphene are those of narcotic overdosage. The patient is usually somnolent but may be stuporous or comatose and convulsing. Respiratory depression is characteristic. Blood pressure and heart rate are usually normal initially, but blood pressure falls and cardiac performance deteriorates, which ultimately results in pulmonary edema and circulatory collapse. (**Ref. 7,** p. 1323)

16. (B) *Key Words:* naloxone, Narcan, artificial respiration
Attention should be directed first to establishing a patent airway and to restoring ventilation. The narcotic antagonist naloxone (Narcan) will markedly reduce the degree of respiratory depression. General supportive measures, in addition to oxygen, include, when necessary, intravenous fluids, vasopressor-inotropic compounds, and, when infection is likely, antibiotics. (**Ref. 7,** p. 1323)

17. (B) *Key Words:* thiamine, Wernicke-Korsakoff syndrome, alcoholism
In addition to being caused by a poor diet, thiamine deficiency in the United States most commonly occurs as a result of alcoholism. The central nervous system manifestations of thiamine deficiency consist primarily of the Wernicke-Korsakoff syndrome. The Wernicke's component is an acute disorder consisting of variable degrees of vomiting, horizontal nystagmus, ophthalmoplegia, fever, ataxic gait, and progressive mental impairment. The Korsakoff syndrome typically has loss of memory and confabulation as prominent features. (**Ref. 2,** p. 1171)

18. (D) *Key Words:* electrical axis, ECG, deviation
The patient has a normal electrical axis of about +50°. Usually axes between 0° and +90° are considered normal. Those between +90° and +180° are considered right axis deviations, and those between 0° and –90° represent left axis deviation. (**Ref. 3,** pp. 168, 187–188)

19. (C) *Key Words:* rheumatoid arthritis, gold, dermatitis, stomatitis
If salicylates and NSAIDs fail to control the inflammation or are not tolerated, alternative therapies such as gold can be tried. Because of the potential toxicity to kidneys and bone marrow, frequent urinalysis and blood counts must be done. Common side effects include pruritic skin rashes and painful mouth ulcers. (**Ref. 2,** p. 1515)

20. (C) *Key Words:* cardiac tamponade, tuberculosis, pericardial effusion, jugular venous distension
Tuberculous pericarditis is less common now that tuberculosis is better controlled and treated. Pulmonary tuberculosis may be present, but often pericardial effusion is an isolated manifestation.

Virtually any pericardial effusion can progress to cardiac tamponade. In extreme cases, arterial blood pressure can fall to shock levels. Abnormal jugular venous pulses and pulsus paradoxus are also manifestations of tamponade. (**Ref. 2,** pp. 344, 346)

21. **(A)** *Key Words:* Kussmaul's sign, cardiac tamponade, paradoxical pulse
In cardiac tamponade a paradoxical pulse may develop in which there is an exaggerated decrease in arterial pulse with inspiration. Neck veins normally collapse during inspiration from the more negative pressure in the thorax and pericardium. In constrictive pericarditis and tamponade, the cervical veins are distended and may remain so even after intensive diuretic treatment, and venous pressure may fail to decline during inspiration (Kussmaul's sign). (**Ref. 5,** p. 1100)

22. **(D)** *Key Words:* tick, louse, pediculosis
Each of the listed illnesses are tick-borne except for pediculosis, which is a louse-borne disease. (**Ref. 2,** pp. 2021–2022)

23. **(C)** *Key Words:* overdose, aspirin, poisoning, convulsions
Manifestations of mild salicylate poisoning include vomiting, tachycardia, hyperpnea, fever, tinnitus, lethargy, confusion, respiratory alkalosis, and an alkaline urine (pH > 6). In severe poisoning, convulsions, coma, and respiratory and cardiovascular failure may occur. Vomiting, poor intake, and hyperventilation may cause severe dehydration, acute renal failure, and acidosis. (**Ref. 5,** p. 2458)

24. **(B)** *Key Words:* intubation, vitamin K, oxygen, intravenous fluids
Emergency and supportive measures should include, first and foremost, protection of the airway, with endotracheal intubation if necessary. Oxygen should be administered as indicated by arterial blood gas analysis. Parenteral fluids should be given to produce a brisk urine flow, though care should be taken to avoid the development of pulmonary edema. Seizures should be controlled with intravenous diazepam. Prolongation of the prothrombin time should be corrected with intravenous vitamin K. The subcutaneous route should not be used in this critically ill patient, given the relatively slow and possibly erratic absorption time inherent in this modality. (**Ref. 5,** p. 2458; **Ref. 6,** pp. 278–279)

25. **(B)** *Key Words:* congestive heart failure, digoxin, furosemide, gout, podagra

It is postulated that uricosuric agents (such as furosemide) may induce acute gouty attacks by lowering synovial fluid urate levels and favoring shedding of synovial crystals during dissolution. An acute attack can be of incapacitating severity, with at least half of them involving the metatarsophalangeal joint of the great toe (podagra). Within minutes to hours the affected joint becomes hot, dusky red, and exquisitely painful. (**Ref. 2**, pp. 1110–1111)

26. **(D)** *Key Words:* negative birefringence, urate crystals, polarizing microscope

Urate crystals are water-soluble, but when tissues are treated with nonaqueous fixatives (e.g., absolute alcohol), the crystals are preserved and are negatively birefringent in compensated light. (**Ref. 2**, p. 1110)

27. **(D)** *Key Words:* colchicine, antiinflammatory agent, allopurinol, nonsteroidal agents

The affected joint should be rested and an antiinflammatory agent administered promptly. Three options are colchicine, nonsteroidals, and glucocorticoids. Allopurinol which is of no value in the treatment of the acute attack, is used in the management of chronic gout. (**Ref. 2**, pp. 1113–1114)

28. **(D)** *Key Words:* Sjögren's syndrome rheumatoid arthritis, keratoconjunctivitis sicca, xerostomia

Corneal inflammation as the result of drying is referred to as keratoconjunctivitis sicca. This, along with a dry mouth (xerostomia) and a connective tissue disorder, constitutes Sjögren's syndrome. This syndrome is common in patients with rheumatoid arthritis, especially middle-aged women. (**Ref. 2**, p. 2276)

29. **(D)** *Key Words:* antinuclear antibodies, autoimmune, rheumatoid factor

The underlying pathophysiology appears to be an autoimmune reaction affecting the lacrimal and salivary glands. Females are affected 10 times more frequently than males. The incidence of lymphoma is increased 44-fold. Extraglandular involvement occurs frequently and can be seen in the lungs, kidneys, and nervous system. Autoantibodies are common; the rheumatoid factor may be found in 75 to 90%. Antinuclear antibodies may be positive in 50 to 80%. (**Ref. 2,** pp. 1535–1536, 2276)

30. (**D**) *Key Words:* Schirmer's test, rose bengal dye, slit-lamp exam, xerostomia
    The presence of dry eyes is suggested by a positive Schirmer's test (less than 5 mm of wetting per 5 min, with the patient unanesthetized), although the frequency of both false-positive and false-negative tests is high. The pattern and intensity of staining with rose bengal dye and slit-lamp examination are more reliable in diagnosis. Diminution in stimulated parotid flow rate (PFR, < 5 ml per gland in 10 minutes) is a sensitive indicator of xerostomia. Ham's test looks for abnormal sensitivity of erythrocytes to complement. (**Ref. 2,** pp. 834, 1536)

31. (**B**) *Key Words:* claudication, arterial insufficiency, ischemia
    The symptoms of chronic arterial occlusive disease are intermittent claudication, pain at rest, and trophic changes in the involved limb. Ischemic damage may cause persistent reddish discoloration, and a dry, scaly, shiny skin may be seen. The hair may disappear and the toenails may become brittle, ridged, and deformed. (**Ref. 2,** pp. 360–361)

32. (**A**) *Key Words:* warfarin, anticoagulation, barbiturate, coumadin
    Barbiturates cause resistance to the effects of warfarin by increasing warfarin metabolism, thus requiring a higher warfarin dose than usual to achieve the same effect. Broad-spectrum antibiotics cause increased sensitivity to warfarin by causing vitamin K deficiency, especially if treatment with the antibiotics is for a prolonged period of time. Aspirin, phenylbutazone, and ibuprofen all cause displacement of albumin binding, thus increasing warfarin sensitivity. (**Ref. 2,** p. 1014)

33. (**E**) *Key Words:* ECG, left ventricular hypertrophy, strain pattern
    T wave inversions are noted laterally in leads I and L, as well as in the precordial leads. Left ventricular hypertrophy with a strain pattern can produce such changes. However, other conditions such as cardiomyopathy, ischemia, drug, and metabolic effects can result in similar changes. (**Ref. 3,** pp. 207–212)

34. (A) *Key Words:* ECG, QRS complex, voltage
Patients with left ventricular hypertrophy frequently have prominent voltage of the QRS complexes. However, obesity can dampen this expected high voltage. In the EKG strip shown, the terminal portion of the P wave is inverted in lead V1, suggesting possible early left atrial enlargement. (**Ref. 3,** pp. 203, 207–208)

35. (C) *Key Words:* hypertension, left ventricular hypertrophy
The patient described had hypertension, which is the most common cause of left ventricular hypertrophy. Numerous studies have shown that control of hypertension decreases morbidity and mortality, even in elderly persons. (**Ref. 2,** pp. 207, 256, 266)

36. (B) *Key Words:* congestive heart failure, quinidine, digoxin, arrhythmia
An important interaction between digoxin and quinidine has been described, leading to a substantial increase in steady-state serum digoxin levels (averaging about twofold) when conventional quinidine doses are added to a maintenance digoxin regimen. (**Ref. 2,** p. 203)

37. (C) *Key Words:* hypothyroidism, fibrositis, myopathy
Aches and stiffness simulating fibrositis may appear early in hypothyroidism; untreated, this may progress to proximal myopathy with elevated creatinine kinase levels. Serum cholesterol and triglycerides, creatine phosphokinase (MM isozyme), aldolase, lactic dehydrogenase, and SGOT may all be elevated in the patient with moderate to severe hypothyroidism. (**Ref. 2,** pp. 1262, 1561)

38. (C) *Key Words:* autoimmune, Hashimoto's thyroiditis, idiopathic myxedema, hypothyroidism
Hashimoto's thyroiditis (an autoimmune process) accounts for the majority of cases of primary hypothyroidism. Idiopathic myxedema (probably a variant of Hashimoto's thyroiditis) and thyroid destruction resulting from radioactive iodine therapy or surgery for hyperthyroidism account for additional cases. (**Ref. 2,** p. 1260)

39. (B) *Key Words:* colorectal cancer (right), anemia
The major symptoms of colorectal cancer are rectal bleeding, pain, and change in bowel habits. The clinical presentation in an indi-

vidual patient is related to the size and location of the tumor. Those on the right side are often asymptomatic, and bleeding may be occult. (**Ref. 2,** p. 718)

40. **(B)** *Key Words:* colorectal cancer, metastasis (liver)
An abdominal mass or symptoms and signs of liver metastasis may be the earliest clinical manifestation of an underlying colorectal cancer. Distant spread to the lungs and bones may be silent until very advanced. (**Ref. 2,** p. 718)

41. **(C)** *Key Words:* overdose, acetaminophen, liver
This readily available analgesic and antipyretic is a classic example of an intrinsic, dose-dependent hepatotoxin causing zonal necrosis and acute liver failure, often associated with renal failure. Significant liver injury usually occurs with doses in excess of 10 to 15 grams, most frequently taken in a suicide attempt. Within a few hours the patient develops nausea, vomiting, and diarrhea; a relatively asymptomatic period ensues. Clinical and laboratory signs of liver damage become evident within 24 to 48 hours. (**Ref. 2,** p. 773)

42. **(A)** *Key Words:* overdose, acetaminophen, acetylcysteine, liver
The initial treatment of acetaminophen overdose consists of supportive measures and gastric lavage. N-acetylcysteine should be administered to high-risk patients, in whom it may significantly reduce the severity of liver necrosis and its attendant mortality. This agent appears to act mainly by providing cysteine for glutathione synthesis and is most effective when given within 10 hours of acetaminophen ingestion. (**Ref. 2,** p. 773)

43. **(C)** *Key Words:* ECG, left bundle branch block
The patient has prolongation of the Q-R-S interval, an RS complex in lead V1, and absent septal Q wave in leads V1 and V6 consistent with a diagnosis of left bundle branch block. (**Ref. 3,** pp. 146–154)

44. **(B)** *Key Words:* ECG, electrical axis, left bundle branch block
The axis is leftward and, because lead V2 is nearly isoelectric, the axis is close to −30°. There have been reports that patients with left bundle branch block and left axis deviation have a poorer prognosis than those with normal axes. (**Ref. 3,** p. 187)

45. (B) *Key Words:* polymyalgia rheumatica, erythrocyte sedimentation rate, normochromic normocytic anemia

Polymyalgia rheumatica (PMR), the most likely diagnosis in this patient, is characterized by aching and morning stiffness in the shoulder and hip girdles, the proximal extremities, the neck, and the torso. Fatigue, sense of weakness, loss of weight, and a low-grade fever may be present. A moderate normochromic normocytic anemia is typical. Usually, the erythrocyte sedimentation rate is elevated. **(Ref. 2,** p. 1544)

46. (D) *Key Words:* temporal arteritis, giant cell arteritis, granuloma, inflammation

This disease affects large and medium-sized arteries, especially those branching from the proximal aorta that supply the neck and the extracranial structure of the head. Temporal artery biopsy shows a granulomatous inflammatory infiltrate. Visual symptoms are present in about one-third of patients. Permanent visual loss may be partial or complete and may occur without warning. **(Ref. 2,** p. 1545)

47. (C) *Key Words:* temporal arteritis, giant cell arteritis, corticosteroids

Although polyarthralgia rheumatica may be treated with nonsteroidal antiinflammatory agents or low-dose steroids, in giant cell arteritis, the recommended dose of prednisone is 40 to 60 mg per day. Vascular complications seldom occur after corticosteroids have been started. **(Ref. 2,** p. 1546)

48. (B) *Key Words:* polycythemia vera, malignancy, iron deficiency anemia

Polycythemia vera is a hematologic malignant disorder characterized by excessive proliferation of erythroid, myeloid, and megakaryocytic elements within the bone marrow, resulting in an increased red blood cell mass and frequently elevated peripheral granulocyte and platelet counts. When iron deficiency anemia develops, as evidenced by the decreased MCV in the patient described, the hematocrit may be within normal range. **(Ref. 2,** p. 925)

49. (C) *Key Words:* splenomegaly, extramedullary hematopoiesis, polycythemia vera

The most useful physical finding terms of differential diagnosis is splenomegaly, which is present in about 75% of patients, and reflects principally the development of extramedullary hematopoiesis. (**Ref. 2,** p. 926)

50. (E) *Key Words:* polycythemia vera, bone marrow, iron stores, hyperplasia, panmyelosis
The bone marrow in P. vera is typically hyperplastic and reveals a panmyelosis. Red cell morphology usually reveals hypochromic microcytic cells with a reduced mean corpuscular volume, suggestive of iron-deficient erythropoiesis. This suggestion is frequently confirmed by a low serum iron level and absence of bone marrow iron stores. (**Ref. 2,** p. 926)

51. (B) *Key Words:* polycythemia vera, phlebotomy, hematocrit
The initial treatment in any newly diagnosed case of polycythemia vera is phlebotomy. Efforts should be made to reduce the hematocrit to approximately 45%, a level at which the complications of hypervolemia and hyperviscosity are minimized. Many patients can be successfully managed with phlebotomy alone; however, thrombotic incidents are slightly increased in the first few years of therapy, compared to the alternative treatment modalities. Radioactive phosphorus and chlorambucil both decrease the thrombotic predilection, and long-term myelosuppression with either of these agents is associated with an increased propensity for malignant transformation of bone marrow, skin, and gastrointestinal mucosa. (**Ref. 2,** p. 928)

52. (D) *Key Words:* ECG, heart rate, QRS complex
Heart rate can be easily determined by dividing the number of large blocks encompassing two QRS complexes into 300. Seven such blocks are noted, giving a rate of about 43. (**Ref. 3,** pp. 58–75)

53. (B) *Key Words:* second-degree heart block, Wenckebach phenomenon, ECG
There are two P waves for each QRS complex with a constant P-R interval (2:1 block). There is borderline prolongation of the P-R interval with no evidence of bundle branch block. Therefore, type I, second-degree AV block, i.e., Wenckebach phenomenon, is the most likely diagnosis. (**Ref. 3,** p. 140)

54. (C) *Key Words:* digoxin, low output heart failure, cardiomyopathy

Digoxin is of value in patients with symptoms and signs of heart failure due to ischemic cardiomyopathy, valvular disease, hypertensive heart disease, many types of congenital heart disease, and dilated cardiomyopathies, all of which represent instances of low-output heart failure. The other listed scenarios represent instances of high-output heart failure; in these cases, attention should be paid to correcting the underlying process. (**Ref. 2,** p. 203)

55. **(D)** *Key Words:* digoxin, bioavailability, absorption
Bioavailability of digoxin in the standard tablet formulation is 55 to 75%. A preparation in which digoxin is dissolved in an encapsulated gel gives higher bioavailability, requiring a slight adjustment in the standard maintenance doses. Previously marketed preparations with poor bioavailability are no longer available in the United States. (**Ref. 2,** p. 203)

56. **(C)** *Key Words:* digoxin, half-life, first-order kinetics
Digoxin is excreted exponentially (i.e., first-order kinetics) with a half-life of about 36 hours in young, healthy, normal subjects. (**Ref. 2,** p. 202)

57. **(C)** *Key Words:* ECG, Wolff-Parkinson-White syndrome, palpitations
The ECG shows a shortened P-R interval. Although the Q-R-S interval is not prolonged above the normal limits, there is a slurring of the initial QRS deflection. These findings are consistent with a diagnosis of Wolff-Parkinson-White syndrome. (**Ref. 3,** p. 157)

58. **(D)** *Key Words:* ECG, QRS complex, delta wave, Wolff-Parkinson-White syndrome
The presence of delta waves is characteristic of Wolff-Parkinson-White syndrome in which a ventricle or its component is activated earlier than normal, i.e., preexcitation occurs. (**Ref. 3,** p. 157)

59. **(A)** *Key Words:* Wolff-Parkinson-White syndrome, carotid artery massage, verapamil, Valsalva maneuver
A vagal maneuver (such as carotid artery massage or the Valsalva maneuver), adenosine, or verapamil is effective in aborting a run of paroxysmal supraventricular tachycardia in about 90% of the cases. If hypotension or heart failure occurs due to the dysrhythmia, DC cardioversion should be employed. Nitroglycerin is not

one of the therapeutic options unless it is part of an overall effort to reduce any ischemia that may be contributing to the arrhythmia. (**Ref. 2,** p. 237)

60. **(E)**   *Key Words:* pitting edema, secondary hyperaldosteronism, renin-angiotensin system
Secondary hyperaldosteronism occurs in edematous states such as congestive heart failure, cirrhosis, or the nephrotic syndrome. Decreased renal blood flow (such as that which occurs in renal artery stenosis) may activate the renin-angiotensin system with resultant increased production of aldosterone. In edematous states total body sodium is increased, and serum albumin is often deceased. (**Ref. 2,** p. 1290)

61. **(B)**   *Key Words:* spironolactone, aldactone, aldosterone antagonist, potassium-sparing diuretic
Spironolactone (aldactone) antagonizes the effect of aldosterone. Unlike the other diuretics listed that cause a kaliuresis, spironolactone administration results in potassium retention. Therefore, its use in patients with kidney failure is dangerous as is concurrent administration of potassium salts in patients receiving spironolactone. (**Ref. 2,** p. 201)

62. **(E)**   *Key Words:* malaria, travel, fever
Most patients with malaria present with recurrent fever and chills (at 48-hour intervals for *Plasmodium vivax* and *P. ovale,* and at 72-hour intervals for *P. malariae*). Patients with *P. falciparum* infection typically have irregular fever and chills and rarely present with a regular 48-hour cycle of symptoms despite the 48-hour cycle of the parasite. (**Ref. 2,** p. 1973)

63. **(D)**   *Key Words:* congestive heart failure, beriberi, high output failure
Congestive heart failure from beriberi results from high output failure. Such patients have low peripheral vascular resistance. Cardiac dilatation, particularly of the right ventricle, and hypertrophy occur in this disorder. (**Ref. 2,** p. 1171)

64. **(A)**   *Key Words:* beriberi, vitamin B1 thiamine
Thiamine deficiency, especially when associated with a high carbohydrate diet, can result in beriberi. Worldwide, this is the most common cause of nutritional cardiac disorders. (**Ref. 2,** p. 1171)

65. **(D)** *Key Words:* atopy, epinephrine, bee sting, resuscitation
Intravenous steroids may be helpful in patients with systemic
reactions to insect stings; however, there is a time delay between
institution and desired effect. The other agents listed would more
likely be indicated in the immediate management of patients with
systemic reactions. The patient's respiratory distress may result
from laryngeal edema or bronchospasm. Wheezing is frequently
present. Immediate hospitalization is required in this life-threatening condition. (**Ref. 2,** p. 1466)

66. **(E)** *Key Words:* nephrotic syndrome, ascites, transudate, serum
albumin
Patients with nephrotic syndrome may develop a transudate-type
ascites. Ascites occurs only when the serum albumin is very low,
usually less than 2 mg per deciliter. The fluid is clear and straw-col-
ored and usually contains less than 100 WBC/mm^3. The protein
content is usually less than 3 g/dL. Bloody ascitic fluid may be
found in patients with tumors or tuberculosis. (**Ref. 2,** pp. 738–739)

67. **(E)** *Key Words:* nephrotic syndrome, proteinuria, hypoalbuminemia, aldosterone
Most patients with nephrotic syndrome develop heavy proteinuria
(over 3 g/day protein loss). Hypoalbuminemia results in decreased
plasma oncotic pressure and fluid transudation into the interstitial
spaces. A decrease in plasma volume results in elevated production of aldosterone. Hyperlipidemia and hypercholesterolemia are
common in the nephrotic syndrome and are inversely proportional to the serum albumin concentration. (**Ref. 2,** pp. 479, 559–560)

68. **(C)** *Key Words:* Marfan's syndrome, connective tissue disorder,
lens dislocation, cardiovascular abnormalities
The Marfan syndrome is a dominantly inherited connective tissue
disorder characterized by musculoskeletal abnormalities (arachno-
dactyly, tall stature, scoliosis, pectus deformities, and ligamentous
laxity), cardiovascular abnormalities (mitral valve prolapse and
regurgitation, aortic valve insufficiency, and aortic dilatation,
aneurysm, and dissection), lens dislocation, and myopia. (**Ref. 2,**
pp. 1122–1123)

69. **(D)** *Key Words:* sarcoidosis, adenopathy, chest x-ray
The x-ray shows bilateral hilar and right paratracheal adenopathy.
The x-ray picture and spontaneous resolution of the abnormalities

are most consistent with a diagnosis of sarcoidosis. Sarcoidosis has been reported to occur in African-Americans with a higher frequency than whites. Organ involvement is usually asymptomatic and the disease most frequently regresses spontaneously, although progression to debilitating disease can occur. (**Ref. 2,** pp. 430–435)

70. **(C)** *Key Words:* sarcoidosis, erythema nodosum, granuloma, lupus pernio
Erythema nodosum may be associated with sarcoidosis as a secondary vasculitic reaction. Sarcoid granulomas also occur directly in the skin to produce a variety of small, asymptomatic macular and papular lesions that are present either superficially or more deeply in the dermis. Lupus pernio, consisting of violaceous plaques over the nose, cheeks, and ears, is the most commonly described skin lesion and may be disfiguring. (**Ref. 2,** p. 431)

71. **(B)** *Key Words:* tuberous sclerosis, mental retardation, shagreen patch, autosomal dominant
The earliest skin lesions in patients with tuberous sclerosis are whitish spots, which develop over the extremities and trunk and which can be visualized using a Wood's lamp as a source of ultraviolet light. A shagreen patch of rough, thickened, yellow skin may develop over the lower back. This disorder is inherited as an autosomal dominant trait but about 80% of cases occur sporadically. (**Ref. 2,** p. 2144)

72. **(A)** *Key Words:* tuberous sclerosis, adenoma sebaceum, angiofibroma, telangiectasia
Rather than being true adenomas, the skin lesions in patients with tuberous sclerosis are actually angiofibromas. They may, on occasion, be vascular with a telangiectasialike appearance. (**Ref. 2,** pp. 2321–2322)

73. **(D)** *Key Words:* tuberous sclerosis, mental deficiency, seizure
The disease is inherited as an autosomal dominant trait, but about 80% of the cases are sporadic, owing to new mutations. Recently, the gene has been mapped to the long arm of chromosome 11. Mental deficiency may be mild or severe, but one-third of affected individuals have normal or even superior intelligence. Seizures occur in 80% of cases, usually starting before age 5.

Calcified cerebral lesions and subependymal nodules are well seen on brain CT, but uncalcified cortical tubers may show up better with MRI. Cystic disease of the lungs, an uncommon complication, mainly affects women over the age of 20; the symptoms include pneumothorax, dyspnea, cyanosis, and cor pulmonale. (**Ref. 2,** p. 2144)

74. (**B**) *Key Words:* priapism, corpus cavernosum, vasoocclusion
Priapism refers to a persistent erection of the penis, which is not necessarily associated with sexual desire. It results from vasoocclusion within the corpus cavernosum. (**Ref. 2,** p. 891)

75. (**B**) *Key Words:* sickle cell anemia, priapism, vasoocclusion
The patient has sickle cell anemia, which is a common cause of priapism. It results from vasoocclusion within the corpus cavernosum. Other vasoocclusive clinical syndromes that may be associated with sickle cell anemia include cerebrovascular accidents, hepatic crises, the acute chest syndrome, and acute renal papillary infarction. (**Ref. 2,** p. 891)

76. (**A**) *Key Words:* sickle cell anemia, vasoocclusion, stroke, cholelithiasis, osteomyelitis, septicemia
Common vasoocclusive clinical syndromes include cerebrovascular accidents (i.e., hemiplegias and seizures) caused by involvement of the cerebral vasculature. Although not directly related to the sickling phenomenon, patients are at increased risk of developing infections and cholelithiasis (caused by chronic hemolysis leading to increased bilirubin production). Childhood infections with encapsulated organisms, such as *Haemophilus influenzae* and *Streptococcal pneumoniae,* are common. Although Salmonella osteomyelitis occurs almost exclusively in this patient population, *Staphylococcal aureus* remains the most common cause of bone infections. (**Ref. 2,** p. 891)

77. (**C**) *Key Words:* marantic endocarditis, metastatic carcinoma, sterile vegetations, systemic lupus erythematosus
Marantic endocarditis or nonbacterial thrombotic endocarditis is most frequently discovered during autopsies of patients with terminal cancer. The sterile vegetations found in a few patients with systemic lupus erythematosus (Libman-Sachs endocarditis) are another type of marantic endocarditis. (**Ref. 2,** p. 1639)

78. **(C)** *Key Words:* secondary polycythemia, intravenous pyelogram, erythropoietin, kidney
This patient is presenting with signs and symptoms consistent with secondary polycythemia. Secondary polycythemia can result from disorders characterized by excessive autonomous production of erythropoietic stimulatory substances (erythropoietin, androgens, adrenal corticosteroids). Increased, autonomous erythropoietin production may occur in certain neoplasms, as a result of nonneoplastic lesions of the kidney (hydronephrosis, cysts, tumors, vascular lesions) that produce local ischemia involving the renal oxygen-sensing mechanism, or in certain rare familial syndromes, without a demonstrable anatomic lesion. (**Ref. 2,** p. 921)

79. **(B)** *Key Words:* chronic pancreatitis, alcoholism, gall bladder
Although most of the causes of acute pancreatitis can lead to a chronic condition, alcoholism is most frequently associated with chronic pancreatitis. Disorders of the gallbladder are more likely to result in repeated attacks of acute pancreatitis. Acute pancreatitis associated with cholelithiasis is actually associated with a higher mortality than that resulting from alcoholism. (**Ref. 2,** pp. 722, 725–726)

80. **(A)** *Key Words:* amyl nitrite, cyanide poisoning, methemoglobin, sodium thiosulfate
As soon as cyanide poisoning is suspected, administration of nitrite—via a 3% solution intravenously or amyl nitrite inhalation—is crucial. It converts hemoglobin to methemoglobin, which selectively binds cyanide. This is followed by administration of sodium thiosulfate to convert cyanide to the less toxic thiocyanate. (**Ref. 2,** p. 112)

81. **(B)** *Key Words:* Charcot's triad, jaundice, biliary pain, fever
Intermittent cholangitis consisting of jaundice, biliary pain, and fever and chills (Charcot's triad) is a common presenting symptom complex in patients (without a prior history of surgery on the biliary tree) of choledocholithiasis. The intermittent nature of the symptoms reflects the presence of intermittent obstruction of the biliary tree. Pruritus can be an important symptom of cholestasis (impaired bile secretion) that may be present in a number of diseases, but it is not part of Charcot's triad. (**Ref. 2,** pp. 753, 812)

82. **(D)** *Key Words:* pellagra, niacin, tryptophan
Niacin can be formed from tryptophan, an essential amino acid. Niacin is an essential component of nicotinamide adenine dinucleotide (NAD) and nicotinamide adenine dinucleotide phosphate (NADP). Endemic pellagra, which can be cured by niacin, occurs in populations consuming large amounts of maize or sorghum. (**Ref. 2,** p. 1174)

83. **(A)** *Key Words:* Gaucher's disease, amino acid metabolism, glucocerebroside
This relatively common familial disorder results from progressive accumulation of glucocerebroside within phagocytic cells of the monocyte-macrophage system involving principally the liver, spleen, bone marrow, and lymph nodes. The rest of the disorders listed are considered inborn errors of amino acid metabolism. (**Ref. 2,** p. 1091)

84. **(D)** *Key Words:* ascorbic acid, vitamin C, collagen
Ascorbic acid (vitamin C) is involved in collagen metabolism, and defects in collagen biosynthesis are believed to be the basis for many of the symptoms of scurvy. These may include pain in bones and joints; development of petechiae and ecchymoses at points of trauma, pressure, and irritation; and poorly healing wounds. (**Ref. 2,** pp. 1176–1178)

85. **(B)** *Key Words:* lead poisoning, lead line, retinal stippling
Among the many manifestations of lead poisoning, formation of a "lead line" along the gum margin may occur. This is caused by deposition of lead sulfide. Retinal stippling near the optic disc may also be an early manifestation of lead toxicity. (**Ref. 2,** p. 2362)

86. **(B)** *Key Words:* Coxsackie group B, myocarditis, pericarditis, hepatitis
In addition to the disorders listed, Coxsackie group B, can cause pleurodynia, hepatitis, and orchitis. In newborns, infection with this virus has resulted in a generalized systemic disorder. (**Ref. 2,** pp. 1858–1859)

87. **(D)** *Key Words:* Swanz-Ganz catheter, pulmonary artery, wedge pressure

A Swan-Ganz is a balloon-tipped catheter useful for obtaining hemodynamic measurements. The catheter is passed into the right atrium, right ventricle, and then into the pulmonary artery. The catheter then floats into a branch of the pulmonary artery and "wedges" there. Blood flow distal to the balloon ceases, and the "wedge" or pulmonary artery occlusion pressure measured by the catheter tip just distal to the balloon reflects the downstream pressure. This pressure usually is equal to the left atrial pressure, which is the same as left ventricular end-diastolic pressure when the mitral valve is open, assuming that pulmonary venous pressure is not higher. (**Ref. 2,** p. 460)

88. **(D)** *Key Words:* syphilis, vasa vasorum, aortitis, aneurysm
Cardiovascular syphilis affects the vasa vasorum, especially of the aortic arch. Aortitis and aortic aneurysm may result. Patients may become symptomatic from 20 to 30 years after acquiring syphilis. These complications occur more frequently and earlier in men, particularly African-American men. (**Ref. 2,** p. 1765)

89. **(C)** *Key Words: Rickettsia,* vasculitis, fever, rash
Most rickettsial diseases produce rashes, usually involving the trunk and extremities. In some of the disorders, such as Rocky Mountain spotted fever, the face may be involved. *Coxiella burnetti* (the agent of Q fever) is unique among the rickettsiae in that it does not produce a rash, despite the similarity of the infection of endothelial cells (vasculitis) as occurs with *Rickettsia rickettsii* (the agent of Rocky Mountain spotted fever). (**Ref. 2,** p. 1794)

90. **(D)** *Key Words:* goiter, iodine deficiency
Iodine deficiency is the most common cause of thyroid disease in the world population, although iodination of salt has eliminated this problem in North America. Areas in which iodine intake remains low include mountainous regions such as the Andes and Himalayas, as well as some areas of central Africa, New Guinea, and Indonesia. Iodine prophylaxis in the form of foodstuffs or the administration of iodinized oil injections has helped this situation in many areas. (**Ref. 2,** p. 1271)

91. **(B)** *Key Words:* Goodpasture's syndrome, autoimmune antibodies, lung, kidney

Goodpasture's syndrome is a disease characterized by anti-glomerular and antialveolar basement membrane antibodies that produces interstitial lung disease with pulmonary hemorrhages, as well as glomerulonephritis with hematuria and renal failure. Unlike Wegener's, upper respiratory tract involvement is not seen. (**Ref. 2,** pp. 557–558)

92. (**A**) *Key Words:* Wegener's granulomatosis, sinusitis, necrosis, lung, kidney
Wegener's granulomatosis is a necrotizing granulomatous process most commonly presenting with evidence of chronic sinusitis, nasal passage, and pulmonary involvement. Like Goodpasture's, renal disease is also common. (**Ref. 2,** pp. 1541–1543)

93. (**C**) *Key Words:* periarteritis nodosa, immune complexes, hepatitis B antigenemia, skin, kidneys
Periarteritis nodosa is a neutrophilic inflammatory disorder of small and medium-sized arteries that has a frequent association with hepatitis B antigenemia with circulating immune complexes. Commonly affected organs are the skin, kidneys, and GI tract. (**Ref. 2,** pp. 1539–1541)

94. (**C**) *Key Words:* Budd-Chiari syndrome, hepatic vein thrombosis, ascites
Thrombosis of the hepatic veins may occur following abdominal trauma or in association with hypercoagulable states induced by oral contraceptives, or hematologic disorders such as polycythemia rubra vera. Its onset may be abrupt, subacute, or chronic. The liver is usually enlarged and tender, and ascites is prominent. (**Ref. 2,** p. 792)

95. (**D**) *Key Words:* chronic pancreatitis, alcoholism, liver disease, abdominal pain
Chronic pancreatitis does not usually present with fever, ascites, or hepatic enlargement unless caused by chronic alcohol ingestion with associated alcoholic liver disease. Chronic pancreatitis most often presents with abdominal pain. If weight loss occurs, it is usually due to efforts to avoid the abdominal pain that often follows eating. (**Ref. 2,** p. 726)

96. (A) *Key Words:* congestive heart failure, gynecomastia, digoxin
Gynecomastia can be associated with the estrogenic activity of various medications besides digitalis glycosides, e.g., cimetidine, spironolactone, diazepam, and ketaconazole. (**Ref. 2,** pp. 1340–1341)

97. (G) *Key Words:* nifedipine, calcium channel blockers, vasodilator effect
Calcium channel blockers (e.g., diltiazem, nicardipine, nifedipine, and verapamil) can all be associated with flushing and headache (vasodilator effects), but these side effects are most commonly seen with nifedipine and nicardipine. Diarrhea is occasionally seen with nifedipine, whereas constipation is more often seen with verapamil. (**Ref. 2,** pp. 264–265)

98. (D) *Key Words:* dysgeusia, cough, ACE inhibitor
Angiotensin-converting enzyme (ACE) inhibitors can all cause altered or absent taste and a nonproductive cough, especially within the first one to two months after initiation. These symptoms respond to decreasing the dose or discontinuing the medication. (**Ref. 2,** pp. 264–265)

99. (E) *Key Words:* Paget's disease, alkaline phosphatase
The major biological change in Paget's disease is an elevated alkaline phosphatase. Because studies have shown that as many as 90% of patients with Paget's disease are asymptomatic, diagnostic chance findings of abnormalities on radiologic examination or blood chemistry screening are invaluable in diagnosing this condition. (**Ref. 2,** pp. 1431–1432)

100. (D) *Key Words:* Wegener's granulomatosis, corticosteroids, cyclophosphamide
The treatment of choice for Wegener's granulomatosis is a combination of corticosteroids and a cytotoxic agent, the most efficacious of which is cyclophosphamide. Irreversible organ system dysfunction can occur if conservative therapy (such as corticosteroid therapy alone) is attempted. Corticosteroids should be administered in an oral daily dose regimen of 1 mg/kg/day of prednisone, for example. (**Ref. 2,** pp. 1542–1543)

101. (B) *Key Words:* osteomyelitis, Staphylococcal aureus, hematogenous spread

Bacteria responsible for hematogenous osteomyelitis reflect essentially their bacteremic incidence as a function of age. Therefore, gram-positive organisms (especially *Staphylococcus aureus*) predominate. The only exception might be in the elderly patient who undergoes a genitourinary manipulation. In this scenario, gram-negative organisms may predominate. (**Ref. 4,** p. 1126)

102. (**D**) *Key Words:* primary biliary cirrhosis, immunosuppression
Corticosteroids are not known to be effective in the treatment of primary biliary cirrhosis and will aggravate the bone disease associated with this condition. D-penicillamine, azathioprine, ursodeoxycholic acid and colchicine have all been used, but none can yet be recommended until further investigations are done. Corticosteroids have a role in the therapy of all of the other conditions listed. (**Ref. 2,** p. 789)

103. (**A**) *Key Words:* systemic lupus erythematosus, rheumatoid factor, cryoglobulins, autoimmune antibodies
Rheumatoid factor occurs in low titer in patients with SLE. Hypergammaglobulinemia may be marked in an untreated patient. Cryoglobulins may be increased. Reduced hemolytic complement levels (CH50) are common in active disease, especially with renal involvement. Antibodies are found that react with DNA, RNA, histones, nuclear ribonucleoprotein, and cytoplasmic antigenic determinants. (**Ref. 2,** p. 1527)

104. (**D**) *Key Words:* Sjogren's syndrome, autoimmune antibodies, rheumatoid factor, hyperglobulinemia
Autoantibodies are common in SS. Rheumatoid factor may be found in 75 to 90%; antinuclear antibodies may be positive in 50 to 80%. Persons with SS manifest B cell hyperactivity. Evidence for this includes the polyclonal hyperglobulinemia seen in more than 50% of patients. Serum hyperviscosity may result from either macroglobulinemia or polymerizing IgG with rheumatoid factor activity. Cryoglobulinemia may be present. (**Ref. 2,** p. 1536)

105. (**C**) *Key Words:* Hutchinson's teeth, congenital syphilis
The permanent dentition of patients with congenital syphilis may show characteristic abnormalities known as Hutchinson's teeth. The upper central incisors are widely spaced, centrally notched, and tapered in a manner of a screwdriver. The molars may show multiple poorly developed cusps (mulberry molars). (**Ref. 2,** p. 1766)

106. (A) *Key Words:* congenital syphilis, cardiovascular abnormalities, saddle nose, saber shins
Cardiovascular alterations have not been observed in congenital syphilis. Neurological manifestations are common, and there may be eighth cranial nerve deafness and interstitial keratitis. Periostitis may result in prominent frontal bones, depression of the bridge of the nose ("saddle nose"), poor development of the maxilla, and anterior bowing of the tibias ("saber shins"). There may be late-onset arthritis of the knees (Clutton's joints). **(Ref. 2, p. 1766)**

107. (B) *Key Words:* myotonic dystrophy, atrophy, myopathy, ptosis, frontal balding
The patient depicted has myotonic dystrophy. Transmission is by dominant inheritance with high penetrance and variable expressivity. The incidence is about 1 in 7500 births. Other manifestations of this disease include mental retardation, cataracts, gonadal atrophy/dysfunction, and cardiac arrhythmias. **(Ref. 2, pp. 2254–2255)**

108. (A) *Key Words: Helicobacter pylori,* gram-negative, microaerophilic, antral gastritis
H. pylori, a gram-negative microaerophilic organism, may be the most common worldwide human infective agent. No reservoir other than the human stomach has been identified and the epidemiology is unknown. The organism is fastidious but can be cultured with careful technique. It is found in nearly all biopsies showing active antral gastritis with polymorphonuclear infiltration, whereas the organism is unusual in the histologically normal stomach. **(Ref. 2, p. 651)**

109. (B) *Key Words:* acute intermittent porphyria, autosomal dominant, abdominal pain
Acute intermittent porphyria is an autosomal dominant disorder. Symptoms rarely occur before puberty. Abdominal pain is the most common symptom. Other manifestations include nausea, vomiting, constipation, tachycardia, hypertension, mental symptoms, and pain in the limbs, head, neck, or chest, etc. Numerous medications, including the barbiturates, can exacerbate an attack. **(Ref. 2, pp. 1127–1129)**

110. (B) *Key Words:* acute intermittent porphyria, pyrrole, heme biosynthesis

The porphyrias result from deficiencies of specific enzymes of the heme biosynthetic pathway. Acute intermittent porphyria is an autosomal dominant disorder that results from an approximately 50% deficiency of PBG deaminase (formerly known as uroporphyrinogen I synthase). The enzyme is deficient in all individuals who inherit the mutant gene and remains fairly constant over time. Most patients with PBG deaminase deficiency remain asymptomatic. (**Ref. 2,** pp. 1126–1127)

111. **(D)** *Key Words:* water, total body weight
Water comprises about 90 lb or 60% of this young man's total body weight. In young adult women, water constitutes about half of their weight. Although there may be a 15% variation in these values in both sexes, there is little variation in the amount of water in healthy subjects. Women have relatively less water because of their higher ratio of fat to lean muscle mass. (**Ref. 2,** p. 500)

112. **(H)** *Key Words: Toxoplasma gondii,* obligate intracellular protozoan, AIDS, central nervous system
Toxoplasmosis is a common disease of birds and mammals caused by *Toxoplasma gondii,* an obligate intracellular protozoan that infects over 500 million humans worldwide. The most common manifestation in patients with AIDS is central nervous system involvement. CT scan usually shows one or more lesions that are contrast enhancing in a ring pattern. Patients can present with such varied symptoms as fever, headache, confusion progressing to coma, focal neurological signs, and seizures. (**Ref. 2,** pp. 1987–1989)

113. **(C)** *Key Words:* AIDS, cytomegalovirus, retinitis, DHPG, ganciclovir, foscarnet
Much of the morbidity and some mortality associated with AIDS has been ascribed to CMV infections of the liver, brain, gastrointestinal tract, lungs, and eyes. Both ganciclovir (DHPG) and foscarnet are effective antiviral agents used in control of CMV infections; therapy is lifelong. (**Ref. 2,** pp. 1836–1837)

114. **(F)** *Key Words: Cryptococcus neoformans,* fungus, meningitis, amphotericin B, fluconazole
Cryptococcus neoformans is a yeastlike round or oval fungus that is the most common etiologic agent of fungal meningitis. Among

HIV-infected individuals, the incidence of cryptococcosis (systemic dissemination) varies from 5 to 10%. Meningitis is the most common manifestation of central nervous system cryptococcosis. In immunocompromised individuals, the mortality rate approaches 30%. Treatment is with amphotericin B. Fluconazole is another effective agent. (**Ref. 2,** pp. 1894–1896)

115. **(E)** *Key Words:* cryptosporidiosis, AIDS, gastrointestinal infection
Cryptosporidiosis is a gastrointestinal infection characterized by watery diarrhea, abdominal cramps, malabsorption, and weight loss. It is usually a severe, unrelenting illness in immunocompromised patients, particularly those with AIDS; it tends to be a self-limited disease in the immunologically normal host. (**Ref. 2,** p. 1991)

116. **(A)** *Key Words: Pneumocystis carinii,* pneumonia, AIDS, prophylaxis, trimethoprimsulfamethoxazole, CD4 count
The most desirable approach to therapy of *Pneumocystis carinii* pneumonia (PCP) is prevention. Two controlled studies have suggested that the attack rate can be reduced by 5- to 10-fold in HIV-infected patients who are at the highest risk: those who have less than 200 CD4 lymphocytes and those who already experienced an episode of PCP. The most widely used agent for prophylaxis is trimethoprimsulfamethoxazole. (**Ref. 2,** p. 1937)

117. **(B)** *Key Words: Mycobacterium avium-intracellulare* complex (MAC), AIDS, CD4 count, chronic diarrhea
Mycobacterium avium-intracellulare complex (MAC) is one of a large number of opportunistic pathogens responsible for chronic diarrhea in AIDS patients. Patients who develop disseminated MAC are usually severely immunocompromised from the standpoint of cellular immune function; therefore, in patients with AIDS, the CD4 count is usually quite low. Diagnosis is most commonly made by biopsy and culture of liver, bone marrow, lymph nodes, and/or blood. (**Ref. 2,** pp. 1743–1745, 1943)

118. **(J)** *Key Words:* Kaposi's sarcoma, neoplasm, AIDS
Kaposi's sarcoma (KS) is the most frequent neoplastic manifestation of HIV infection. It forms one of the Centers for Disease Control and Prevention's criteria that define an individual as hav-

ing AIDS. Although classically an indolent cutaneous neoplasm in HIV-negative individuals, in AIDS patients lymphatic involvement is not unusual and visceral involvement (particularly trachea, lungs, and GI tract) may occur. Unlike "classic" KS, which is usually confined to the lower extremities, cutaneous KS in AIDS patients can form large, confluent plaques anywhere on the body. (**Ref. 2,** pp. 1949–1950)

119. **(D)** *Key Words:* diabetes mellitus, proteinuria, glomerulopathy, glomerular filtration rate (GFR)
The first stage of occult renal (glomerular) damage cannot be diagnosed by conventional laboratory techniques and lasts for approximately 10 years. The patient is devoid of clinical symptoms and signs of glomerulopathy. The most striking laboratory finding is a 20 to 40% increase in the glomerular filtration rate (GFR), possibly due to generalized hypertrophy of glomeruli. It is followed by two clinically evident stages of increasingly severe glomerular injury. Both are identified by the presence of proteinuria. (**Ref. 2,** p. 590)

120. **(E)** *Key Words: Chlamydia trachomatis,* acute urethral syndrome, dysuria, frequency
Dysuria and frequency in the absence of significant bacteriuria (presence of significant numbers of bacteria in the urine to denote active infection rather than contamination) are common problems among young women. This entity has been called the acute urethral syndrome, and in 25% of patients is caused by *Chlamydia trachomatis.* (**Ref. 2,** pp. 593–594)

121. **(A)** *Key Words:* multiple myeloma, bone pain, normocytic normochromic anemia
Bone pain, particularly in the back or chest and less often in the extremities, is present at the time of diagnosis in more than two-thirds of patients. The cause of multiple myeloma is unknown, although radiation may play a role in some cases. A normocytic, normochromic anemia is present initially in two-thirds of patients but eventually occurs in nearly every patient. (**Ref. 2,** pp. 972–973)

122. **(C)** *Key Words:* ulcerative colitis, proctitis, rectal bleeding, tenesmus

The symptoms of ulcerative colitis depend on the extent and severity of inflammation within the colon. UC always involves the rectum; patients with proctitis present with rectal bleeding, tenesmus, and passage of mucopus. (**Ref. 2,** p. 701)

123. (**B**) *Key Words:* Crohn's disease, gastroduodenum, peptic ulcer disease
The symptoms and signs of Crohn's disease are also determined by the site and extent of inflammation. Gastroduodenal CD mimics peptic ulcer disease, with nausea, vomiting, and epigastric pain. (**Ref. 2,** p. 702)

124. (**B**) *Key Words:* Crohn's disease, weight loss, malabsorption
Weight loss is more common in CD than in UC due to small bowel–related malabsorption or a reduced intake of food to minimize postprandial symptoms. (**Ref. 2,** p. 702)

125. (**C**) *Key Words:* ulcerative colitis, continuous superficial inflammation, Crohn's disease, asymmetric transmural inflammation
Ulcerative colitis encompasses a spectrum of diffuse, continuous, superficial inflammation of the colon, which begins within the rectum and extends to a variable proximal level. The inflammatory features are constant within the involved segment and, once established, the inflammation's upward margins usually remain constant in the individual. Crohn's disease is characterized by focal, asymmetric, transmural inflammation. (**Ref. 2,** p. 699)

126. (**B**) *Key Words:* nongonococcal urethritis, *Chlamydia trachomatis, Trichomonas vaginalis,* Herpes simplex
A large number of studies have established *Chlamydia trachomatis* as a cause of approximately 40% of cases of nongonococcal urethritis (NGU). A very small proportion of cases of NGU in men is due to *Trichomonas vaginalis* or Herpes simplex infection. *Phthirus pubis* is the ectoparasite that causes pubic lice infestation. *Candida albicans* is a common cause of vaginitis and balanitis. (**Ref. 2,** p. 1752)

127. (**A**) *Key Words:* cystic fibrosis, autosomal recessive inheritance, biliary cirrhosis, allergic aspergillosis
Cystic fibrosis is a heritable disease that follows an autosomal recessive pattern of transmittance. A child born to two heterozy-

gous carriers has a 1:4 risk of having the disease, a 1:2 chance of being a carrier, and a 1:4 chance of neither being a carrier nor having the disease. All of the other statements concerning cystic fibrosis are true. (**Ref. 2,** pp. 418–420)

128. **(A)** *Key Words:* breast cancer, estrogen receptor protein, mammography
Increased monitoring should be given to patients with prior curative treatment for breast cancer, since they have a 10 to 15% lifetime chance of developing a second primary breast cancer. Annual mammography examinations are recommended for women with a prior breast cancer regardless of age. ERP is found in 60% of postmenopausal patients vs. 30 to 40% of premenopausal women. ERP-positive tumors are also more likely to respond to hormonal therapy. (**Ref. 2,** pp. 1381–1383)

129. **(E)** *Key Words:* prostate-specific antigen, digital rectal exam, VDRL, prostatitis, urine culture, urinalysis
The serum VDRL will tell you only if the patient has been exposed to the agent of syphilis (*Treponema pallidum*) in the past, since it is an antibody test. It cannot tell you if the current symptoms are caused by untreated syphilis. The digital rectal examination will give you an idea if there is prostatic enlargement (of either benign or malignant origin), which can certainly cause these symptoms (though this will provide only a rough estimate of size). The prostate-specific antigen can be elevated in either benign or malignant disease; however, a normal value does not necessarily exclude these possibilities. Both a urinalysis and urine culture are useful for detecting bacterial prostatitis. (**Ref. 2,** pp. 1351–1353)

130. **(A)** *Key Words:* prostate-specific antigen, prostate cancer, benign prostatic hypertrophy
Measurements of serum prostate-specific antigen (PSA) are not sufficiently accurate to diagnose men with early prostate cancer. Approximately 15 to 20% of men with benign prostatic hypertrophy (BPH) have PSA values greater than 10 ng/ml. Symptoms due to BPH can be of an obstructive (hesitancy, straining, dribbling, and retention) or irritative (frequency, nocturia, dysuria, urgency, and incontinence) in origin. Early carcinoma of the prostate is asymptomatic. As the disease spreads into the urethra, it may cause symptoms of urinary obstruction indistinguishable from

those caused by BPH. Statement D is true. The etiology of prostatic carcinoma is unknown, though the disease does not occur in men castrated before puberty. Multiple factors, including viral and environmental, have been postulated. (**Ref. 2, pp.** 1352–1353)

131. **(E)** *Key Words:* skin cancer, ultraviolet radiation, immunosuppression, sunburn
The cancers are more common in patients living in southern latitudes of the northern hemisphere and in Australia and in those with light complexions who sunburn easily. These cancers are more common on areas of the body exposed to sunlight. They are more common in immunosuppressed patients, attesting to the importance of the immune surveillance system in the etiology of cancer. (**Ref. 2, p.** 2315)

132. **(B)** *Key Words:* osteoporosis, bone density, estrogen replacement therapy
Insufficient accumulation of bone mass during skeletal growth predisposes to fractures later in life as age-related bone loss ensues. All of the other statements concerning osteoporosis are true. (**Ref. 2, pp.** 1426–1427)

133. **(A)** *Key Words:* osteoporosis, bone resorption, estrogen, calcium, vitamin D, calcitonin
Estrogen effectively reduces bone resorption, as does calcitonin; however, calcitonin therapy must be accompanied by calcium supplements in order to prevent secondary hyperparathyroidism. Calcium, which may act by decreasing parathyroid hormone secretion, is a safe, well-tolerated, and inexpensive therapy. Vitamin D treatment should probably be reserved for patients with a documented or suspected impairment in calcium absorption. It should be used judiciously, since the dose that increases calcium absorption is not much smaller than the dosage that increases bone resorption. (**Ref. 2, pp.** 1429–1430)

134. **(D)** *Key Words:* multiple sclerosis, myelin, epidemiology
Multiple sclerosis is more common farther from the equator in North America, Europe, Australia, and New Zealand. There have been reported clusters of cases in small areas such as in pockets in Switzerland. The rest of the statements concerning multiple sclerosis are true. (**Ref. 2, pp.** 2196–2197)

135. (E) *Key Words:* multiple sclerosis, unilateral vision loss, paresthesias
The first four options are common initial problems of multiple sclerosis. Urinary frequency, retention, hesitancy, or incontinence; hearing loss; vertigo; pain in the extremities, face, or trunk; and dysarthria, along with diminished intelligent functioning are all less common initial features. **(Ref. 2,** pp. 2197–2198)

136. (C) *Key Words:* infectious mononucleosis, Epstein-Barr virus (EBV), rapid heterophile test, rash, ampicillin
The constellation of complaints and physical findings is most consistent with the diagnosis of infectious mononucleosis. In most cases this is caused by primary Epstein-Barr virus (EBV) infection. Although this infection occurs during the first decade of life in less developed countries, among middle and higher socioeconomic groups in industrialized countries, primary infection occurs in the adolescent and postadolescent groups, usually as a result of kissing. Rashes occur significantly more often if ampicillin is given to a patient with acute EBV infection, but they are not usually vesicular in nature, as is the rash of varicella infection. Recurrent streptococcal infection of the throat is not usually accompanied by hepatosplenomegaly and does not give a highly positive heterophile test (which is 95% specific and 95% sensitive in the adolescent population). Acute HIV infection can certainly cause a monolike syndrome and should always be part of your differential diagnosis. However, it should be suspected if the heterophile is negative or only positive at a low level. The incubation period for hepatitis B (assuming the patient has an illness similar to his girlfriend) is too long to be the cause of his complaints. **(Ref. 2,** pp. 1838–1839)

137. (A) *Key Words:* Epstein-Barr virus, viral capsid antigen, nuclear antigen, early antigen
Specific serologic testing for EBV infection involves measuring antibodies to latently infected (anti-EBNA), early replication cycle (anti-EA), or late replication cycle (anti-VCA) viral proteins, usually by enzyme-linked immunoassay or indirect immunofluorescence microscopy. With acute primary infection, EA and IgM VCA titers are high, and EBNA and IgG VCA titers are low. Patients recovering from recent primary infection have lower IgM VCA or EA titers, a low EBNA titer and a higher IgG VCA titer. After sev-

eral months, IgM VCA and EA titers are low or negative, but EBNA and IgG VCA titers are high. (**Ref. 2,** p. 1839)

138. (C) *Key Words:* infectious mononucleosis, ruptured spleen, intraabdominal bleeding

No treatment is necessary for most cases of infectious mononucleosis. Rest during the acute symptomatic period and gradual return to normal activities as tolerated are advised. Patients with splenomegaly should restrict their involvement in sports until the spleen returns to normal size, as they run the risk of traumatic rupture. The patient's signs and symptoms are consistent with intraabdominal bleeding, and his spleen must be removed. (**Ref. 2,** p. 1839)

139. (C) *Key Words:* vaccines, pregnant women, cholera

All of the choices except cholera are live attenuated vaccines and are theoretically contraindicated in pregnant women due to the concern that they could potentially harm the developing fetus. The cholera vaccine is inactivated. Inactivated vaccines are generally felt to be safe for pregnant women. (**Ref. 2,** pp. 56–61)

140. (A) *Key Words:* influenza vaccine, antibody, health care workers, immunosuppression

As a general rule, doctors should avoid vaccinating patients at the onset of a serious acute illness, as the ability to mount an effective antibody response may be impaired. Health care workers are also included on the list of persons who should receive annual influenza vaccinations, even if they themselves are not members of high-risk groups. This is to minimize transmission to compromised patients who may suffer serious illness (including death) from a bout of the flu. Additionally, household contacts of immunocompromised patients should also be vaccinated. (**Ref. 2,** p. 60)

141. (D) *Key Words:* Lyme disease, erythema chronicum migrans, tick, spirochete

Erythema chronicum migrans is the unique clinical marker for Lyme disease, a tick-borne spirochetal illness. The rash (when it occurs, which is not all of the time) begins as a red macule or papule at the site of the tick bite. As the area of redness expands, there is often central clearing as depicted. Dermatophytosis of the trunk (tinea corporis) can be caused by several species of

Trichophyton and result in annular inflamed patches with elevated scaling and, at times, vesicular borders with a tendency for central clearing. Nummular eczema does not have a definitive cause, although dry skin or underlying infections may play a role. It manifests by coin-shaped patches on the extensor areas of the extremities or trunk. The most common cutaneous manifestations of a drug reaction are hives or morbilliform rashes, although lesions similar in appearance to erythema migrans can occur. Drugs often implicated in cutaneous reactions include trimethoprim-sulfamethoxazole, penicillin G (and semisynthetic penicillins), and quinidine, among others. (**Ref. 2,** pp. 1773, 2297, 2299–2302)

142. **(B)** *Key Words:* Lyme disease, acrodermatitis chronica atrophicans
Acrodermatitis chronica atrophicans is a chronic skin lesion associated with late (years later) Lyme disease. It is rare in the United States, though common in Europe. It appears as violaceous infiltrated plaques or nodules that eventually atrophy. It is most common on extensor surfaces. The other items listed are all potential early manifestations of Lyme disease. (**Ref. 2,** pp. 1774–1775)

143. **(A)** *Key Words:* Lyme disease, doxycycline, amoxicillin, ceftriaxone
Doxycycline or amoxicillin are considered by most physicians to be the drugs of choice for the treatment of Lyme disease. Doxycycline is contraindicated in young children. Ceftriaxone is used to treat serious complications of Lyme such as meningitis and arthritis resistant to oral agents. Trimethoprim-sulfamethoxazole has no place in the treatment of Lyme disease. (**Ref. 2,** p. 1776)

144. **(A)** *Key Words:* acute interstitial nephritis, pyelonephritis, penicillin, rifampin, systemic lupus erythematosus
Acute bacterial pyelonephritis is a common cause of AISN. The clinical presentation of fever, chills, flank pain, and bacteriuria is characteristic. Several penicillin cogeners may cause AISN but methicillin has been responsible for most of the cases. Although rifampin, isoniazid, para-aminosalicylic acid, and ethambutol have all been implicated as causing AISN, rifampin appears to be related to more severe cases and recurs with rechallenge. Glomerulonephritis is usually the primary renal lesion in patients with SLE, but AISN can be found as well. (**Ref. 2,** pp. 570–571)

145. **(B)** *Key Words:* Wilson's disease, hepatolenticular degeneration, autosomal recessive inheritance, hepatitis, dementia
Wilson's disease (hepatolenticular degeneration) is a hereditary disease (inherited in an autosomal recessive pattern) characterized by an accumulation of copper, primarily in the corneas, liver, kidney, and brain. It can cause intermittent hepatic dysfunction, which can be mistaken for hepatitis of a viral etiology. Neurological signs may be subtle, and tremor and deterioration of handwriting may be among the earliest manifestations. Schizophreniform symptoms and bizarre behavior may appear, but the mental status examination almost always shows signs of organic dementia. The other diseases listed are not consistent with the presentation as outlined. (**Ref. 2,** pp. 1132–1133)

146. **(D)** *Key Words:* Kaysher-Fleischer rings, cornea, copper, slit-lamp exam
Kaysher-Fleischer rings are golden brown or greenish rings or arcs in Descemet's membrane at the limbus of the cornea in patients with Wilson's disease. They are made of copper-containing granules and develop primarily after redistribution of liver copper. Present in nearly all patients with neurological or psychiatric symptoms, they may be seen with the naked eye but slit-lamp exam is preferred. In patients with scarlet fever, Pastia's lines are linear striations of confluent petechiae; Rumpel-Leede sign refers to the development of petechiae distal to an obstruction (such as a blood pressure cuff) in patients also with scarlet fever. There is no such thing as a von Willebrand ring. (**Ref. 2,** pp. 1132–1133, 1628–1629)

147. **(B)** *Key Words:* Wilson's disease, copper excretion, liver biopsy
In Wilson's disease, biliary excretion of copper is impaired, and as a result total body copper is progressively increased. The specific nature of the metabolic abnormality that causes this defect is not known. As for the liver biopsy, the changes are not characteristic for Wilson's disease. Stains for copper are unreliable, since they are often negative most frequently during early disease when they are most useful. The rest of the statements are true. (**Ref. 2,** pp. 1132–1133)

148. **(C)** *Key Words:* Wilson's disease, D-penicillamine, prednisone
D-penicillamine remains the drug of choice; a year or more of therapy may be required before a response is noted. Exacerbation

of symptoms may occur at the beginning of therapy and should not be misconstrued as indicative of an erroneous diagnosis. Prednisone may be used to manage adverse side effects of penicillamine until they have cleared. Trientine or zinc can be tried if side effects of penicillamine are unmanageable. (**Ref. 2,** pp. 1132–1133)

149. **(A)** *Key Words:* cigarette smoking, nicotine gum, cessation
The use of nicotine gum increases the chance of successful short-term smoking cessation when used with an appropriate behavioral intervention program. All the remaining statements are true. (**Ref. 2,** pp. 36–37)

150. **(B)** *Key Words:* gastroesophageal reflux, lower esophageal sphincter pressure
There is a tendency for mean LES pressure to be significantly lower in subjects with GERD than in persons without GERD. The most common event associated with reflux appears to be an inappropriate relaxation of the LES. Thus, two abnormalities of LES may be associated with reflux: a sphincter with very low tone, as measured by LES pressure, or inappropriate relaxation of a normally competent sphincter. All the other statements are correct. (**Ref. 2,** pp. 344, 346, 640–641)

References

1. Barker, LR, Burton JR, Zieve PD: *Principles of Ambulatory Medicine,* 4th ed. Baltimore, Williams & Wilkins, 1995.

2. Wyngaarden JB, Smith LH, Bennett: *Cecil Textbook of Medicine,* 19th ed. Philadelphia, W. B. Saunders, 1992.

3. Dubin: *Rapid Interpretation of EKGs.* Rest TK.

4. Gorbach, Bartlett, Blackwell: *Infectious Diseases.* Philadelphia, W. B. Saunders, 1992.

5. Isselbacher, Braunwald, Wilson, Martin, Fauci, Casper: *Harrison's Principles of Internal Medicine,* 13th ed. New York, McGraw-Hill, 1994.

6. Olsen KR: *Lange Poisoning and Drug Overdose,* 2nd ed. Stamford, CT, Appleton & Lange, 1994.

7. *Physician's Desk Reference,* 49th ed. Montvale, NJ, Medical Economics Data Production Co., 1995.

3

Psychiatry

Carlyle Chan, MD

DIRECTIONS: Each of the questions or incomplete statements below is followed by a list of suggested answers or completions. Select the **one** that is best in each case.

---

1. Tics that involve multiple muscle groups would **MOST LIKELY** be seen in
   A. Huntington's chorea
   B. Tourette's disorder
   C. Parkinson's disease
   D. Alzheimer's disease
   E. malingering disorders

2. Bowlby described a sequential pattern of protest, despair, and detachment as a reaction to
   A. separation
   B. deprivation
   C. sensory bombardment
   D. narcotic withdrawal
   E. PCP intoxication

3. According to Erikson, the psychosocial task of the adolescent years is the achievement of
   A. basic trust, basic mistrust
   B. sense of ego identity; identity confusion
   C. generativity; stagnation
   D. integrity; despair
   E. sense of autonomy; pervasive sense of shame and doubt

4. The psychosocial task of the Oedipal period, according to Erikson, is the achievement of
   A. basic trust; basic mistrust
   B. autonomy; shame and doubt
   C. initiative; a sense of guilt
   D. industry; a sense of inferiority
   E. sense of ego identity; identity diffusion

5. Sensorimotor intelligence (Piaget) ends with the attainment of
   A. object constancy
   B. concrete operations
   C. formal operations
   D. rapprochement
   E. autism

6. In operant conditioning, negative reinforcement
   A. decreases the probability that a negative stimulus will recur
   B. strengthens the response
   C. is the same as punishment
   D. is not contingent on the response of the organism
   E. reinforces successively closer approximations to the desired behavior

7. The period defined in psychoanalysis as "latency" is roughly contemporaneous with the Piagetian stage of
   A. sensorimotor stage
   B. formal operations
   C. concrete operations
   D. preoperational thought
   E. logical thought

8. The most rapid acquisition of a behavior is found in
   A. partial reinforcement
   B. positive reinforcement
   C. negative reinforcement
   D. continuous reinforcement
   E. Pavlovian conditioning

9. Splitting is
   A. primitive idealization
   B. projective identification
   C. division of the self and external objects into "all good" and "all bad"
   D. ambivalence
   E. none of the above

10. Defense mechanisms
    A. are unconscious
    B. are not ego functions
    C. are not used by normal adults
    D. develop after the resolution of the Oedipal conflict
    E. include suppression

11. The hypothesis that a depressed person may maintain his depression by how he thinks is a tenet of
    A. Heinz Kohut
    B. Aaron Beck
    C. Margaret Mahler
    D. Otto Kernberg
    E. Fritz Perls

12. The WISC
    A. is a projective test
    B. includes only verbal tests
    C. tests only innate intellectual ability
    D. includes only nonverbal tests
    E. is the child equivalent of the WAIS

13. The optimal serum concentration of lithium for the treatment of bipolar disorder is
    A. 0–0.3 mEq/L
    B. 0.4–0.7 mEq/L
    C. 0.8–1.2 mEq/L
    D. 1.3–1.6 mEq/L
    E. 1.7–2.0 mEq/L

14. The following are different levels of IQ scores. Patients falling within which range would be reported as having "moderate mental retardation"?
    A. IQ level below 20 or 25
    B. IQ level 20–25 to 35–40
    C. IQ level 35–40 to 50–55
    D. IQ level 50–55 to approximately 70
    E. IQ level 71–85

15. The chemical formula in Figure 3-1 depicts which of the following?
    A. A hydrazine MAO inhibitor
    B. A tricyclic derivative
    C. A butyrophenone
    D. A phenothiazine derivative
    E. A thioxanthene derivative

16. Of the following psychotropic drugs, which is the MOST LIKELY to produce pigmentary retinopathy?
    A. Lithium
    B. Thioridazine
    C. Maprotiline HCl
    D. Haloperidol
    E. Amitriptyline

17. In the use of the multiaxial system for evaluation of patients with suspected psychiatric disorders, which of the following refers to the physical conditions?
    A. Axis I
    B. Axis II
    C. Axis III
    D. Axis IV
    E. Axis V

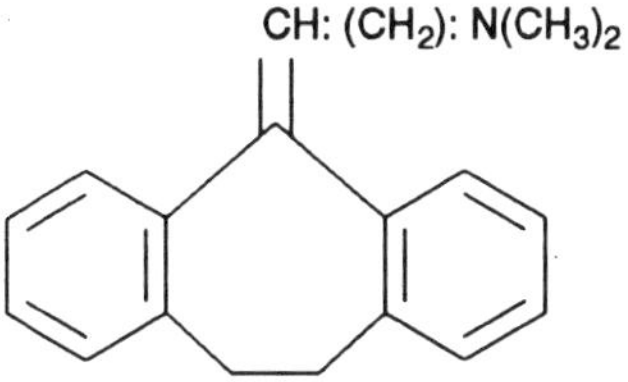

CH: (CH$_2$): N(CH$_3$)$_2$

Figure 3-1

18. In prescribing a benzodiazepine to an elderly patient, which of the following would be expected to have a half-life of less than one day?
    A. Chlordiazepoxide
    B. Diazepam
    C. Clonazepam
    D. Oxazepam
    E. Phenobarbital

19. Which of the following is a piperidine phenothiazine?
    A. Haloperidol
    B. Stelazine
    C. Mellaril
    D. Trilafon
    E. Prolixin

20. Chlordiazepoxide exerts its therapeutic effects **MOST QUICK-LY** when it is administered
    A. orally
    B. intramuscularly
    C. subcutaneously
    D. with anticholinergics
    E. with stimulants

21. An absolute contraindication to electroconvulsive therapy (ECT) is
    A. brain tumor
    B. increased intracerebral pressure
    C. hypertension
    D. myocardial disease
    E. none of the above

22. Which of the following drugs will tricyclic antidepressants block?
   A. Haldol
   B. Griseofulvin
   C. Reserpine
   D. Lithium
   E. Guanethidine

23. **TRUE** statements concerning grief and bereavement include
   A. the initial physical symptoms may be indistinguishable from depression
   B. widowers and widows have an increased death rate in the first year following the death of a spouse
   C. identification phenomenon may occur
   D. grief may extend from one to two years
   E. all of the above

24. In the Midtown Manhattan Study, what percentage of questionnaire respondents were considered "less than well"?
   A. 10%
   B. 24%
   C. 23.4%
   D. 81.5%
   E. 87%

25. In negligence,
   A. a standard of care must exist
   B. a duty must be owed by the defendant or someone for whose conduct he or she is answerable
   C. the duty must be owed the plaintiff
   D. there must be a breach of duty
   E. all of the above

Questions 26–60: Each of the numbered items or incomplete statements in this section is negatively phrased, as indicated by a capitalized word such as **NOT, LEAST,** or **EXCEPT.** Select the **one** lettered answer or completion that is best in each case.

26. A patient who is taking disufiram daily and who begins to drink alcohol is likely to experience all the following symptoms **EXCEPT**
   A. nausea and vomiting
   B. dyspnea

   C. tachycardia
   D. skin flushing
   E. bradycardia

27. Forms of brief dynamic psychotherapy include all the following **EXCEPT**
   A. broad-focused short-term dynamic
   B. cognitive
   C. time limited
   D. short-term anxiety provoking
   E. short-term interpersonal

28. Neuroimaging techniques include all the following **EXCEPT**
   A. magnetic resonance
   B. positron emission tomography
   C. computed tomography
   D. electromyogram
   E. cerebral angiography

29. The diagnostic criteria for psychological factors affecting medical conditions include all the following **EXCEPT**
   A. there is a temporal relationship between meaningful stimulus and initiation or exacerbation of condition
   B. a general medical condition is present (Axis III)
   C. psychological factors interfere with medical treatment
   D. stress-related responses precipitate or exacerbate medical symptoms
   E. symbolism is the principal diagnostic criterion

30. Which of the following is **NOT TRUE** with regard to informed consent?
   A. To perform any procedure or any touching of a patient in a medical center without consent constitutes battery
   B. The consent process contains three elements: information, competence, and voluntariness
   C. It requires the physician to relate sufficient information to the patient to allow him or her to decide if the procedure is acceptable in light of its risks and benefits
   D. It is never added in the claim of malpractice
   E. Consent forms must not substitute for a physician–patient dialogue

31. Dementia includes all the following **EXCEPT**
    A. aphasia
    B. memory impairment
    C. delirium
    D. disturbances in executive functioning
    E. agnosia

32. In the DSM IV classification of mood disorders, which of the following is **NOT** included?
    A. Dysthymic disorder
    B. Substance-induced mood disorder
    C. Bipolar affective I disorder
    D. Minor depression
    E. Cyclothymic disorder

33. Manic episodes are characterized by all the following **EXCEPT**
    A. duration of one week or longer
    B. elevated, expansive, or irritable mood
    C. distractibility
    D. increased talkativeness
    E. deflated self-esteem

34. Diagnostic criteria for conduct disorder include all the following **EXCEPT**
    A. has deliberately engaged in fire setting
    B. often lies (other than to avoid physical or sexual abuse)
    C. exhibits conduct disturbance lasting at least three weeks
    D. has been physically cruel to animals
    E. has broken into someone else's house, building, or car

35. Anorexia nervosa is characterized by all the following **EXCEPT**
    A. intense fear of becoming obese
    B. weight loss to less than 85% of expected weight
    C. disturbance of body image
    D. onset in early latency years
    E. amenorrhea

36. The affect of schizophrenia is **NOT**
    A. blunted
    B. flat

C. inappropriate
D. infectious
E. restricted

37. Anticholinergic side effects include all the following **EXCEPT**
   A. peripheral vasodilation
   B. delirium
   C. dry mucous membranes
   D. impaired visual accommodation
   E. peripheral neuropathy

38. Causes of mental retardation include all the following **EXCEPT**
   A. too much early stimulation
   B. hereditary disorders
   C. pregnancy problems and premarital morbidity
   D. acquired childhood diseases
   E. unknown causes

39. The mental status examination includes all the following **EXCEPT**
   A. general appearance, manner, and attitude
   B. affect, thought processes
   C. memory
   D. judgment
   E. personal history

40. Which of the following is **NOT** considered an example of primary prevention?
   A. Genetic counseling of persons with a family history of PKU (phenylketonuria)
   B. Intensive intervention with blind infants
   C. Competency training in preschool settings
   D. Widow-to-widow self-help groups
   E. Lithium clinics

41. Which of the following is **NOT TRUE**?
   A. There is a disproportionate number of schizophrenic patients in lower socioeconomic classes in industrialized nations
   B. The lifetime prevalence for schizophrenia in the United States is about 6.5%
   C. Part of the homeless problem in large cities may be related to inadequate follow-up of deinstitutionalized schizophrenic patients
   D. In the northern hemisphere, more schizophrenic patients are born in the winter months of January to April
   E. Approximately 90% of patients in treatment for schizophrenia are between 15 and 54 years of age

42. Which of the following has the **LEAST** anticholinergic side effects?
   A. Desipramine
   B. Amitryptiline
   C. Nortriptyline
   D. Trazodone
   E. Imipramine

43. The following are early symptoms of lithium toxicity **EXCEPT**
   A. heightened auditory sensitivity
   B. dysarthria
   C. ataxia
   D. coarse tremor
   E. neuromuscular irritability

44. The following are all criteria for establishing testamentary capacity **EXCEPT**
   A. knowing that one is making a will
   B. knowing the objects of one's bounty
   C. knowing the extent of one's property
   D. no undue influence
   E. knowing the difference between right and wrong

45. Which of the following statements is **NOT TRUE**?
   A. Confidentiality is the obligation of the professional to keep in confidence (i.e., from third parties) whatever information is shared by the patient in the absence of permission to disclose

B. Privilege is the right of patients to ban or exclude from judicial or quasijudicial settings testimony about material that has been revealed within the professional relationship

C. Breaching confidentiality may be a liability issue

D. Privilege belongs to the doctor, who may decide to exercise it or not

E. Tarasoff holds that a therapist has a duty to warn intended victims

46. Which of the following is **NOT** characteristic of posttraumatic stress disorder?
    A. Numbing of responsiveness
    B. Increased arousal
    C. Impairment of memory of an important aspect of the trauma
    D. Voices commenting
    E. Reexperiencing of past trauma

47. The borderline personality disorder is characterized by all the following **EXCEPT**
    A. unstable, intense relationships
    B. inappropriate intense anger
    C. potentially self-damaging impulsiveness
    D. social withdrawal
    E. disturbances in identity

48. Which of the following is **NOT** characteristic of the schizotypal personality disorder?
    A. Magical thinking
    B. Relatives with schizophrenic disorder
    C. Illusions
    D. Odd speech
    E. Delusions

49. Which of the following is **NOT TRUE** of the dementia of the Alzheimer's type?
    A. Marked atrophy of basal ganglia
    B. No gross neurological deficits, except possible aphasia
    C. Generalized cortical atrophy
    D. Neurofibrillary tangles
    E. Misdiagnosis may run as high as 50%

50. Alcohol-induced psychotic disorder (formerly alcohol halluci-
   nosis) is characterized by all the following **EXCEPT**
   A. high incidence in people in their early twenties
   B. voices discussing patient in the third person
   C. auditory hallucinations
   D. duration of less than one week
   E. occurrence within a few days of alcohol withdrawal

51. "Primary process" is a psychoanalytic term used to describe a cer-
   tain kind of thinking that is **NOT**
   A. primitive, dominated by emotions
   B. characteristic of the infant
   C. prominent in dreams and psychoses
   D. taking into consideration external reality
   E. typical of psychotic states

52. The following statements about the physician's feelings toward
   the patient are **TRUE EXCEPT**
   A. the feelings may be based in the reality of the patient's
      appearance, character, and conflicts
   B. the feelings may be based on what the patient represents to
      the therapist's unconscious, in terms of early important fig-
      ures
   C. strong negative feelings toward a patient will always interfere
      with treatment
   D. it is important to determine if negative feelings stem from
      reality or transferred aspects of the relationship
   E. most patients have some unlikable qualities

53. Which of the following is **NOT** characteristic of major depressive
   episode with melancholic features?
   A. Early morning awakening
   B. Psychomotor agitation
   C. Quality of mood different from mourning
   D. Mood worse in early morning
   E. Trouble falling asleep

54. All the following are **TRUE** of minor tranquilizers **EXCEPT**
   A. they are occasionally useful in treating transient situational
      reactions
   B. they exert their effect on the cerebral cortex

C. they can reduce patients' understanding of their environment
D. they are very useful in preventing paranoid reactions in the elderly, even when used at low doses
E. elderly patients usually require reduced dosages

55. Of the following medications, which would be **LEAST LIKELY** to result in extrapyramidal side effects?
   A. Haloperidol
   B. Loxapine
   C. Chlorpromazine
   D. Perphenazine
   E. Fluphenazine

56. Neuroleptic induced Parkinsonism may include all the following **EXCEPT**
   A. pill-rolling-type tremor
   B. masked facies
   C. cogwheel rigidity
   D. hunch-backed appearance
   E. decreased salivation

57. The following statements about neuroleptic malignant syndrome are **TRUE EXCEPT**
   A. it occurs in 10% of patients on antipsychotic medication
   B. it is a potentially life-threatening disorder
   C. patients display rigidity and sometimes catatonia
   D. creatinine phosphokinase (CPK) levels are elevated
   E. symptoms also include fever and hypertension

58. Common side effects of serotonin specific reuptake inhibitors (SSRIs) include all the following **EXCEPT**
   A. nausea and vomiting
   B. headaches
   C. sweating
   D. nervousness
   E. insomnia

59. Neuropsychiatric complications of HIV infection include all the following **EXCEPT**
   A. delirium
   B. vascular myelopathy
   C. peripheral nervous system involvement
   D. amnesia
   E. dementia

60. The following statements about risperidone (Risperdal) are **TRUE EXCEPT** it
   A. is useful in the treatment of schizophrenia
   B. is effective in reducing negative symptoms of schizophrenia
   C. is useful in the treatment of psychotic disorders
   D. has fewer extrapyramidal side effects
   E. has numerous neurological adverse effects

Questions 61–65: This section consists of clinical situations, each followed by a series of questions. Study each situation and select the **one** best answer to each question following it.

61. A 25-year-old man has a six-month history of believing that "people" are trying to put "bad thoughts" into his head and to make him do "bad things." He finds special messages from them in TV news reports and in the newspaper. He is agitated, pacing constantly. His affect is inappropriate, and he laughs as he tells of his persecution. Physical examination is within normal limits. Drug screen is negative. The pharmacologic treatment of choice is
   A. clorazepate (Tranxene) 30 mg/d
   B. lorazepam (Ativan) 20 mg/d
   C. haloperidol (Haldol) 5 to 20 mg/d
   D. amitryptiline (Elavil) 150 mg/d
   E. imipramine (Tofranil) 25 mg/d

62. A 30-year-old resident is noted to be especially frugal, rigid, and punctual. In most areas of his life he is meticulous, but his desk and bedroom are very messy. He tends to be obsequious with superiors and rather sadistic with the medical students in his control. Occasionally he has temper tantrums. From a psychodynamic point of view, these characteristics are derivatives of which stage of development?
   A. Oral
   B. Anal

C. Phallic
D. Oedipal
E. Latency

63. A 34-year-old alcoholic has previously undergone therapy unsuccessfully in an attempt to discontinue alcohol abuse. He then went to a behavioral therapist who, after counseling, allowed him to drink but gave him an emetic agent every time he drank. Which of the types of therapy was being used?
A. Retrogression
B. Confrontation
C. Psychoanalytic
D. Aversion
E. Masochism

64. A 24-year-old woman is reported to the police as a missing person by her parents. Her fiance has recently broken their engagement, and she had been extremely despondent. When found by police in another state, she was noted to be suffering from amnesia. Which of the following **BEST** characterizes her situation?
A. Extinction
B. Fugue
C. Autosuggestion
D. Schizoid personality
E. Introversion

65. A psychiatric consult is requested for a 63-year-old woman to determine the etiology of her dementia. She had been admitted to the hospital appearing extremely malnourished and emaciated. She had already been evaluated by a dermatologist and a gastroenterologist for some of her medical problems. Which of the following vitamin deficiencies did the psychiatrist suspect?
A. Vitamin A deficiency
B. Vitamin B1 (thiamin) deficiency
C. Vitamin B2 (riboflavin) deficiency
D. Vitamin B3 (niacin) deficiency
E. Vitamin C deficiency

66. A 34-year-old Vietnam veteran with considerable combat experience, on questioning by a psychiatrist, appeared to have forgotten and was reluctant to discuss certain events. With the help of a psychiatrist, he was able to recall these experiences. He felt relieved after some previously repressed incidents were recalled. The emotional release the patient underwent is called
   A. abreaction
   B. acting out
   C. adaptation
   D. compensation
   E. parapraxis

67. A 78-year-old woman is brought to the emergency room because the family felt "she was going crazy." On examination, she has a deep voice, her face is somewhat puffy, her skin is dry, her hair is thin with loss of lateral eyebrow, and she is hard of hearing. Which of the following is the **MOST LIKELY** diagnosis?
   A. Hyperthyroidism
   B. Hypothyroidism
   C. Hyperparathyroidism
   D. Hypoparathyroidism
   E. Addison's disease

68. A 60-year-old male schizophrenic had been taking large doses of a phenothiazine for several years. On examination, his muscles are rigid, and he is tremulous. He walks with a shuffling gait. On occasion, drooling is noted. The patient **MOST LIKELY** is displaying
   A. organic brain syndrome
   B. catatonia
   C. a pyramidal system disorder
   D. an extrapyramidal system disorder
   E. an irreversible side effect of his medication

69. A young woman who is being treated with medication for an atypical depression goes to a party where she eats chicken liver paté and cheese. She develops a severe headache. Her physical examination is normal, except for a blood pressure reading of 200/130 mmHg. The woman probably has been taking
   A. a butyrophenone
   B. a phenothiazine
   C. a monoamine-oxidase inhibitor

D. a tricyclic antidepressant
E. lithium carbonate

70. A 34-year-old Malaysian man suddenly bursts into a wild rage and kills an innocent bystander. Which of the following conditions would **BEST** describe the episode?
    A. Susta
    B. Acute paranoia
    C. Amok
    D. Amentia
    E. None of the above

71. A patient receiving a potent antipsychotic drug is noted to be extremely and uncontrollably restless. Which of the following is he **MOST LIKELY** to have?
    A. Automatism
    B. Akinesia
    C. Akathisia
    D. Agitated depression
    E. Apraxia

72. A 26-year-old woman suffers from three or four panic attacks a week. The **MOST APPROPRIATE** pharmacological choice would be
    A. imipramine (Tofranil) 25 mg/d, increasing the dose gradually if necessary
    B. imipramine (Tofranil) 150–300 mg/d
    C. oxazepam (Serax) 30 mg/d
    D. clorazepate (Tranxene) 30 mg/d
    E. chlordiazepoxide (Librium) 100 mg/d

73. You admit to the hospital a patient with a six-month history of marked thought disorder, inappropriate affect, and auditory hallucinations. His level of consciousness is clear, his orientation and memory good. Making a diagnosis of schizophrenic disorder, you prescribe trifluoperazine (Stelazine) 5 mg/qid. The next day he develops a painful spasm of the sternocleidomastoid muscle, which twists his head to the right. He has developed
    A. muscular dystonia
    B. tardive dyskinesia
    C. akathisia
    D. akinesia
    E. Parkinsonism

Questions 74–75: A 28-year-old man has had repeated conflicts with the law, and frequently gets into arguments. He has a poor employment history.

74. Which of the following might **BEST** describe him?
    A. Autistic
    B. Antisocial personality disorder
    C. Obsessive-compulsive personality
    D. Type B personality
    E. None of the above

75. Which of the following would be **LEAST EXPECTED** in this patient?
    A. Impulsive behavior
    B. Masochism
    C. Rejection of authority
    D. Low tolerance to frustration
    E. Irresponsibility

Questions 76–77: A 24-year-old man is admitted from the emergency room complaining of severe abdominal pain. On examination, multiple surgical scars are noted. The patient feels he needs emergency surgery. Except for the patient's complaints, no objective evidence of an acute abdomen is observed. Review of previous hospitalizations elsewhere indicates that, despite multiple abdominal explorations, no pathology has been discovered. When told of these facts, the patient signs out against medical advice.

76. His **MOST LIKELY** diagnosis is
    A. Munchausen's syndrome
    B. psychogenic fugue
    C. Korsakoff's disease
    D. hysteria
    E. Tourette's syndrome

77. The previous patient is later readmitted to another hospital. After thorough questioning, a psychiatrist determines that the subject is being untruthful during the interview. It is noted that he is able to present his medical complaints in considerable detail in a matter that arouses the interest of the interviewer. Which of the following

would **BEST** describe the patient's presentation of his purported medical history and problems?

A. Logorrhea
B. Perseveration
C. Pseudologia phantastica
D. Dissociation
E. Echolalia

Questions 78–80: You are asked to evaluate a 46-year-old alcoholic man who was admitted to the hospital two days previously for pancreatitis. He had become markedly tremulous and began to experience hallucinations. A clouded state of consciousness is noted.

78. Which of the following is **LEAST LIKELY** concerning this patient?
    A. Alcohol withdrawal delirium is the most likely diagnosis
    B. The patient probably has autonomic hypoactivity
    C. His hallucinations are most likely visual
    D. His disorder has been referred to as delirium tremens
    E. The patient probably has a rapid heart rate

79. Which of the following would **LEAST LIKELY** occur in patients with this disorder?
    A. Frightening illusions
    B. Delusions
    C. Ataxia
    D. Hypothermia
    E. Convulsions

80. Upon being questioned, the patient states that "bugs are crawling all over my body." Which of the following would **MOST PROPERLY** describe this manifestation?
    A. Formication
    B. Trichotillomania
    C. Akathesia
    D. Confabulation
    E. None of the above

Questions 81–83: On careful questioning of a severely anemic 14-year-old girl, you obtain the history that for several years she has been ingesting a substance shown in Figure 3-2, which she refers to as "sour dirt." There is no history of any previous mental or physical disorder.

81. Which of the following would **BEST** describe her practice?
 A. Schafer syndrome
 B. Pica
 C. Rumination
 D. Anorexia nervosa
 E. Malingering

82. Which of the following would **MOST LIKELY** be observed in an infant who practices this activity?
 A. Pervasive developmental disorder
 B. Lead poisoning
 C. Morbid obesity
 D. Retinopathy
 E. Moon facies

Figure 3-2

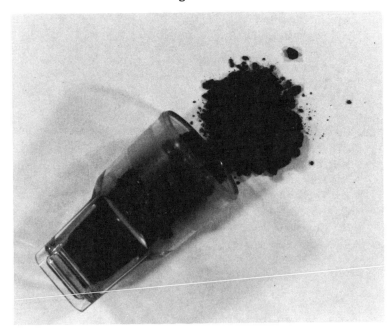

83. To diagnose this disorder, a substance without nutritive value must be ingested for how long a period of time?
    A. 1 week
    B. 2 weeks
    C. 1 month
    D. 3 months
    E. 1 year

Questions 84–87: A 38-year-old white married woman comes to her family physician with a history of vague abdominal pains. She is certain she has cancer. Exhaustive medical examinations and general hospitalizations have failed to reveal any abnormality other than "spastic colitis." Yet she continues to believe she has cancer, but, as she says, "The doctors just haven't found it yet." She wakes up early in the morning (about 4 A.M.). She has lost at least 15 pounds in the past six weeks (a fact she attributes to cancer). Her speech is monotonous and slow. Tears come to her eyes as she talks about how her youngest child joined the Navy five months ago. Since then she has felt useless, and she has found no pleasure in anything. Although she never feels good, she believes she feels worse in the morning. She previously had been well. She denies any previous history of similar symptoms. She has received no prior psychiatric help.

84. Which of the following is the **MOST LIKELY** Axis I diagnosis?
    A. Hypochondriasis
    B. Major depression, single episode
    C. Bipolar disorder
    D. Cancer of the pancreas
    E. Somatoform disorder

85. Which of the following is the **MOST LIKELY** Axis II diagnosis?
    A. Compulsive personality disorder
    B. Borderline personality disorder
    C. Diagnosis deferred
    D. Problems related to the social environment
    E. GAF-45

86. The woman
    A. should not be asked about suicide
    B. should be asked about suicide
    C. may make a suicidal manipulative gesture
    D. is very unlikely to attempt suicide
    E. none of the above

87. Which of the following would allow the therapist to be **LESS** concerned about the suicide?
- **A.** Family history of suicide
- **B.** Patient's mood improves
- **C.** Patient tells about her suicidal ideas
- **D.** Patient made a suicidal gesture two weeks ago
- **E.** None of the above

88. A 30-year-old woman has a several-year history of multiple somatic complaints for which she has been "worked up" and treated by many competent physicians. However, all their efforts have failed to influence her chronic but fluctuating history of malaise and somatic distress. She now complains of an array of symptoms: dyspareunia, irregular and painful menses, back pains, chest pains, lightheadedness, nausea, heartburn, painful urination, "weak spells," and "twitching legs"—all in a vague but dramatic manner. Physician examination and laboratory testing again disclose no abnormality. The **MOST LIKELY** diagnosis is
- **A.** Munchausen's syndrome
- **B.** factitious disorder
- **C.** malingering
- **D.** hypochondriasis
- **E.** somatization disorder

89. Which of the following is **NOT** correct?
- **A.** Brain norepinephrine is metabolized to 3,4 MHPG
- **B.** Norpramin blocks the reuptake of norepinephrine
- **C.** Amitryptiline blocks the reuptake of only norepinephrine
- **D.** Some cases of depression are associated with low brain levels of norepinephrine
- **E.** Urinary levels of 3,4 MHPG are low in some groups of depressed people

Questions 90–121: Each group of the following questions consists of lettered headings followed by numbered words, phrases, or statements. For **each** numbered word, phrase, or statement, select the **one** lettered heading that is most closely associated with it. Each lettered heading may be selected once, more than once, or not at all.

Questions 90–93:

> **A.** Fear of pain
> **B.** Fear of heights
> **C.** Fear of strangers
> **D.** Fear of leaving home

90. Acrophobia

91. Algophobia

92. Agoraphobia

93. Xenophobia

Questions 94–97:

> **A.** Preoperational stage of cognitive development
> **B.** Formal operations stage
> **C.** Sensorimotor stage
> **D.** Concrete operations stage

94. Birth to roughly 18 months

95. Roughly 18 months to 7 years

96. Roughly 7 years to 11–13 years

97. 11–13 years

Questions 98–100: Match the following psychosexual development stage with the appropriate age groups.

> **A.** 1–3 years
> **B.** Birth to 12 months
> **C.** 2½–6 years

98. Oral

99. Anal

100. Phallic

Questions 101–104:

    A. Repression
    B. Denial
    C. Displacement
    D. Projection
    E. Reaction-formation
    F. Dissociation

101. Involuntary banishment of feelings, ideas, or impulses from awareness

102. Consciously intolerable facts or thoughts are ignored

103. Attribution of one's own wishes or attitudes to another

104. Feeling or impulse originally directed toward one person is transferred to another

Questions 105–107:

    A. "Bonnie rule"
    B. Durham decision
    C. M'Naghten

105. Judge David Bazelon

106. Attempted assassination of Sir Robert Peel

107. Incorporated into the Insanity Defense Reform Act of 1985

Questions 108–110:

    A. Pica
    B. Bulimia nervosa
    C. Anorexia nervosa

108. Self-induced starvation

109. Repeated consumption of nonnutritive substance

110. Poor dentition

Questions 111–114: For each type of personality test, indicate its **MOST APPROPRIATE** use.

    A. Draw-a-Person Test
    B. Sentence Completion Test
    C. Thematic Apperception Test (TAT)
    D. Rorschach Test

111. Most useful for judging motivational aspects of behavior

112. May be used to tap specific conflict areas; generally reveals more conscious, overt attitudes and feelings

113. Useful for detecting psychomotor difficulties correlated with brain damage

114. Especially revealing of personality structure; most widely used projective technique

Questions 115–118: Usual dose range of antidepressants.

    A. 75–300 mg/d
    B. 50–150 mg/d
    C. 10–40 mg/d
    D. 200–600 mg/d

115. Fluoxetine (Prozac)

116. Trazodone (Desyrel)

117. Nortriptyline (Pamelor)

118. Imipramine (Tofranil)

Questions 119–121:

    A. Paroxetine (Paxil)
    B. Venlafaxine (Effexor)
    C. Fluoxetine (Prozac)
    D. Sertraline (Zoloft)

119. Long half life

120. Both serotonin and norepinephrine reuptake inhibitor

121. Short half life, no active metabolites

122. Information learned from the National Institute of Mental Health Epidemiologic Catchment Area Program includes
    A. as a group, anxiety disorders were the most prevalent, with a lifetime prevalence rate of 14.6%
    B. substance abuse is more prevalent in older age groups
    C. prevalence of affective (mood) disorders was equal to that of schizophrenia
    D. men were found to have higher overall rates of mental disorders than women
    E. women had higher prevalence rates of alcoholism than men

123. Among people who have attempted suicide, which of the following groups would be at the **HIGHEST** risk for completed suicide?
    A. Women
    B. Those under the age of 45
    C. The employed
    D. Those living with relatives
    E. Those with previous attempts by violent methods

124. A middle-aged man comes to you because he fears his wife will leave him. He tells you that his wife has moved out of the house, that he ejaculates prematurely, and that he does not satisfy her. He drinks some wine before dinner and three or four gin and tonics afterward. He states that for the past several weeks he has had trouble sleeping, awakening early. He is not hungry and has lost about five pounds. He is not able to concentrate on his work and finds pleasure in nothing, saying, "Things just don't look good."

He sighs deeply and pauses. At this point, it would be **MOST HELPFUL** to say, "Tell me more about

A. your drinking problem"
B. what's wrong at work"
C. your wife's moving out"
D. your sexual problems"
E. things not looking good"

125. Which of the following is **TRUE** of patients with amnestic syndrome?
    A. They may be oriented and alert, but cannot remember what happened a few hours earlier
    B. They are able to remember recent events
    C. They have delusional psychoses
    D. Alcohol abuse and deficiency of niacin combine to cause the clinical picture
    E. Tactile hallucinations are often found in the syndrome

126. Which of the following is the **MOST FREQUENT** irreversible cause of dementia in the United States?
    A. Folate deficiency
    B. Alzheimer's disease
    C. Normal pressure hydrocephalus
    D. HIV infection
    E. Hypothyroidism

127. The largest diagnostic group among suicide completers is
    A. depression
    B. alcoholism
    C. schizophrenia
    D. anxiety disorders
    E. drug dependence

128. Which of the following terms describes the thought pattern marked by speech that is indirect and tedious in detail, but eventually arrives at a coherent goal?
    A. Tangentiality
    B. Word salad
    C. Circumstantiality
    D. Derailment
    E. Klang associations

129. Which of the following statements is **TRUE** regarding the prognosis of anorexia nervosa and bulimia nervosa?
   A. Some cases may remit spontaneously and never come to the attention of a physician
   B. Long-term studies have consistently shown negligible mortality rates
   C. Upon remission of the eating disorder symptoms, associated affective disorder symptoms remit as well
   D. Recent studies have documented full-blown symptomatology persisting into middle and late adulthood, and even into old age
   E. Bulimia nervosa has a greater mortality rate than anorexia nervosa

130. Stages of response in the dying patient, according to Elisabeth Kubler-Ross include
   A. denial, anxiety, depression, acceptance
   B. anger, intellectualization, bargaining, acceptance
   C. isolation of affect, bargaining, depression, acceptance
   D. fear, denial, depression, acceptance
   E. anger, bargaining, depression, acceptance

131. Priapism is **MOST COMMONLY** associated with which of the following medications?
   A. Fluoxethine
   B. Pimozide
   C. Tranylcypromine
   D. Trazodone
   E. Chlorazepate

132. Which of the following has been found effective in the treatment of nocturnal enuresis in children?
   A. Pemoline
   B. Imipramine
   C. Dextroamphetamine
   D. Temazepam
   E. Methylphenidate

133. During the orgasm phase of the human sexual response cycle
   A. there is involuntary dilation of internal and external sphincters
   B. blood pressure increases by 20 to 40 mm
   C. heart rate decreases by 20 to 40 bpm

D. there is a flaccid paralysis of large muscle groups
E. breast size in the woman increases 25%

134. The borderline personality is **NOT** characterized by
  A. unpredictability
  B. unstable and intense interpersonal relationships
  C. inappropriate, intense anger
  D. social withdrawal
  E. disturbances in identity

135. Predisposing causes for subdural hematoma include all the following **EXCEPT**
  A. age over 60 years
  B. alcoholism
  C. residence in suburbia
  D. epilepsy
  E. renal dialysis

136. Which of the following is **NOT** characteristic of delirium?
  A. Disorientation
  B. Memory impairment
  C. Disturbance of sleep–wake cycle
  D. Perceptual disturbances
  E. Normal level of arousal

137. A psychosocial formulation includes each of the following **EXCEPT**
  A. an assessment of the patient's mental function
  B. an assessment of the patient's behavior
  C. an assessment of the patient's social circumstances
  D. an assessment of the patient's personality
  E. an emphasis on how one patient is similar to others

138. All the following would mitigate against a diagnosis of paranoid schizophrenia **EXCEPT**
  A. inappropriate affect
  B. marked loosening of associations
  C. catatonic behavior
  D. disorganized behavior
  E. preoccupation with a systematized delusion

139. Which of the following does **NOT** produce physical dependence?
   A. Alprazolam
   B. Buspirone
   C. Ethanol
   D. Lorazepam
   E. Chlorazepate

140. Each of the following statements is correct **EXCEPT**
   A. testamentary capacity refers to competency to make a will
   B. every person of legal age is assured competent to make a will unless judged otherwise
   C. a person may be ruled incompetent to handle his money if mental illness makes him incapable of rationally dealing with finances
   D. commitment automatically includes adjudication of incompetence and loss of civil rights
   E. *competency* is a legal, not a medical, term

141. Postconcussional disorder is characterized by all the following **EXCEPT**
   A. headache aggravated by stooping or sudden movement
   B. vertigo aggravated by stooping or sudden movement
   C. emotional lability
   D. hypersensitivity to sensory stimuli
   E. dilated pupils

142. Obsessive compulsive disorder is characterized by all the following **EXCEPT**
   A. recurrent ideas, thoughts, and images
   B. repetitive behaviors
   C. distress about the symptoms
   D. *la belle indifference*
   E. attempts to ignore or suppress symptoms

Questions 143–147: The following group of questions consists of lettered headings followed by a list of numbered words, phrases, or statements. For each number word, phrase, or statement, select the **one** lettered heading that is most closely associated with it. Each lettered heading may be selected once, more than once, or not at all.

A. Confabulation
B. Hallucination
C. Illusion
D. Depersonalization
E. Obsession

143. Misinterpretation of sensory experience

144. Production of stories to fill in gaps in memory

145. Sense of one's own unreality

146. Sensory perception in the absence of an identifiable external stimulus

147. Recurrent idea that one fights against

Psychiatry

Answer Key

1. B	27. B	53. E	79. D
2. A	28. D	54. D	80. A
3. B	29. E	55. C	81. B
4. C	30. D	56. E	82. B
5. A	31. C	57. A	83. C
6. A	32. D	58. C	84. B
7. C	33. E	59. C	85. C
8. D	34. C	60. E	86. B
9. C	35. D	61. C	87. E
10. A	36. D	62. B	88. E
11. B	37. E	63. D	89. C
12. E	38. A	64. B	90. B
13. C	39. E	65. D	91. A
14. C	40. E	66. A	92. D
15. B	41. B	67. B	93. C
16. B	42. D	68. D	94. C
17. C	43. A	69. C	95. A
18. D	44. E	70. C	96. D
19. C	45. D	71. C	97. B
20. A	46. D	72. A	98. B
21. E	47. D	73. A	99. A
22. E	48. E	74. B	100. C
23. E	49. A	75. B	101. A
24. D	50. A	76. A	102. B
25. E	51. D	77. C	103. D
26. E	52. C	78. B	104. C

105. B	116. D	127. A	138. E
106. C	117. B	128. C	139. B
107. A	118. A	129. A	140. D
108. C	119. C	130. E	141. E
109. A	120. B	131. D	142. D
110. B	121. A	132. B	143. C
111. C	122. A	133. B	144. A
112. B	123. E	134. D	145. D
113. A	124. E	135. C	146. B
114. D	125. A	136. E	147. E
115. C	126. B	137. E	

Psychiatry

Answers and Comments

1. **(B)** Tourette's disorder is a relatively rare syndrome that involves multiple muscle groups (also referred to as multiple tics). Additionally, at some point, there must be at least one vocal tic, and the possible tics could include hiccuping, sighing, whistling, inpiration, belching, sucking and smacking sounds, throat clearing, yawning, sniffing and blowing through the nostrils. Criteria for diagnosis include the presence of symptoms for more than a year. **(Ref. 1,** pp. 1080–1085)

2. **(A)** Bowlby described the sequential pattern of protest, despair, and detachment as a reaction to separation from their mother in children between 6 months and 3 years of age. Attachment is important for healthy physical and emotional development. Separation is tolerable only in moderation. Overly long separation in early life can produce complications. **(Ref. 2,** p. 31)

3. **(B)** The major task of adolescence is the attainment of a sense of identity. Erik Erikson's schema of eight sequential psychosocial tasks has been a major contribution to our understanding. Erikson's psychosocial tasks should be distinguished from the traditional psychoanalytic stages of psychosexual development (oral, anal, phallic, Oedipal, etc.). **(Ref. 2,** pp. 23–26)

4. **(C)** The major psychosocial task of the Oedipal period is the development of a sense of initiative. This mode of operation con-

trasts with traditional psychoanalysis's psychosexual zones and phases and shows how these modes of behavior continue throughout life. (**Ref. 2,** pp. 23–26)

5. (**A**) For Piaget, intelligence is biological. The first stage (the stage of sensorimotor intelligence) begins with the reflex arc and ends with the attainment of object constancy. That is, the infant (about 18 months) knows an object continues to exist even if he cannot see it. (**Ref. 2,** p. 22)

6. (**A**) Negative reinforcement is not punishment. It is a process whereby an action that tends to a removal of a negative stimulus increases that action. For example, an adolescent will take out the garbage to avoid his parents' harangue. (**Ref. 1,** pp. 165–169)

7. (**C**) The phase of concrete operations (ages 6–12) generally is achieved during the latency stage, supplanting the intuitive phase (4–7 years), during which concepts of space and time are acquired. Impressionistic intuition is replaced by small logical steps in reasoning, and data used is concrete. (**Ref. 2,** pp. 23–25)

8. (**D**) Instrumental or operant conditioning is a form of learning in which relatively spontaneous behavior is punished or rewarded. Partial reinforcement consists of different forms of intermittent reward of which fixed-ratio scheduling is one. In fixed-ratio scheduling, a specific number of responses must occur before a reward is given. Continual reinforcement, where every response is reinforced, produces the most rapid acquisition of behavior. In classical or Pavlovian conditioning, in contrast, a stimulus that once had no ability to bring on a specific response becomes able to do so. (**Ref. 1,** pp. 165–169)

9. (**C**) Borderline and psychotic conditions are typified by the predominance of primitive defenses such as splitting. Splitting refers to the process of experiencing the self or others as "all good" or "all bad," rather than having both good and bad properties. (**Ref. 1,** p. 250)

10. (**A**) Defense mechanisms are unconscious. They function automatically, out of our awareness, to reduce conflict and anxiety. Coping mechanisms include both the defense mechanisms and

conscious mechanisms such as suppression and fact finding. (**Ref. 5,** pp. 48–49)

11. **(B)**   Aaron Beck's work on the cognitive theory of depression is now quite accepted. A similar approach can be found in transactional analysis (see Allen, *Psychiatry: A Guide,* New York, Medical Examination Publishing Company, 1984) and in Albert Ellis, *The Practice of Rational Emotive Theory* (New York, Springer Publishing Co., 1987). However, these ideas go back to the Greek philosopher Heraclitus of Ephesus. Heinz Kohut is most famous for his work on narcissism and disorders of the self. Kernberg has brought object-relations theory into the mainstream of modern psychiatry. Margaret Mahler's work on the separation-individuation stage of child development is already classic. These three have revitalized psychoanalysis. Fritz Perls developed gestalt therapy. (**Ref. 1,** pp. 20–23, 254–260, 540–545)

12. **(E)**   The WISC (Weschler Intelligence Scale for Children) is the child version of the WAIS. Like the WAIS, it includes verbal and performance tests. (**Ref. 2,** pp. 126–127)

13. **(C)**   Lithium carbonate is felt to be prophylactic for episodes of depression as well as mania and bipolar illness. Carbamazepine is also being used in bipolar illness for effects on manic and depressive phases, particularly in patients who appear to be resistant to lithium. Doses of lithium should be adjusted to reach serum levels between 0.8–1.2 mEq/L during the acute phase. Episodes are usually managed initially with antipsychotic agents until the lithium can begin to take effect. (**Ref. 7,** p. 139)

14. **(C)**   According to the American Association on Mental Deficiency's classification, the degree of mental retardation depicted in items A to D would be reported as being profound, severe, moderate, and mild, respectively. Patients are no longer reported as having "borderline" deficiency. (**Ref. 1,** p. 1026)

15. **(B)**   The drug depicted is the tricyclic derivative, amitriptyline. This frequently used antidepressant is long-acting and is often given at bedtime to decrease its sedative effect during the daytime. It may take several weeks before maximal antidepressant activities occur after initiating amitriptyline therapy. (**Ref. 1,** pp. 991–992)

16. **(B)** The physician should be aware of potential side effects of psychotropic drugs before prescribing them. Phenothiazines, especially chlorpromazine and thioridazine, can result in pigmentation of the lens. Pigmentary retinopathy is more likely to occur in patients receiving thioridazine at doses over 800 mg/d. (**Ref. 1,** p. 949)

17. **(C)** In DSM IV, mental disorders are included in Axes I or II and physical disorders are classified in Axis III. Psychosocial and environmental problems are classified in Axis IV. Axis V registers the clinician's global assessment of the functioning of the patient. (**Ref. 4,** pp. 29–31)

18. **(D)** Oxazepam (Serax) has a half life of about 5 to 18 hours. This short half life may benefit elderly patients who are more vulnerable to the cumulative effects of agents such as hypnotics or sedatives. Oxazepam has a relatively short half life in younger patients also. The half life of diazepam may be roughly estimated by adding 20 hours to the number of years the patient is above the age of 30. Phenobarbital, of course, is not a benzodiazepine. (**Ref. 1,** p. 913)

19. **(C)** Phenothiazines can be subdivided chemically into three groups: aliphatics, piperazines, and piperidines. All these groups, like nonphenothiazine antipsychotics such as butyrophenones, share one property: They block dopamine receptors. (**Ref. 8,** pp. 110–111)

20. **(A)** Chlordiazepoxide (Librium) is poorly and erratically absorbed when given intramuscularly. When treating alcohol withdrawal, oral dosages are thus the preferred method of administration. (**Ref. 1,** pp. 405–406)

21. **(E)** There are almost no absolute contraindications for ECT, given under modern anesthesia and with a modern machine. All the conditions listed can increase the risk of complications of ECT. However, in many cases, measures can be taken to reduce the risk. It should be noted that, with modern methods, ECT is really safer than the use of tricyclic medication. (**Ref. 1,** p. 1010)

22. **(E)** The blockage of a rather nonspecific transport system by the tricyclics will block the access of guanethidine to its site of action in the sympathetic nerve terminals. (**Ref. 8,** p. 193)

23. **(E)** Grieving is a dynamic state, with its symptoms lasting until the person has had the opportunity to experience the entire calendar year at least once without the lost person. The bereaved person may take on the qualities, mannerisms, or characteristics of the deceased to perpetuate that person in some way. (**Ref. 3,** pp. 595–598)

24. **(D)** This study was conducted in 1954, sampling 1660 adults from New York City. More precise data was obtained in the NIMH Epidemiologic Catchment Area survey in the late 1970s and 1980s. (**Ref. 1,** pp. 193–195)

25. **(E)** *Malpractice* is the term referring to professional negligence. An expert must establish the four Ds of malpractice: "A Dereliction of a Duty that Directly leads to Damages." In negligence: (1) a standard of care must exist; (2) the person who is answerable for his/her conduct must owe a duty; (3) the plaintiff must be owed the duty; (4) a breach of the duty is the legal cause for injury or damage. (**Ref. 1,** p. 1183)

26. **(E)** Disulfiram (Antabuse) inhibits the enzyme acetaldehyde dehydrogenase, resulting in acetaldehyde poisoning. The usual dose is 250–500 mg/d. Patients should be aware that they may react to even small amounts of alcohol present in food, mouthwash, and over-the-counter medicines. (**Ref. 3,** p. 321)

27. **(B)** Cognitive therapy is generally not considered a dynamic psychotherapy. However, increasingly cognitive therapies are becoming integrated with psychodynamic theory and practice. (**Ref. 2,** pp. 400–407, 408–416)

28. **(D)** Electromyogram is used for the electrodiagnosis of peripheral nerve and muscle disease. The remaining techniques provide images of the central nervous system. (**Ref. 1,** pp. 112–125)

29. **(E)** The diagnostic criteria for a diagnosis of psychosocial factors affecting medical conditions are important in DSM IV. In DMS II, in contrast, psychosocial factors were considered important only in initiating disorders. Symbolism is not a diagnostic criterion, but rather a psychodynamic mechanism. (**Ref. 4,** p. 678)

30. (D) A claim in regard to informed consent is not usually added to charges of malpractice. Informed consent must be based on adequate information concerning therapy, available alternatives, and known and unknown collateral risks. It must be freely given, and not induced in a frenzied situation. (**Ref. 1**, pp. 1178–1179, 1191–1192)

31. (C) Multiple cognitive deficits are the essential feature of dementia. Memory, judgment, abstract thought, and other higher cortical functions decline. The diagnosis is not made if these features are due to a reduced ability to maintain or shift attention to external stimuli, as in delirium. (**Ref. 4**, p. 135)

32. (D) In mood disorders the primary feature is a mood disturbance, whereas abnormalities in behavior and thinking are considered secondary processes. Major depression is classified under mood disorders. Minor depression is classified under dysthymic and cyclothymic disorders. (**Ref. 4**, pp. 317–319)

33. (E) Manic patients display inflated self-esteem, often to the point of grandiosity. They appear to require decreased sleep, and often get involved in activities with potentially painful consequences. Symptoms may be severe enough to cause considerable impairment in functioning at work or social activities in relation with others. The patient may require hospitalization and may exhibit psychotic features. (**Ref. 4**, pp. 328–332)

34. (C) A disturbance of conduct is a persistent or repetitive behavior pattern. There are a total of 15 behaviors, of which at least three must be present in the past 12 months, with at least one in the past 6 months. (**Ref. 4**, p. 90)

35. (D) Although it may occur in the latency years, anorexia nervosa typically occurs during adolescence. The essential features of this disorder are that the persons involved refuse to maintain a minimally normal body weight, are intensely afraid of gaining weight, and display a perceptual distortion of the shape and size of their bodies. Anorexia may be a misnomer as appetite is rarely lost. (**Ref. 4**, pp. 539–545)

36. (D) An infectious affect is more characteristic of mania. Affect refers more to fluctuations in emotional "weather," whereas mood is a more sustained and pervasive emotion. (**Ref. 3**, p. 27)

37. **(E)** The peripheral syndrome is characterized by mydriasis, dry mouth, cycloplegia, flushing, and tachycardia. Sometimes, however, sweating may occur with the tricyclic antidepressants. (**Ref. 8,** pp. 38–39)

38. **(A)** Mental retardation can be clarified according to prenatal, perinatal, and postnatal causes. Prenatal causes are chromosomal, biochemical, environmental, or unknown. Perinatal causes are associated with the birth process. Postnatal causes include traumatic, metabolic, infectious, toxic, and other causes of brain damage. (**Ref. 2,** pp. 362–365)

39. **(E)** Personal history is not part of the mental status examination. Indeed, the mental status examination is a description of a person's mental state at one point in time, much like the still photos advertising a movie. The mental status does not tell where persons have been or where they are going. (**Ref. 3,** pp. 25–33)

40. **(E)** Primary prevention is prevention in the layman's use of the word. Secondary prevention is early diagnosis and treatment. Reducing the residual effects of a disorder is the goal of tertiary prevention. (**Ref. 1,** p. 203)

41. **(B)** Despite the severity of the disorder, only half the affected population has a history of treatment. The actual lifetime prevalence is about 1%. (**Ref. 2,** p. 205)

42. **(D)** Trazodone (Desyrel) has the weakest anticholinergic properties. Anticholinergic side effects include palpitations, loss of visual accommodation, dry mouth, aggravation of narrow-angle glaucoma, urinary retention, and paralytic ileus, as well as delirium. (**Ref. 8,** p. 179)

43. **(A)** Early symptoms of toxicity include vomiting, slurred speech, dizziness, ataxia, mystagmus, and muscle weakness. Patients in acute mania can usually tolerate quite high doses of lithium, but the dosage must be rapidly reduced to maintenance levels when the acute attack has subsided. More severe intoxication may present as delirium, myoclonus, impaired consciousness, seizures, coma, and death. (**Ref. 8,** p. 143)

44. **(E)** Testamentary capacity refers to the capacity to make a will. Knowledge as to whether the particular act was right or wrong is one of the M'Naghten criteria for insanity. The student should note that terms such as *insanity* and *competence* have specific legal definitions. These are not medical terms. (**Ref. 1,** pp. 1179–1183)

45. **(D)** Even under threat of subpoena, privilege is the right to maintain confidentiality. The belief that privilege somehow belongs to the doctor is one of the most widely held misconceptions. Privilege belongs to the patient and hence can be waived only by the patient. (**Ref. 1,** pp. 1172–1174)

46. **(D)** Voices commenting is a Schneiderian criterion for schizophrenia and was chosen as one of the diagnostic criteria for schizophrenic disorder in DSM IV. The other symptoms are part of diagnostic criteria for posttraumatic stress disorder (PTSD). (**Ref. 1,** pp. 458–459)

47. **(D)** The borderline personality is characterized by general instability of mood, identity, and interpersonal relationships. Psychodynamically, these people use much denial and splitting, experiencing themselves as either "all good" or "all bad." Developmentally, they seem fixated at the "rapproachment stage" of separation-individuation (Mahler). (**Ref. 4,** pp. 650–654)

48. **(E)** Schizotypal personality disorder criteria contain no frank psychotic symptoms and occur over an extended period of time. Hence, they are an Axis II diagnosis. Delusions constitute one of the A criteria for schizophrenic disorders in the DSM IV classification. (**Ref. 4,** pp. 641–645)

49. **(A)** Dementia of the Alzheimer's type is the most common of the presenile dementias. Pathologically, we cannot currently distinguish it from senile dementia. Histologically, it is characterized by diffuse neural loss, neurofibrillary tangles, especially in the hippocampal gyrus, and senile plaques in the gray matter. There is no destruction of the basal ganglia, as occurs in Huntington's chorea and Jakob-Creuzfeldt's disease. The student should distinguish the reversible forms of dementia, such as vitamin deficiency (e.g., B12), normal pressure hydrocephalus, and the pseudodementia of depression in the elderly. (**Ref. 1,** pp. 1159–1160)

50. **(A)** The typical age for the onset of alcohol hallucinations is about 40, after 10 or more years of heavy drinking. Alcohol-induced psychotic disorder can occur during intoxication or withdrawal and from delirium tremens. There is, however, a clear state of consciousness; the patient has auditory, as opposed to visual and tactile, hallucinations. (**Ref. 1,** p. 408)

51. **(D)** Primary process is the illogical mode of thinking that is typical of the unconscious. It is the type of thinking found in dreams and in psychosis. Secondary process, in contrast, refers to orderly mental activity that gives due regard to everyday logic. (**Ref. 5,** pp. 148–149)

52. **(C)** The tendency for physicians to displace feelings from earlier figures in their life onto the patient is called countertransferance. Understanding countertransferance feelings may help avoid interference in proceeding with treatment. (**Ref. 1,** p. 7)

53. **(E)** Trouble falling asleep is not typical of melancholia, in contrast to early morning awakening. Patients with symptoms of melancholia seem more likely to respond to tricyclic medications. (**Ref. 4,** pp. 383–384)

54. **(D)** Major tranquilizers, such as chlorpromazine, thioridazine, and haloperidol, are useful in the treatment of paranoid reactions in the elderly. The minor tranquilizers actually can reduce patients' understanding of their surroundings because of their effect on the cerebral cortex. However, the minor tranquilizers are sometimes useful in controlling the transient situational reactions. (**Ref. 1,** pp. 906–914, 945–947)

55. **(C)** Although high-potency, low-anticholinergic drugs are more likely to cause symptoms, all antipsychotics can cause extrapyramidal side effects. Chlorpromazine, which has only about 2% of the relative potency of haloperidol, would be expected to have the lowest incidence of such effects. (**Ref. 1,** p. 950)

56. **(E)** Nearly all the antipsychotic medications can result in extrapyramidal effects including acute dystonic reactions, akathisia, and neuroleptic-induced Parkinsonism. The latter is characterized by increased salivation as well as other features listed. (**Ref. 1,** pp. 949–950)

57. **(A)** Neuroleptic malignant syndrome (NMS) is a potentially life-threatening disorder associated with potentially any antipsychotic medication. All medication should be discontinued upon recognition of the disorder. In addition to IV fluids, antipsychotic agents, and cooling agents, electroconvulsive therapy may also be useful. It may occur in 1% of patients on antipsychotic medications. (**Ref. 3**, pp. 516, 560)

58. **(C)** Serotonin-specific reuptake inhibitors (SSRIs) have a separate side effect profile from tricyclic antidepressants. Sweating is more common in tricyclics such as imipramine. SSRIs can cause insomnia in some patients and drowsiness in others. (**Ref. 1**, pp. 976–981)

59. **(C)** Delirium in HIV infection can be caused by many factors including infections and metabolic, medication, and intracranial lesions. Chronic sequelae of these causes of delirium can result in dementia. Cerebral HIV infection accounts for a large percentage of the dementia in AIDS patients. Vascular myelopathy is less frequent and similar to cobalamin deficiency. Peripheral nerve involvement is often the result of local infections, neoplasms, or HIV polyneuropathy. (**Ref. 3**, pp. 612–616)

60. **(E)** Risperidone is chemically different from all other antipsychotics. Its benzisoxazole structure also has antagonist properties at serotonin type 2 (5-HTs) receptors. It has been reported to have fewer neurological adverse effects than other drugs in its class. (**Ref. 1**, pp. 944, 946)

61. **(C)** This man is exhibiting psychotic symptoms. Consequently, a major tranquilizer is the treatment of choice. (**Ref. 8**, pp. 109–118)

62. **(B)** Frugality, punctuality, meticulousness, sadistic rage, problems with control, submission, and defiance are common with people fixated at the anal stage. Because of their use of reaction-formation, these characteristics may exist side-by-side with their opposites. In psychoanalytic theory, fixation at any stage of early development is believed to lead to particular personality characteristics. The fixation may occur either because of excessive gratification or because of deprivation, as experienced by the child in terms of individual needs. (**Ref. 5**, pp. 14–15)

63. **(D)** The patient was undergoing aversion therapy in which the subject's undesirable behavior, i.e., drinking alcohol, was being couple with an unpleasant stimulus, i.e., an emetic agent. This is a form of behavior therapy. Disulfiram (Antabuse) is frequently used to establish an aversive reaction to alcohol by inducing nausea and other untoward effects when alcohol is consumed. Antabuse blocks the oxidation of alcohol at the acetaldehyde stage. During alcohol metabolism, which follows Antabuse intake, the acetaldehyde blood concentration may be 5 to 10 times higher than that found during metabolism of the same amount of alcohol alone. (**Ref. 1,** pp. 937–938)

64. **(B)** A fugue is defined as a state of dissociation, or a personality separation during which normal life patterns are totally repressed. The state may last for days or months, even years, during which the individual may initially have total amnesia, leaving home and wandering about for days. The subject may appear quite normal, or may be confused and disoriented. (**Ref. 1,** p. 307)

65. **(D)** Although pellagra psychosis formerly resulted in a relatively high incidence of admissions to mental hospitals, its occurrence is uncommon at present. Patients with niacin deficiency invariably are deficient in other vitamins as well. Both delirium and seizures may occur early, with motor abnormalities developing later. In addition to dementia, diarrhea and dermatitis are frequent manifestations. (**Ref. 1,** p. 372)

66. **(A)** Becoming aware of previous unpleasant incidents, which the patient has repressed, can result in an emotional release or abreaction. This discharge of unpleasant emotion can assist patients and allow them to gain insight into the problem areas, with some resultant desensitization. (**Ref. 5,** p. 1)

67. **(B)** Many endocrinopathies, including hypothyroidism, can result in mental changes, and the possible presence of such disorders should be considered in patients presenting with psychiatric manifestations. Severe cases of hypothyroidism have resulted in what has been referred to as "myxedema madness." (**Ref. 1,** p. 371)

68. **(D)** The use of psychotropic medications, especially phenothiazines, may result in extrapyramidal syndrome that may be

manifested by the Parkinsonian symptoms exhibited by the patient. Dystonia, i.e., abnormal involuntary posturing, as well as restlessness and motor inertia may also occur. The disorder is caused by the overgrowth of bone as well as connective tissue and viscera. Soft tissue overgrowth is mainly responsible for enlargement of the patient's hands, requiring a larger wedding band. Psychological complaints including loss of libido are frequent in this disorder. (**Ref. 3**, pp. 512–517)

69. **(C)** When a person who is taking a monoamine oxidase inhibitor eats food containing the amino acid tyramine, he or she may have a hypertensive crisis. Some of the foods to be avoided include chianti and other red wines, beer, fava beans, aged cheeses, smoked meats, liver, and yeast. In addition, over-the-counter medicines containing pseudoephedrine or similar sympathomimetics can also cause problems. (**Ref. 2**, p. 374)

70. **(C)** The etiology of the phrase "to run amok" derives from the culturally disapproved disorder that has been associated with Malaysian men. Physicians should be aware of practices found among different cultures in addition to their own. (**Ref. 1**, p. 493)

71. **(C)** Akathisia is one of the three major extrapyramidal side effects of antipsychotic medications. These extrapyramidal side effects may be confused with psychotic agitation. Although akathisia is often referred to as an extrapyramidal side effect, its cause is actually unknown. It often does not respond to anti-Parkinsonian agents used in treatment of other extrapyramidal side effects, which is one reason it is such a troublesome side effect. Some researchers cite the effectiveness of beta blockers (e.g., propranolol) in treating this side effect as evidence that it is related to catecholamine rather than dopamine receptor activation. (**Ref. 3**, pp. 513–514)

72. **(A)** Imipramine (Tofranil), starting at a low dose, can prevent panic attacks. Some patients require antidepressant doses. MAOIs, SSRIs, and high-potency benzodiazepines have also shown efficacy. New evidence shows that patients may respond to low and moderate dosages of benzodiazepines. To treat any "anticipatory anxiety" (the fear of having a panic attack), an antianxiety agent will probably be necessary. (**Ref. 1**, pp. 589–591)

73. (A) Muscular dystonia is the most common extrapyramidal side effect within the first few days after beginning treatment with a major tranquilizer, accounting for about 6% of extrapyramidal symptoms. Akathisia, however, is the most common side effect overall. (**Ref. 8**, pp. 122–123)

74. (B) Individuals with antisocial personality disorders have difficulty getting along with others and often have problems such as those experienced by this person. Such individuals are usually egocentric and disregard the rights of others. The essential manifestation of an antisocial personality disorder is a pervasive pattern in which others' rights are violated or disregarded. This behavior usually begins before the age of 15. (**Ref. 4**, pp. 645–650)

75. (B) Antisocial subjects are hedonistic rather than masochistic. In addition to lacking a sense of responsibility, they have a stunted development of conscience and often exploit others. (**Ref. 4**, pp. 645–650)

76. (A) Munchausen's syndrome is a condition characterized by continued and habitual presentation for surgery and/or hospitalization for an imagined acute illness. The patient gives a meticulous history, all of which is false, but insists on medical attention. This syndrome is a chronic, fictitious disorder with physical symptoms. (**Ref. 3**, pp. 294–299)

77. (C) In this condition, the patient displays uncontrollable lying in which he voluntarily presents involved and elaborate fantasies. This form of habitual, pathological lying may not just involve the patient's medical problems but often involves other areas of the patient's life. (**Ref. 1**, p. 306)

78. (B) Alcohol withdrawal delirium results from discontinuation or decreasing alcohol intake after having been drinking for a protracted period. In this syndrome, a coarse, irregular tremor usually occurs and may involve the hands, tongue, and eyelids. Hyperactivity of the autonomic nervous system with diaphoresis, tachycardia, or hypertension often occurs. Occasionally, orthostatic hypotension may develop. (**Ref. 4**, pp. 129–132, 197–199)

79. **(D)** Such patients may exhibit all the manifestations listed with the exception that fever rather than hypothermia is more likely to be present. Patients with alcohol withdrawal can experience seizures, or the so-called rum fits. (**Ref. 4,** pp. 129–132, 197–199)

80. **(A)** Patients with alcohol withdrawal delirium may experience hallucinations of all modalities of sensation. Although visual hallucinations are most common, tactile hallucinations, such as described by the patient, are not uncommon. The description of insects crawling over the subject's body would be referred to as fomication. (**Ref. 2,** pp. 478–479)

81. **(B)** Pica, which consists of ingestion of nonnutritive substances, can start in infancy. A wide variety of substances may be ingested including paint, plaster, string, hair, or cloth. Older children may consume insects, pebbles, leaves, sand, or animal droppings. Adolescents and adults may eat soil or clay. The exact roles played by social influences, nutritional status, and possible psychopathology in this practice are complex and have not been fully delineated. (**Ref. 4,** pp. 95–96)

82. **(B)** The diagnosis of pica can occur during the course of another mental disorder, such as schizophrenia, pervasive developmental disorder, or a physical condition, such as Kleine-Levin syndrome. Lead poisoning with possible resultant mental deficiency can result from chronic ingestion of lead-containing substances such as old paint. Infants and children living in old housing are more likely to suffer serious consequences from pica. (**Ref. 4,** pp. 95–96)

83. **(C)** According to DSM IV, the subject must have been ingesting the substance for a period of a month or more. Those who practice pica lack any food aversion. Occasionally, a mineral deficiency, such as a lack of iron or zinc, may contribute to this practice. (**Ref. 4,** pp. 95–96)

84. **(B)** She meets the criteria for a major depressive episode. She has melancholia, early morning awakening, anorexia, weight loss, and psychomotor retardation. Cancer of the pancreas and retroperitoneal lymphoma are notorious for causing depression. At this point, however, there is no evidence she has cancer. (**Ref. 4,** pp. 320–327)

85. **(C)** It is not possible to make an Axis II diagnosis from the incomplete history given. This does not mean there is not an Axis II disorder. It is important to note that DSM IV uses five axes. Axis II is for the diagnosis of personality (or, in children, developmental) disorder. Axis III is for a traditional medical diagnosis. Axis IV reports psychosocial and environmental problems affecting diagnosis, prognosis, and treatment. Axis V is a global assessment of functioning (GAF) on a 100-point scale. (**Ref. 4,** p. 26)

86. **(B)** It's a myth that asking a depressed patient about suicide may "plant" the idea. Quite the opposite is true. If a patient does have thoughts of suicide, it may be beneficial to discuss what no one else wants to hear. Every depressed patient should be asked about suicide. (**Ref. 3,** p. 216)

87. **(E)** Suicidal risk increases with depressed mood, especially if vegetative signs are present, as in this case. The risk may become even greater as she improves and becomes more energetic. Indeed, if she decides to kill herself, her mood may improve remarkably. (**Ref. 1,** pp. 803–811)

88. **(E)** Somatization disorder usually begins in the twenties and runs a fluctuating course, although the patient is rarely free of symptoms. These people do not have symptoms of melancholia. Although they may include conversion phenomena in their list of complaints, the diagnosis of conversion disorder should be reserved for those in whom conversion symptoms are primary. Hypochondriasis is characterized by unrealistic interpretations of physical signs and symptoms, and by an obsessive fear that one is ill. (**Ref. 4,** pp. 446–450)

89. **(C)** Amitryptiline also blocks the reuptake of serotonin. It should be noted that, in some groups of severely depressed patients, norepinephrine levels seem normal, but serotonin and its breakdown product 5HIAA in the spinal fluid are low. In other groups, the biochemistry seems normal. (**Ref. 8,** p. 184)

90. **(B)** This series of questions defines certain fears. Specific phobias (previously called simple phobias) can lead to avoidance behavior. Although quite prevalent in the general population, many phobias are not severe enough or cause sufficient distress to war-

rant a diagnosis. Agoraphobia can occur in the context of panic disorder or without a history of panic disorder. The fear of high places is referred to as acrophobia. (**Ref. 4**, pp. 393–417; **Ref. 7**, p. 9)

91. (**A**) The fear of pain is termed algophobia. (**Ref. 4**, pp. 393–417; **Ref. 7**, p. 24)

92. (**D**) Literally fear of the marketplace, agoraphobia is the fear of leaving the familiar setting of the home. (**Ref. 7**, p. 106)

93. (**C**) The fear of strangers is referred to an xenophobia. (**Ref. 7**, p. 692)

94. (**C**) According to Piaget, the sensorimotor stage (birth to 18 months) is where the infant uses senses and motor activity to interface with environment. The focus is coordination of the senses and the motor acts. (**Ref. 1**, p. 158)

95. (**A**) In the preoperational stage (18 months to 7 years) the child relies on perception and intuition in thought processes to comprehend the world. (**Ref. 1**, p. 158)

96. (**D**) From 7 to 11–13 years (concrete operations stage) the child starts to abstract commonalities from tangible objects. When the child can see, touch, or gain images from objects, similarities between them can be extracted. (**Ref. 1**, p. 158)

97. (**B**) The last stage of cognitive development, according to Piaget, is the formal operations stage. This stage is characterized by the capacity to indulge in abstract, conceptual thinking in which tangible objects are not necessary for the conceptualization to occur. (**Ref. 1**, p. 158)

98. (**B**) The following three answers relate to Freud's theory of psychosexual development. He suggested that the choice and nature of love and other interpersonal relationships depended on the nature and quality of relationships early in life. Awareness of the world is a developmental process that is initially focused on psychosexual stages as described by Freud. The oral stage, from birth to 12 months, is the earliest stage of infant psychosexual development. (**Ref. 1**, pp. 244–249)

99. (A) The period of pregenital psychosexual development, the anal stage, is usually from 1 to 3 years. (**Ref. 1,** p. 249)

100. (C) The period from about 2½ to 6 years is referred to as the phallic stage. (**Ref. 1,** p. 249)

101. (A) This series of questions involves descriptions of defense mechanisms. By definition, defense mechanisms act automatically, out of our awareness (unconscious) to alleviate anxiety and handle conflict. We all use defense mechanisms. Certain ones, however, especially if overused, will distort reality or produce symptoms. It is most important that the student understand defense mechanisms well. (**Ref. 1,** pp. 250–252)

102. (B) Repression, which is a form of forgetting, should be distinguished from denial and from suppression. Repression protects against drive derivatives and affects, while denial extinguishes external reality. Suppression is a conscious coping mechanism, as when a person consciously decides not to think of something. (**Ref. 1,** pp. 250–252)

103. (D) It is important to distinguish projection from displacement. Projection is more primitive and develops during the oral stage of development. It distorts reality and is seen in paranoid conditions. Unacceptable internal feelings are perceived and reacted to as though they are coming from outside. (**Ref. 1,** pp. 250–252)

104. (C) In displacement, the shift permits the original symbolism to be less emotionally charged manner. For example, a patient may feel more comfortable expressing anger at the therapist than at the boss. (**Ref. 1,** pp. 250–252)

105. (B) The Durham rule, once regarded as breakthrough in forensic psychiatry, has now been abandoned. It stated "that an accused is not criminally responsible if his unlawful act was the product of mental disease or mental defect." (**Ref. 2,** pp. 462–464)

106. (C) The M'Naghten rule is the traditional rule for determining insanity. It addresses itself to whether the defendant knew the nature and quality of his or her act and that it was wrong. In many states it is now supplemented by the American Law Institute criteria. (**Ref. 2,** pp. 462–464)

107. (A) The "Bonnie rule" holds that a person is not responsible if, because of mental disease, that person is unable to appreciate wrongfulness of his or her conduct. (**Ref. 2,** pp. 462–464)

108. (C) Anorexia nervosa presents with all the physiological findings of what is, in effect, self-induced starvation. However, self-induced starvation is not its sole characteristic. It is more common in adolescent girls than boys, and is not related to a known physical illness. (**Ref. 4,** pp. 539–544)

109. (A) Pica refers to the eating of nonnutritive substances repeatedly for at least 1 month. (**Ref. 4,** pp. 95–96)

110. (B) Bulimia nervosa refers to repeated episodes of binge eating of large quantities of food, often with termination by self-induced vomiting, which can destroy tooth enamel; repeated attempts to lose weight by restrictive diets; marked weight changes; knowledge that the eating pattern is abnormal; and a fear of being unable to stop, together with depression and self-deprecatory thoughts. (**Ref. 4,** pp. 545–550)

111. (C) The TAT contains a series of 30 pictures and one blank card that the subject uses to create a story. TAT cards have different stimulus value and can be assumed to elicit data pertaining to different areas of functioning. The TAT is most useful as a tool for judging motivational aspects of behavior. (**Ref. 1,** p. 229)

112. (B) The Sentence Completion Test responses have been shown to be useful in creating a level of confidence in regard to predictions of overt behavior and may be used to tap specific conflict areas of interest to the psychologist. (**Ref. 1,** p. 229)

113. (A) The Draw-a-Person test was initially used to measure intelligence in children. It is now also used in adults. The test assumes that the person drawn represents the expression of the body of the person in the environment. Many clinicians use the drawings as a screening technique for the detection of brain damage. (**Ref. 1,** p. 229)

114. (D) The Rorschach Test is a standard set of 10 ink blots that serve as the stimuli for associations, and is especially helpful as a diagnostic tool. The thinking and associational patterns of the subject are brought more clearly into focus chiefly because the ambiguity of the stimulus provides comparatively few cues for what may be conventional or standard responses. Surveys have shown this to be one of the most commonly used individual tests in clinical settings throughout the country. (**Ref. 1,** pp. 227–228)

115. (C); 116. (D); 117. (B); 118. (A)   Most antidepressants require that doses be titrated. Improvement in sleep and energy may be observed within the first week of drug treatment while improvement in mood may not respond until the fourth week. Medications should be continued through at least 4 or 5 symptom-free months. (**Ref. 3,** pp. 518–526)

119. (C); 120. (B); 121. (A)   Fluoxane (Prozac), paroxetine (Paxil), and sertraline (Zoloft) are the three serotonin-specific reuptake inhibitors (SSRIs) currently available in the United States. Fluvoxamine and citalopram are SSRIs in use in Europe. Venlafaxine (Effexor) blocks reuptake of serotonin, norepinephrine, and dopamine and has no activity at muscarinic, histaminic, or adrenergic receptors. (**Ref. 1,** pp. 976–979, 1002–1004)

122. (A)   Anxiety disorders had the highest prevalence rates: 8.9% for 6 months and 14.6% for lifetime. Six-month and lifetime prevalence rates for affective (mood) disorders were 5.8% and 8.3%, respectively, compared to 0.8% and 1.3% for schizophrenia. Males were more likely to have alcohol dependence than females. Female depression rates were twice as high as for males. Substance abuse is more common among individuals under 30 than in older adults. (**Ref. 1,** pp. 194–195)

123. (E)   Factors associated with subsequent suicide in those who attempt suicide include: age 45 years, male sex, unemployed or retired, living alone, poor physical health, medical treatment within the last six months, having a psychiatric disorder, and having made previous attempts by violent methods. Eight of ten individuals who successfully suicide have given warnings of their intent. (**Ref. 1,** p. 809)

124. (E)   It is important to pick up on the patient's feeling tone and on the fact that he or she may be hinting about suicide. Every depressed patient should be asked about suicide at the first visit. There is time for investigation and treatment for premature ejaculation, alcoholism, and marital conflict—but not if the patient is already dead. (**Ref. 9,** pp. 31–34, 398–400)

125. **(A)** Amnestic syndrome is most often caused by a combination of alcohol abuse and thiamine deficiency, known as Korsakoff's syndrome. Although patients with the syndrome may in fact be oriented and alert, they cannot express any memory of events more than a few hours old. (**Ref. 9,** p. 153)

126. **(B)** Although infection and metabolic disorders are important causes of irreversible dementia, Alzheimer's disease, the cause of which is not clearly understood, is responsible for 50 to 60% of all cases of dementia in the United States. (**Ref. 9,** pp. 146–147)

127. **(A)** One-half of suicide completers suffer from depression, compared to 30% who suffer from alcoholism and a smaller percentage who suffer from other illnesses. Nevertheless, physicians should not overlook the possibility of suicide in other disorders. (**Ref. 9,** pp. 394–395)

128. **(C)** Circumstantiality is marked by long-windedness that is goal-directed. Tangentiality is a type of speech reflecting thoughts that may be related to the question in an oblique way, but in which the goal of speech is never reached. Word salad is a pattern of speech that is incomprehensible. Derailment consists of a pattern of thought resulting in speech in which ideas slip off the track onto a completely different track. Klang associations involve associations of similar sounding or rhyming words. (**Ref. 9,** pp. 50–53)

129. **(A)** Long-term studies have reported mortality rates ranging from 0 to 20%. Even after eating disorder symptoms have subsided, depressive symptoms and bizarre eating patterns frequently persist. It is rare to see the full syndrome of either disorder after the age of 40. (**Ref. 4,** pp. 543, 548)

130. **(E)** Kübler-Ross conceptualized five stages experienced by people when they receive news of a fatal illness: shock and denial, anger, bargaining, depression, and acceptance. Individuals do not

172 / 3: Psychiatry

necessarily experience all stages, nor do reactions necessarily follow a strict sequence. (Ref. 1, pp. 76–77)

131. (D) Priapism, the symptom of prolonged erection in the absence of sexual stimuli, is a rare but serious side effect of trazodone. It has also been associated with the use of the antipsychotic drugs chlorpromazine and thioridazine. A patient experiencing priapism while taking trazodone (Desyrel) should discontinue the medicine and contact his physician immediately. (Ref. 8, p. 179)

132. (B) Tricyclic antidepressants, especially imipramine, have been found to have a beneficial antianuretic effect in children. The usual dosage is 50 to 100 mg at bedtime. (Ref. 8, pp. 185, 189)

133. (B) There is an involuntary contraction of sphincters. Heart rate actually increases to 160 beats per minute. There are involuntary and voluntary movements of large muscle groups, including carpalpedal spasm and facial grimacing. An increase in breast size occurs during the excitement phase. (Ref. 1, p. 655)

134. (D) The borderline personality is characterized by instability in identity, interpersonal relationships, and affect. Intense and unstable interpersonal relationships do not constitute social withdrawal. (Ref. 4, pp. 650–654)

135. (C) Subdural hematomas are caused by disruption of the veins that bridge the brain parenchyma and meninges, and usually follow falls. Illnesses leading to falls or weakened blood vessels are likely to predispose to subdural hematomas. Residence in suburbia is irrelevant. (Ref. 9, p. 149)

136. (E) Consciousness is almost always clouded; there are perceptual disturbances; and agitation or stupor is present in delirium. These symptoms cannot be accounted for by a preexisting or evolving dementia. Disturbances can develop over a short period of time (hours or days) and can fluctuate during the course of a day. (Ref. 4, pp. 123–124)

137. (E) Unlike the diagnostic process, which emphasizes the similarity of one patient to others with the same diagnosis, the psychosocial formulation emphasizes the uniqueness of each patient.

Psychodynamic formulation is based on psychoanalytic theory and is just one aspect of the psychosocial formulation. Psychodynamic formulations are the most common formulation encountered in clinical psychiatry. (**Ref. 2,** p. 92)

138. **(E)** In paranoid schizophrenia, none of the following can be prominent: incoherence, marked loosening of associations, flat or grossly inappropriate affect, catatonic or grossly disorganized behavior. The essential feature is the presence of prominent delusions or auditory hallucinations in the context of relatively intact cognitive functioning and affect. (**Ref. 4,** p. 287)

139. **(B)** The use of any benzodiazepine can result in physical dependence. The risk of dependence is increased by long-term use and the use of high-potency agents. Physiological dependence after chronic alcohol use is well known. Buspirone, an antianxiety agent of the azospirodecanedione class, does not appear to produce dependence. (**Ref. 8,** pp. 71–72)

140. **(D)** Comptency is a legal concept and is judged by the court; it is not a medical concept. The establishment of incompetency is a process separate from commitment. (**Ref. 6,** pp. 820–821)

141. **(E)** Postconcussional disorder is most frequently associated with a closed head injury where signs of localized brain damage are slight or absent. The principal symptomatic features include headache, fatigue, insomnia, emotional lability, a marked intolerance to physical and mental exertion, hypersensitivity to stimuli, and hypochondriacal preoccupation. Objective signs of physical illness such as dilated pupils should warrant further investigation. (**Ref. 1,** pp. 326, 368–369)

142. **(D)** *La belle indifference* is characteristic of conversion disorders. It refers to the patient's inappropriately cavalier attitude towards a serious symptom. If the conversion mechanism effectively deals with anxiety and conflict, it is not surprising that the patient is unconcerned. Obsessions or compulsions cause marked distress. (**Ref. 1,** pp. 601–603, 622)

143. **(C)** A genuine external stimulus is misinterpreted as an illusion. (**Ref. 9,** p. 46)

144. **(A)** Korsakoff's syndrome is characterized by confabulation, which occurs when patients invent stories to fill in memory gaps. (**Ref. 9,** p. 298)

145. **(D)** Depersonalization is characterized by periods in which persons have a strong and unpleasant sense of their own unreality, which may be associated with a sense that their environment is also unreal. (**Ref. 9,** p. 289)

146. **(B)** Hallucinations, which may be experienced in any sensory modality, are false perceptions occurring in the absence of an identifiable external stimulus. (**Ref. 9,** p. 46)

147. **(E)** Obsession are persistent ideas, thoughts, or impulses that are unpleasant and difficult for patients to ignore. (**Ref. 9,** p. 65)

References

1. Kaplan HI, Sadock BJ, Grebb JA: *Kaplan and Sadock's Synopsis of Psychiatry: Behavioral Sciences, Clinical Psychiatry,* 7th ed. Baltimore, Williams and Wilkins, 1994.

2. Goldman HH: *Review of General Psychiatry,* 3rd ed. Norwalk, CT, Appleton and Lange, 1992.

3. Stoudemire A: *Clinical Psychiatry for Medical Students,* 2nd ed. Philadelphia, J. B. Lippincott Company, 1994.

4. American Psychiatric Association: *Diagnostic and Statistical Manual of Mental Disorders,* 4th ed. Washington, D.C., American Psychiatric Association, 1994.

5. Moore BE, Fine, BD: *Psychoanalytic Terms and Concepts.* New Haven, CT, The American Psychoanalytic Association and Yale University Press, 1990.

6. Nicholi, AM: *The New Harvard Guide to Psychiatry.* Cambridge, MA, The Belknap Press of Harvard University Press, 1988.

7. Campbell RJ: *Psychiatric Dictionary,* 5th ed. New York, Oxford University Press, 1981.

8. Kaplan HI, Sadock, BJ: *Pocket Handbook of Psychiatric Drug Treatment.* Baltimore, Williams and Wilkins, 1993.

9. Andreasen, NC, Black, DW: *Introductory Textbook of Psychiatry.* Washington, D.C., American Psychiatric Press, 1991.

4

Surgery

Michael Metzler, MD

DIRECTIONS: Each of the questions or incomplete statements below is followed by a list of suggested answers or completions. Select the **one** that is best in each case.

Questions 1–3: Refer to Figure 4-1.

1. The test shown in Figure 4-1 is of importance in the diagnosis of
    A. Addison's disease
    B. hypoparathyroidism
    C. hyperthyroidism
    D. carcinoid syndrome
    E. hyperparathyroidism

2. The examiner is attempting to elicit which of the following signs?
    A. Chvostek's
    B. Bell's
    C. Trousseau's
    D. Trendelenberg's
    E. None of the above

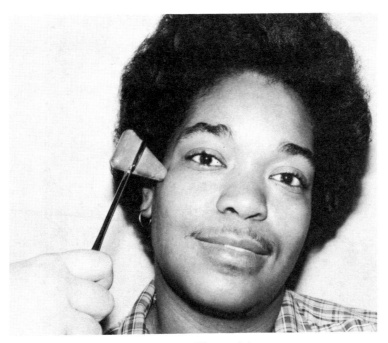

Figure 4-1

3. This patient's condition resulted from a surgical complication. Which of the following operations was the patient **MOST LIKELY** to have undergone?
   A. Nephrectomy
   B. Esophageal dilation
   C. Thyroidectomy
   D. Carotid endarterectomy
   E. Vocal cord tumor biopsy

4. The point depicted by the X in Figure 4-2 represents
   A. Sudeck's critical point
   B. McBurney's point
   C. McEwen's point
   D. Boas' point
   E. none of the above

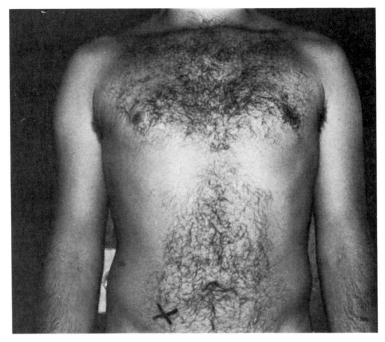

Figure 4-2

5. Which of the following is **NOT TRUE** of appendicitis?
   A. It is the most common acute abdominal surgical condition
   B. It is the most frequent in the fifth and sixth decades
   C. The amount of lymphoid tissue in the appendix is roughly related to the likelihood of developing the condition
   D. The incidence has been declining
   E. Obstruction of the appendiceal lumen is the fundamental inciting mechanism

6. The following are all indications for urgent laparotomy **EXCEPT**
   A. visceral perforation suspected as the cause of pneumoperitoneum
   B. continuing, significant solid organ hemorrhage
   C. ruptured corpus luteum cyst diagnosed by laparoscopy
   D. peritonitis from unknown source
   E. paracentesis yielding bile

7. This 52-year-old African-American male underwent extensive surgical procedures for relief of intestinal obstruction (Figure 4-3). Raised dense lesions developed around the patient's sites of surgical incision. These lesions

A. represent development of squamous cell carcinoma
B. represent development of basal cell carcinoma
C. are areas of chronic fungal inflammation
D. are keloids
E. none of the above

Figure 4-3

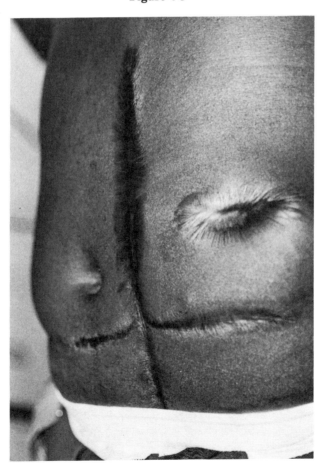

8. A 78-year-old man has had longstanding epidermoid carcinoma of the penis, shown in Figure 4-4. He sought medical attention only after pronounced hematuria developed. Which of the following is **NOT TRUE** of the patient's condition?
   A. Penile cancer develops in squamous epithelium of the foreskin or glans penis
   B. Carcinoma of the glans is a rapidly growing malignancy whose incidence is unrelated to circumcision or hygiene
   C. The chance of this condition developing would be markedly decreased by circumcision as a child
   D. Elderly subjects are more likely to develop this disorder
   E. The lesion is slow-growing

Questions 9–12: After an operation for a perforated bowel, a 63-year-old man developed hypotension and oliguria. Despite appropriate treatment for gram-negative sepsis and support of blood pressure, urine volume remained low. An EKG and blood chemistries were ordered.

Figure 4-4

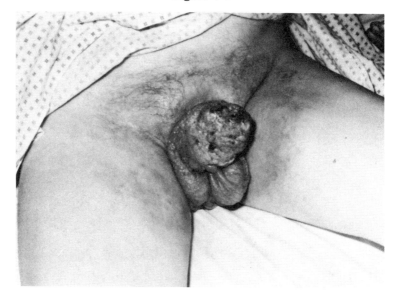

9. The patient's EKG (Figure 4-5) is **MOST CONSISTENT** with
   A. anterior myocardial infarction
   B. inferior myocardial infarction
   C. hypocalcemia
   D. hyperkalemia
   E. atrial flutter

10. In such patients, all the following EKG changes may be noted **EXCEPT**
    A. shortened P-R interval
    B. depression of the ST segment
    C. prolongation of the Q-R-S interval
    D. loss of P waves
    E. ventricular fibrillation

11. Which of the following would **NOT** be appropriate therapy in this patient?
    A. Sodium bicarbonate
    B. Sodium polystyrene sulfonate cation exchange resin
    C. Glucose
    D. Spironolactone
    E. Insulin

12. Should the patient's oliguria become anuria despite diuretic therapy, and cardiac irritability and congestive failure develop, all the following may be useful **EXCEPT**
    A. peritoneal dialysis
    B. hemodialysis
    C. calcium
    D. hydrochlorothiazide
    E. continuous arteriovenous hemodialysis (CAVHD)

Questions 13–15: The x-ray shown in Figure 4-6 is that of a 58-year-old man with a long history of cigarette smoking.

13. Which of the following is **MOST LIKELY** in the patient?
    A. Bronchiectasis
    B. Pancoast tumor
    C. Tuberculosis
    D. Sarcoidosis
    E. Bronchial adenoma

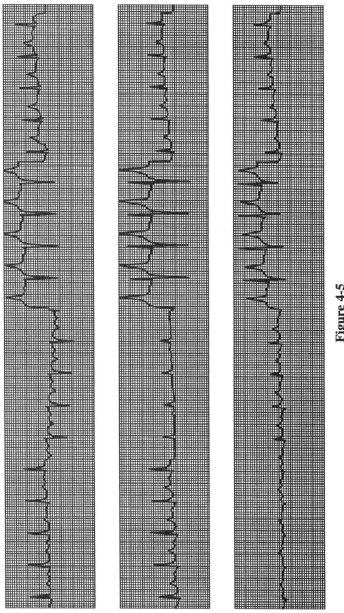

Figure 4-5

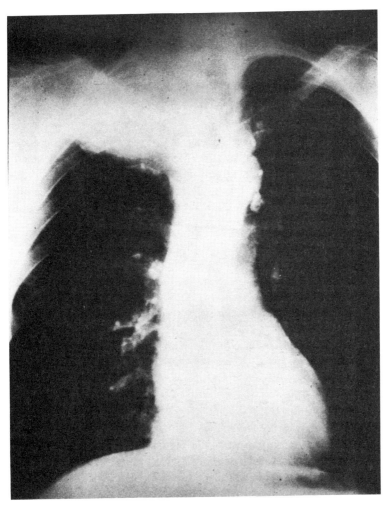

Figure 4-6

14. To which of the following structures is the patient's tumor **LEAST LIKELY** to result in early metastasis?
    A. The brachial plexus
    B. Pleura
    C. Pancreas
    D. Bone
    E. Chest wall

15. Should this patient's cervical sympathetic plexus become involved by tumor spread, all the following may result **EXCEPT**
    A. ptosis
    B. Horner's syndrome
    C. mydriasis
    D. anhidrosis
    E. enophthalmos

Questions 16–17: A 64-year-old man developed septicemia and congestive heart failure after surgery. Medications prescribed included ethacrynic acid and an aminoglycoside antibiotic.

16. For which of the following is the subject at **GREATEST** risk?
    A. Hemolytic anemia
    B. Neuropathy
    C. Ototoxicity
    D. Ocular toxicity
    E. Hepatitis

17. The preceding toxic reaction is **MORE LIKELY** to occur in patients with
    A. hepatic insufficiency
    B. renal insufficiency
    C. malabsorption
    D. anemia
    E. dementia

18. The gangrenous foot shown in Figure 4-7 occurred in a patient with endocarditis who developed widespread emboli to numerous organs. Which of the following would be **LEAST EXPECTED** to have occurred in this patient?
    A. Pain
    B. Paresthesia
    C. Pink extremity
    D. Paralysis
    E. Loss of pulse

19. In about what percent of subjects with arterial emboli is origin of the embolus from the heart?
    A. Less than 5%
    B. 10%

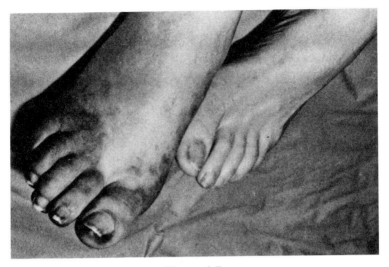

Figure 4-7

C. 24%
D. 50–70%
E. 80–90%

Questions 20–21: The x-ray of the tibia (Figure 4-8) was obtained in a 58-year-old man with an 80-pack-per-year history of cigarette smoking. Several years previously, his hemoglobin was noted to be elevated.

20. The **MOST LIKELY** diagnosis is
    A. metastatic bronchogenic carcinoma
    B. multiple myeloma
    C. polycythemia rubra vera
    D. metastatic prostatic carcinoma
    E. pulmonary hypertrophic osteoarthropathy

21. Which of the following would be **MOST HELPFUL** to alleviate the patient's bone pain?
    A. Corticosteriods
    B. Radiotherapy
    C. Sedatives
    D. Calcitonin
    E. Surgery

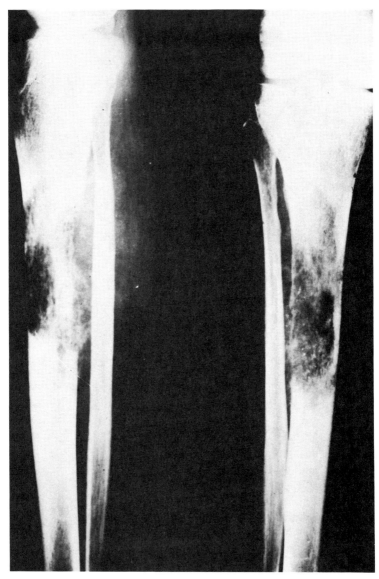

Figure 4-8

22. Which of the following paraneoplastic syndromes is **LEAST LIKELY** to be associated with bronchogenic carcinoma?
A. Myasthenic syndrome
B. Hypocalcemia
C. Inappropriate antidiuretic hormone (ADH) syndrome
D. Dermatomyositis
E. Peripheral neuropathy

23. In the patient depicted in Figure 4-9, if only the posterior half of his left upper extremity were burned, about what percent of his total body surface would be involved?
A. 1.125%
B. 2.25%
C. 4.5%
D. 9.0%
E. 18.0%

Questions 24–27: Match the following choices with the numbered statements. Each answer may be used once, more than once, or not at all.

A. Fine needle aspiration cytology
B. Ultrasound examination
C. Excisional biopsy without needle localization
D. CT scan
E. Needle-directed excisional biopsy

24. Test you would recommend for diagnosis of a palpable 2-cm mass in a 42-year-old woman who had a negative mammogram and physical exam two months ago

25. Test you would recommend for diagnosis of a 0.5-cm breast lesion that has an irregular margin, microcalcifications, and spiculations by mammography. The mass is not palpable on physical exam

26. Test you would recommend if results of fine needle cytology of a palpable breast mass were read as "suspicious for malignancy"

27. Test you would recommend to confirm cystic nature of nonpalpable breast lesion with smooth borders seen on routine screening mammography

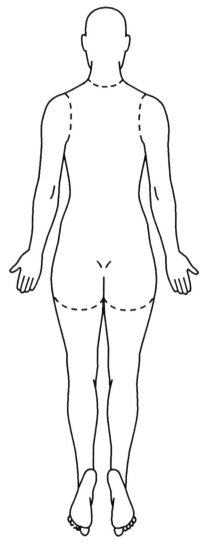

Figure 4-9

Questions 28–32: Match the following choices with the numbered statements. An answer may be used once, more than once, or not at all.

    A. Computed tomographic (CT) scan
    B. Diagnostic peritoneal lavage (DPL)
    C. Plain x-rays of the abdomen
    D. Arteriography
    E. None of the above

28. Useful in abdominal evaluation of hemodynamically unstable trauma victim who has a closed head injury and is unresponsive to painful stimuli

29. Allows rational nonoperative management of intraabdominal solid organ injury

30. Considered the definitive study for evaluation of possible traumatic aortic disruption

31. Always reliable for diagnosis of ruptured diaphragm

32. Use may result in operation for intraabdominal injury not requiring operative repair

Questions 33–34: The hand shown in Figure 4-10 is that of a 48-year-old man with chronic arthritis.

33. Which of the following is **MOST LIKELY** to have occurred in this patient?
    A. Development of boutonnière deformity
    B. Development of a swan-neck deformity
    C. Extensor tendon erosion
    D. Metacarpal fracture
    E. None of the above

34. Definitive treatment of this condition involves
    A. splinting only
    B. nonsteroidal antiinflammatory agents (NSAIDs)
    C. a cast
    D. surgical repair of ruptured tendon
    E. cytotoxic therapy

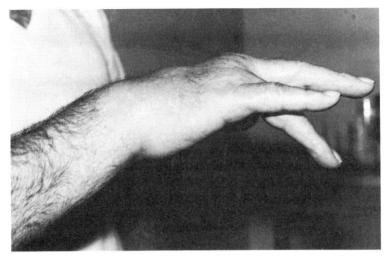

Figure 4-10

Questions 35–37: After undergoing a thoracotomy, a 65-year-old woman with no prior history of palpitations or heart disease developed the rhythm shown in Figure 4-11. The electrocardiogram was recorded at a paper speed of 25 mm/sec.

35. The patient's ventricular rate is
    A. 75
    B. 100
    C. 125
    D. 150
    E. 250

36. The patient's atrial rate is
    A. 75
    B. 150
    C. 300
    D. 600
    E. indeterminate

37. Treatment of this arrhythmia might include all the following **EXCEPT**
    A. beta-blockade therapy
    B. vagal maneuvers

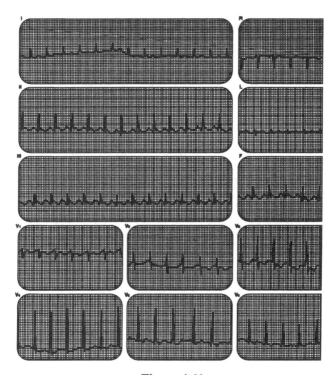

Figure 4-11

C. correction of electrolyte abnormalities
D. digoxin
E. B-agonist therapy

Questions 38–40: The sexually active man depicted in Figure 4-12 developed painful left inguinal adenopathy. The overlying skin became violaceous and adherent. The matted nodes were fluctuant in some areas and indurated in others.

38. The **MOST LIKELY** diagnosis is
    A. condyloma acuminatum
    B. condyloma latum
    C. lymphogranuloma venereum
    D. primary syphilis
    E. secondary syphilis

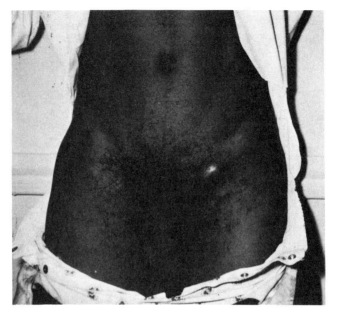

Figure 4-12

39. The causative organism in this patient's condition is
A. *Neisseria gonorrhoeae*
B. *Chlamydia trachomatis*
C. *Chlamydia psittaci*
D. herpes genitalis
E. herpes febrilis

40. Which of the following antibiotics are frequently used in treatment?
A. Gentamicin
B. Doxycycline
C. Penicillin G
D. Amphotericin
E. Nystatin

Questions 41–42: Refer to Figure 4-13.

41. Which of the following is present in Figure 4-13?
A. Fracture of the first metatarsophalangeal joint
B. Osteomyelitis

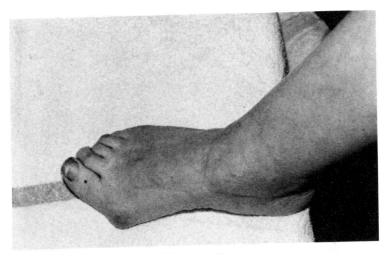

Figure 4-13

   C. Hallux valgus
   D. Hallus varus
   E. None of the above

42. This patient also has evidence of which of the following?
   A. Vasculitis
   B. Bunion formation
   C. Onycholysis
   D. Ankle sprain
   E. None of the above

Questions 43–44: The x-ray shown in Figure 4-14 is that of a 72-year-old demented man brought in complaining of left chest pain. He is a poor historian, but complains of tenderness to palpation over the left lateral chest.

43. Which of the following is **MOST LIKELY** in this patient?
   A. Cardiac tamponade
   B. Fractured ribs
   C. Aortic dissection
   D. Pulmonary sequestration
   E. Pleural effusion

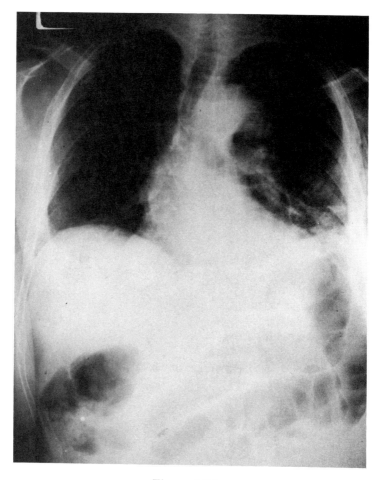

Figure 4-14

44. Complications, which may occur in patients with this condition, would **LEAST LIKELY** include
   A. tension pneumothorax
   B. intrathoracic bleeding
   C. atelectasis
   D. pulmonary embolism
   E. flail chest

Questions 45–47: Refer to Figures 4-15a and 4-15b. The following list contains responses which may be used once, more than once, or not at all.

A. Sliding hiatal hernia
B. Paraesophageal hiatal hernia
C. Morgagni (parasternal) hernia
D. Bochdalek (pleuroperitoneal) hernia
E. Spigelian (lateral ventral) hernia

45. Figure 4-15a shows a diagram of which type of diaphragmatic hernia?

46. Figure 4-15b shows a diagram of which type of diaphragmatic hernia?

47. Surgical repair is indicated if medical management does not relieve symptoms

48. Congenital lung cysts tend to do all the following **EXCEPT**
    A. become infected
    B. resemble a pneumothorax or emphysema on chest x-ray
    C. compress normal lung tissue
    D. undergo malignant change
    E. fill with fluid

49. The finding that is associated with the need for operative correction of tetralogy of Fallot is
    A. squatting
    B. cyanotic spells
    C. dyspnea on exertion
    D. polycythemia
    E. leukocytosis

50. Hemoptysis is associated with all the following **EXCEPT**
    A. mitral stenosis
    B. bronchiectasis
    C. pneumonia
    D. empyema
    E. bronchogenic carcinoma

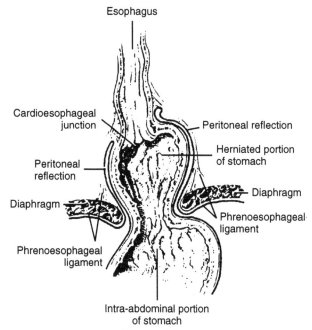

Figure 4-15a

Figure 4-15b

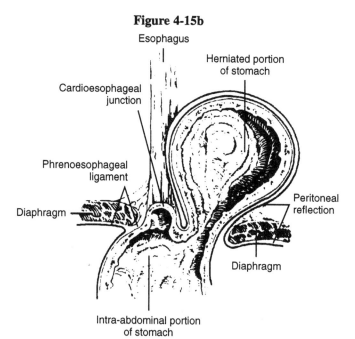

Questions 51–53: A 64-year-old postal worker has an asymptomatic, palpable, pulsatile mass noted in his abdomen during a retirement physical examination. An abdominal aortic aneurysm (AAA) is suspected.

51. The test you would order to confirm your diagnosis is
    A. abdominal aortogram
    B. ultrasound
    C. computed tomographic (CT) scan
    D. Doppler pressure indices
    E. magnetic resonance imaging (MRI)

52. Complications of abdominal aortic aneurysms include all the following **EXCEPT**
    A. dyspepsia
    B. rupture
    C. fistula formation
    D. thrombosis
    E. embolization

53. Of patients who present with aneurysmal disease, what percent die of causes unrelated to vascular disease?
    A. <5%
    B. 20%
    C. 30%
    D. 50%
    E. 65%

Questions 54–58: Match the following choices of abdominal pain patterns with the numbered statements. An answer may be used once, more than once, or not at all.

    A. Pain pattern suggestive of early acute appendicitis
    B. Pain pattern suggestive of urolithiasis
    C. Pain pattern suggestive of perforated viscus
    D. Pain pattern suggestive of cholecystitis
    E. Pain pattern suggestive of pancreatitis

54. Acute onset of severe flank pain radiating to the groin, crescendo in nature; patient cannot seem to be still during examination; pain not increased by anterior abdominal palpation

55. Acute onset sharp pain in left lower quadrant spreading to entire infraumbilical area over 1–2 hours; abdomen rigid to examination, bowel sounds absent, rebound tenderness over left lower quadrant

56. Several hours of vague, poorly localized epigastric pain and anorexia, which recently gave way to well localized right lower quadrant pain and tenderness to palpation

57. Epigastric pain radiating through to the midback; pain made better with seated position, leaning slightly forward

58. Pain that awakens patient at night; steady pain or pressure sensation boring through to back in right upper quadrant; it lasts several hours and gradually disappears; it is frequently accompanied by nausea

59. Hyperacute organ rejection following transplantation is characterized by all the following **EXCEPT**
    A. presence of preformed antibodies to donor cells
    B. graft destruction by 24–48 hours
    C. tolerance to a second transplant from the same donor
    D. no effective method for treatment
    E. may be eliminated by pretransplant crossmatch testing

60. A patient presents with acute pancreatitis. From the list of causes that follow, which is the **MOST COMMON**?
    A. Cholelithiasis
    B. Spider bites
    C. Estrogen therapy
    D. Diuretic use
    E. Trauma

61. All the following criteria are predictive for the severity of an episode of pancreatitis **EXCEPT**
    A. age
    B. amylase level
    C. blood glucose
    D. white blood cell count
    E. PaO_2

Questions 62–64: A 45-year-old male has a right inguinal mass that extends into his scrotum on standing and disappears when supine. This has been present for years, but he is now concerned because it is getting worse.

62. He **MOST LIKELY** has
    A. lymphogranuloma venereum (LGV)
    B. an incarcerated inguinal hernia
    C. a femoral artery aneurysm
    D. an indirect inguinal hernia
    E. inguinal adenopathy

63. Arrangements are made to treat the patient on an elective basis, but he returns the next day with a painful right groin mass that no longer disappears on assuming the supine position. It has been this way for the last 8 hours. Direct manual pressure does not help. He **MOST LIKELY** has
    A. lymphogranuloma venereum
    B. an incarcerated inguinal hernia
    C. a femoral artery aneurysm
    D. an indirect inguinal hernia
    E. inguinal adenopathy

64. The **MOST APPROPRIATE** treatment would be
    A. admission and observation
    B. elective repair
    C. emergent repair if reduction is not possible
    D. a truss
    E. needle aspiration biopsy

Questions 65–70: Match the following choices of skin problems with the numbered statements relating to them. An answer may be used once, more than once, or not at all.

    A. Ischemic extremity ulcer
    B. Venous stasis extremity ulcer
    C. Decubitus ulcer
    D. Puncture wound
    E. Cellulitis

65. May develop as a consequence of deep vein thrombosis (DVT)

66. Treated by compressive dressing

67. Associated with "rest pain"

68. Usually induced by immobilization and prolonged pressure in areas of decreased sensation

69. Requires tetanus immunization to be up-to-date

70. Cured by antibiotic therapy

71. A 23-year-old motorcycle accident victim is brought to the ER. He is combative, complaining of chest pain, refuses to lie flat, and is yelling obscenities (in short breaths). His BP is 80/50; pulse is 140/min. He is ashen in color. His trachea is deviated to the right; there are no breath sounds over the left chest. He has an obvious femur fracture that the EMT says has no distal pulse. His greatest **IMMEDIATE** need is
   A. endotracheal intubation
   B. 2 IV lines
   C. needle decompression left chest
   D. needle decompression right chest
   E. immediate transfer

Questions 72–73: A 46-year-old accident victim is brought to the ER following ejection from the auto as the result of a head-on auto accident. His initial BP was 90/palpation; pulse was 120. He postures symmetrically to painful stimuli and has alcohol on his breath. You intubate his trachea, place him on a ventilator, and insert bilateral chest tubes because of bilateral pneumothoraces seen on chest x-ray (CXR). Follow-up CXR shows multiple bilateral rib fractures, and both lungs reinflated with chest tubes in good position. His pelvis x-ray shows no fractures. His extremities show no obvious fracture to clinical exam. He has had 4 L of crystalloid and BP is now 80/p with 140 pulse. His neck veins have become distended, as are those of his upper extremities. His heart tones are not well heard. A diagnostic peritoneal lavage is negative for bleeding.

72. The **MOST IMMEDIATE** life-threatening problem is
   A. tension pneumothorax
   B. impending cerebral herniation

    C. hypovolemic shock
    D. pericardial tamponade
    E. ethanol intoxication

73. IMMEDIATE therapy requires
    A. needle thoracentesis
    B. CT scan
    C. uncrossmatched blood
    D. pericardiocentesis
    E. thiamine injection

74. A 38-year-old female was an unrestrained back seat occupant in an accident in which she sailed into the windshield. She is awake and alert, has facial lacerations, but no obvious fractures. She complains of severe left shoulder pain on inspiration. Her abdomen has some left upper quadrant tenderness to palpation, and bowel sounds are absent. The nasogastric tube you placed appears to be in the stomach, but above the left diaphragm on CXR. There is also fluid in the left chest. Your **MOST PRESSING** concern is to
    A. place a left chest tube to drain the fluid
    B. obtain surgical consultation for immediate abdominal exploration
    C. obtain a CT scan of the chest and abdomen
    D. admit for observation and serial examinations
    E. transfer to the care of a plastic surgeon for repair of facial lacerations

Questions 75–80: Match the following choices with the numbered statements. An answer may be used once, more than once, or not at all.

    A. Prothrombin time (PT)
    B. Partial thromboplastin time (PTT)
    C. Platelet count
    D. Bleeding time
    E. Euglobulin clot lysis

75. Test used to determine the competency of platelets when an adequate platelet number is present

76. Indicates increased fibrinolytic activity

77. Low in patients with disseminated intravascular coagulation (DIC)

78. Used to follow patient on continuous infusion heparin therapy for thrombosis

79. Used to follow patient taking coumarin

80. Likely abnormal in patients taking high-dose aspirin therapy

Questions 81–85: Match the following choices with the numbered statements. An answer may be used once, more than once, or not at all.

    A. Fresh frozen plasma (FFP)
    B. Cryoprecipitate (Cryo)
    C. Factor VIII concentrate
    D. Prothrombin complex
    E. Desmopressin (DDAVP)

81. Used to prepare patients with hemophilia A for surgery and during the postoperative period

82. Used to treat patients with factor IX deficiency

83. Increases release of von Willebrand factor VIII from vascular endothelium in patients with von Willebrand's disease

84. Used to replace clotting factors impaired by coumarin therapy

85. Used to replace fibrinogen

Questions 86–90: A 56-year-old woman is admitted after two weeks of frequent vomiting. She is dehydrated. Work-up shows complete gastric outlet obstruction due to longstanding peptic ulcer disease. Her serum chloride is 90 mEq/dL (low), sodium 134 mEq/dL (low), bicarbonate 35 mEq/dL (high), and her urine pH is low (acidic).

    86. The explanation for the alkalotic serum and acidic urine is
        A. renal bicarbonate loss
        B. use of aluminum-based antacids

C. vomiting of hydrogen and chloride ions with paradoxic aciduria

D. diarrhea

E. use of diuretics

87. The fluid you would use to restore intravascular volume would be
   A. normal saline
   B. ½ normal saline
   C. albumin
   D. Ringer's lactate
   E. blood

88. She eventually undergoes operation during which the distal two-thirds of her stomach is removed (without truncal vagotomy) and reconstructed via a gastrojejunostomy. Long-term nutritional risks include
   A. morbid obesity
   B. pernicious anemia
   C. hypercalcemia
   D. hyperchloremia
   E. postvagotomy diarrhea

89. The patient returns two years later without interim follow-up complaining of fatigue, malaise, and weakness. She is eating without difficulty. Upper gastrointestinal endoscopy shows unremarkable postoperative changes. Her blood smear shows a megaloblastic anemia with hypersegmented neutrophils. Treatment should include
   A. calcium supplement
   B. H-2 blockers
   C. parenteral vitamin B12
   D. oral vitamin B12
   E. iron only

90. The disorder affecting this patient may also be seen in patients with
   A. sigmoid colectomy
   B. severe Crohn's disease
   C. appendectomy
   D. splenectomy
   E. segmental jejunal resection

91. All the following factors increase the likelihood of infection after operation **EXCEPT**
   A. age over 70 years
   B. advanced cancer
   C. remote synchronous infection
   D. obesity
   E. clipping hair in the operative field just prior to operation

92. Regarding the use of perioperative prophylactic antibiotics, all the following statements are true **EXCEPT**
   A. they should be administered within one hour before skin incision
   B. they should be appropriate spectrum for organisms frequently implicated in wound infections following the procedure being performed
   C. they should be continued at least 5 days postoperatively
   D. their usefulness is diminished if started postoperatively
   E. they may be unnecessary (in retrospect) on some trauma cases

93. All the following cases would be classified as clean or class I **EXCEPT**
   A. tonsillectomy
   B. mastectomy
   C. thyroidectomy
   D. breast biopsy
   E. cataract removal

94. All the following cases would be classified as clean-contaminated or class II **EXCEPT**
   A. pneumonectomy
   B. routine cholecystectomy
   C. hysterectomy
   D. abscess drainage
   E. incidental appendectomy

95. Select the **TRUE** statement regarding antibiotic therapy from the list that follows.
   A. Prophylactic antibiotics are frequently used in major burn patients
   B. Prophylactic antibiotics have decreased wound infections in cases of elective colon surgery

C. Antibiotics are useful in preventing infectious complications of pancreatitis

D. A first-generation cephalosporin is useful for *Pseudomonas* infections

E. Penicillin is not indicated in most β-strep infections

96. A 2-week-old male infant is admitted for evaluation of vomiting. All the following would support a diagnosis of hypertrophic pyloric obstruction **EXCEPT**

A. first-born child

B. bilious vomitus

C. palpation of an olive-shaped mass in the right upper abdomen

D. ultrasound confirmation of "olive"

E. prior history of occasional emesis

97. Intestinal obstruction of the newborn is caused by all the following **EXCEPT**

A. hernias

B. volvulus

C. intussusception

D. adhesions secondary to prior operations

E. vascular accidents

98. Hirschprung's disease is caused by

A. absence of ganglia in the colon

B. meconium plug

C. malrotation

D. intussusception

E. vascular abnormality

99. The diagnosis of Hirschprung's disease is confirmed by

A. barium enema

B. chromosome analysis

C. suction rectal biopsy

D. blood test

E. endoscopy

100. The first stage of treatment of Hirschprung's disease is
   A. laxatives
   B. high fiber diet
   C. colostomy
   D. enemas
   E. total parenteral nutrition (TPN)

Questions 101–103: A 19-month-old is admitted with a 6-hour history of abdominal pain. It apparently started abruptly while she was playing. She had a slightly bloody bowel movement one hour before admission. Figure 4-16 demonstrates the pathologic process.

101. The diagnosis is
   A. internal hernia
   B. malrotation
   C. intussusception
   D. appendicitis
   E. intestinal duplication

102. Nonsurgical therapy frequently effective in treating this problem is
   A. barium enema
   B. observation and hydration
   C. cathartics
   D. ultrasound
   E. colonoscopy

103. Intussusception in adult patients differs from that in children in that it
   A. more frequently involves a mural bowel lesion
   B. is not accompanied by bloody stool
   C. may also occur in the esophagus
   D. frequently occurs with gallstone ileus
   E. is more frequent in adults

104. In adults, the **MOST COMMON** cause of colonic obstruction is
   A. diverticulitis
   B. cancer
   C. volvulus
   D. Crohn's disease
   E. foreign body

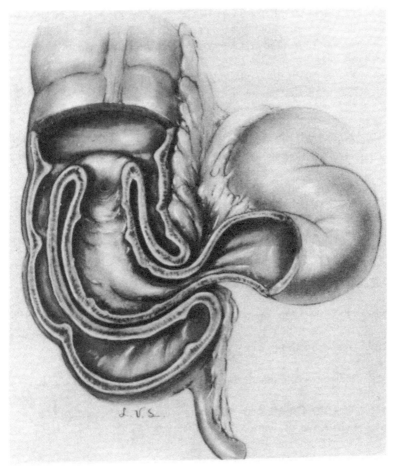

Figure 4-16

105. The **MOST COMMON** location of colon cancer is
   A. cecum
   B. transverse colon
   C. rectosigmoid
   D. splenic flexure
   E. descending colon

106. A patient who has a Stage III rectal cancer resected with no evidence of remaining disease has the best chance of survival if s/he
   A. is followed by quarterly sigmoidoscopic exams
   B. eats a high fiber diet postoperatively
   C. is followed by quarterly colonoscopic exams
   D. has radiation therapy
   E. checks stool occult blood quarterly

Questions 107–110: Match the following choices with the numbered statements. An answer may be used once, more than once, or not at all.

   A. Right colon cancer
   B. Left colon cancer
   C. Rectal cancer
   D. Epidermoid anal cancer
   E. Cancer of the appendix

107. Treated primarily by radiation and chemotherapy

108. Often found incidentally during another procedure

109. May grow to large size and not obstruct bowel lumen

110. May cause colonic perforation remote from the site of tumor

111. The **BEST** method for determining the depth of insertion of a central venous pressure (CVP) catheter is
   A. 15 cm from the tip
   B. 17 cm from the tip
   C. 20 cm from the tip
   D. 15 cm from right subclavian insertion point; 17 cm from left subclavian insertion point
   E. distance from insertion point to 2nd intercostal space

112. The **BEST** surface landmark for approximating the distal superior vena cava above the pericardial reflection is
   A. the sternomanubrial joint (angle of Louis)
   B. 4th intercostal space
   C. 5th intercostal space
   D. sternal notch
   E. sternoclavicular joint

113. The test that **BEST** tells whether or not a catheter tip is in an intravascular position is
    A. chest x-ray
    B. ultrasound
    C. aspiration of blood
    D. ability to flush easily
    E. ability to easily pass a guide wire

114. **TRUE** statements concerning peripherally inserted central (PIC) catheters include all the following **EXCEPT** they
    A. are useful for long-term infusion
    B. have a lower serious complication rate
    C. are good for high-volume fluid resuscitation
    D. are usually placed via antecubital vein
    E. should be considered in long-term vascular access planning

115. Tips of central venous catheters not parallel to the axis of the vessel containing them risk
    A. perforation
    B. arrhythmia
    C. no increased risk
    D. intravascular migration
    E. patient discomfort

Questions 116–120: Match the following choices with the numbered statements. An answer may be used once, more than once, or not at all.

    A. Figure 4-17a
    B. Figure 4-17b
    C. Both
    D. Neither

116. Which figure represents a patient who **LIKELY** had healthy bone that sustained severe axial trauma?

117. Which figure represents a patient who **LIKELY** had osteoporosis and minor trauma?

118. With which injury is neurologic deficit **MORE LIKELY** to be associated?

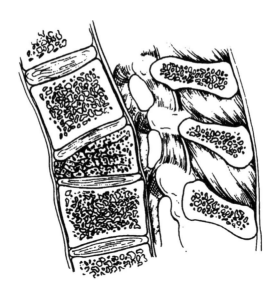

Figure 4-17a

Figure 4-17b

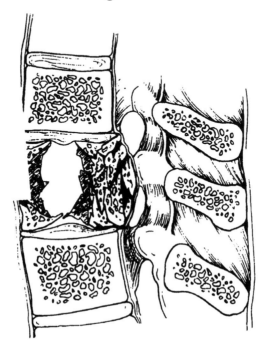

119. Which injury is **MORE LIKELY** to be treated by rest and corset brace?

120. Which figure represents the **MOST COMMON** type of spinal fracture?

Questions 121–125: Match the appropriate postgastrectomy syndrome with its description.

    A. Dumping syndrome
    B. Gastric atony, delayed emptying of solids
    C. Afferent loop obstruction
    D. Blind loop syndrome
    E. Alkaline gastric reflux

121. Crushing upper abdominal pain occurring within 45 minutes of eating; the pain abates suddenly accompanied by vomiting of dark fluid without food

122. Weakness, anemia, and malabsorption of vitamin B12 and folate associated with bacterial overgrowth

123. Anxiety, diaphoresis, tachycardia, palpitations, weakness, and fatigue occurring either within 15 minutes or about 3 hours after eating

124. May be the most frequent complication of gastric resection

125. Weakness, weight loss, persistent nausea, upper abdominal pain radiating to the back; diagnosis suggested by endoscopic appearance of the stomach and confirmed by gastric biopsies

Questions 126–129: A 6-year-old falls from a swing striking his head. He is briefly unconscious, then awakens, and is crying. His pupils are equal. He is taken to the ER. While there he complains of headache, becomes lethargic, then comatose. He vomits and is noted to have unequal pupils (right pupil dilated and nonreactive to light). A CT scan shows a skull fracture of the temporal bone along the course of the middle meningeal artery.

126. Which figure shows the **MOST LIKELY** lesion?
   A. Figure 4-18a
   B. Figure 4-18b
   C. Both
   D. Neither

127. The dilation of the pupil is caused by
   A. injury to the eye
   B. elevated intracranial pressure effect on a cranial nerve
   C. direct nerve injury in the accident
   D. hyperventilation treatment
   E. a congenital lesion

128. **IMMEDIATE** treatment for an epidural hematoma includes all the following **EXCEPT**
   A. intubation and hyperventilation
   B. mannitol
   C. neurosurgical consultation
   D. admission for observation only
   E. operation

129. Intracranial pressure may be decreased by all the following **EXCEPT**
   A. increasing $PaCO_2$
   B. removing brain tissue
   C. removing cerebrospinal fluid (CSF)
   D. decreasing cerebral blood flow
   E. decreasing $PaCO_2$

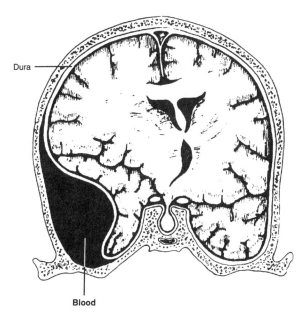

Figure 4-18a

Figure 4-18b

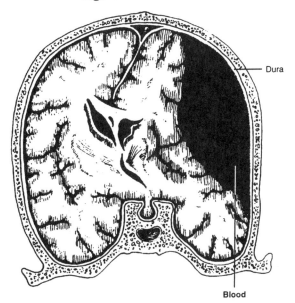

Questions 130–133: A 47-year-old male has developed a mass in his left groin over the last several months. It has become painful on standing. Physical examination indicates an inguinal hernia that appears not to be within the spermatic cord. It is above the inguinal ligament.

130. At operation, the hernia described would **LIKELY** appear like
    A. Figure 4-19a
    B. Figure 4-19b
    C. both
    D. neither

131. If the bulge had extended beneath the inguinal ligament, it would **LIKELY** be a
    A. spigelian hernia
    B. femoral hernia
    C. epigastric hernia
    D. sliding hernia
    E. Richter's hernia

132. The common denominator of all hernias is a
    A. fascial defect
    B. history of lifting
    C. history of operation
    D. history of infection
    E. family history

133. The area in Figures 4-19a and 4-19b labeled "?" is the
    A. spermatic cord
    B. internal ring
    C. hernia sac
    D. external ring
    E. conjoint tendon

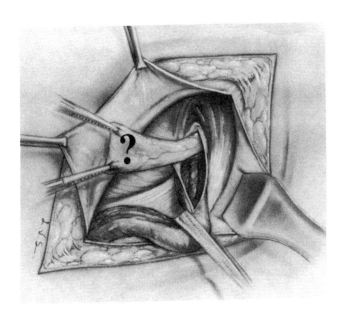

Figure 4-19a

Figure 4-19b

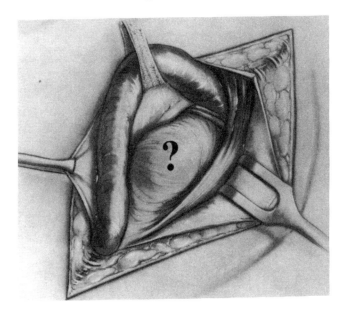

Questions 134–136: Match the following choices with the numbered statements. An answer may be used once, more than once, or not at all.

    A. Linea alba
    B. Contains a Meckel's diverticulum
    C. Linea semilunaris
    D. Lumbar triangle
    E. Pelvic floor

134. Littre's hernia includes this structure

135. Spigelian hernia occurs through this structure

136. An epigastric hernia occurs through this structure

Questions 137–145: Figure 4-20 is a diagram of a gastric parietal cell. The left side of the figure represents the cell in the resting state; the right in the stimulate or secreting phase. **G** is the gastrin receptor, **Ach** is the acetylcholine receptor, **H** is the histamine receptor. Match the following choices with the numbered statements. An answer may be used once, more than once, or not at all.

    A. Gastrin receptor
    B. Acetylcholine receptor
    C. (H-2) histamine receptor
    D. Sodium-potassium-ATP pump
    E. Acid product (HCL), luminal surface

137. When a hungry person sees or smells food, this pathway stimulates acid secretion

138. Food in the stomach (primarily protein) activates this site primarily, but also has effects that are mediated by acetylcholine

139. Stimulation of this receptor facilitates acid production; it is inhibited by cimetidine

140. This secretory mechanism is blocked by omeprazole

141. Gastric mucus at this area of the cell protects from autodigestion

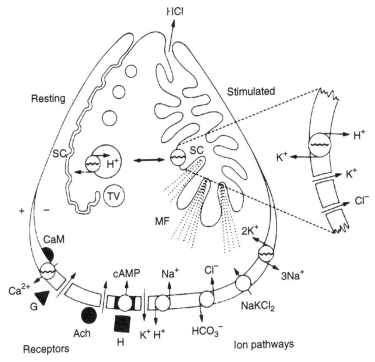

Figure 4-20

142. A partial gastrectomy with gastrojejunostomy reconstruction (Billroth II), leaving a segment of antrum (excluded antrum), may cause recurrent ulceration via this receptor

143. A truncal vagotomy decreases function at this receptor area

144. Zollinger-Ellison syndrome acts through this receptor site

145. Antacids act at this area

Questions 146–152: Match the following choices with the numbered statements. An answer may be used once, more than once, or not at all.

A. Glutamine
B. Arginine
C. ω-3 fatty acids
D. ω-6 fatty acids
E. Water-soluble vitamins

146. Nonessential amino acid (AA) whose levels decline more than any other AA during injury and continues to be depressed during recovery

147. Diets high in this cause depression of the immune system via increased prostaglandin synthesis

148. Cold water fish are a source of this

149. Vegetable oils are a good source of this

150. This amino acid enhances T-cell activation

151. This is the major energy substrate for the gut enterocyte

152. Serve as enzyme cofactors and facilitate reactions involving energy transfer

153. A 45-year-old man is admitted with his third episode of upper gastrointestinal hemorrhage. He has had two prior ulcer operations. You suspect Zollinger-Ellison syndrome. All the following would support your suspicions **EXCEPT**
   A. a fasting gastrin level of 450 pg/mL
   B. suppression of hypergastrinemia by secretin given IV
   C. past operative notes detailing ulcers in the duodenum and jejunum
   D. liver metastases on CT scan
   E. a history of diarrhea

154. The following statements concerning multiple endocrine neoplasia type-2a (Sipple's) syndrome are all true **EXCEPT**
  A. 20–40% of all patients have pheochromocytomas
  B. 17–60% have parathyroid hyperplasia
  C. some have medullary thyroid cancer
  D. 70% of pheochromocytomas are bilateral
  E. hyperparathyroidism is rarely symptomatic

Surgery

Answer Key

1. B	27. B	53. A	79. A
2. A	28. B	54. B	80. D
3. C	29. A	55. C	81. C
4. B	30. D	56. A	82. D
5. B	31. E	57. E	83. E
6. C	32. B	58. D	84. A
7. D	33. C	59. C	85. B
8. B	34. D	60. A	86. C
9. D	35. D	61. B	87. A
10. A	36. C	62. D	88. B
11. D	37. E	63. B	89. C
12. D	38. C	64. C	90. B
13. B	39. B	65. B	91. E
14. C	40. B	66. B	92. C
15. C	41. C	67. A	93. A
16. C	42. B	68. C	94. D
17. B	43. B	69. D	95. B
18. C	44. D	70. E	96. B
19. E	45. A	71. C	97. D
20. A	46. B	72. D	98. A
21. B	47. A	73. D	99. C
22. B	48. D	74. B	100. C
23. C	49. D	75. D	101. C
24. A	50. D	76. E	102. A
25. E	51. B	77. C	103. A
26. C	52. A	78. B	104. B

105. C	118. B	131. B	144. A
106. D	119. A	132. A	145. E
107. D	120. A	133. C	146. A
108. E	121. C	134. B	147. D
109. A	122. D	135. C	148. C
110. C	123. A	136. A	149. D
111. E	124. B	137. B	150. B
112. A	125. E	138. A	151. A
113. C	126. A	139. C	152. E
114. C	127. B	140. D	153. B
115. A	128. D	141. E	154. C
116. B	129. A	142. A	
117. A	130. B	143. B	

Surgery

Answers and Comments

1. **(B)** In patients with hypocalcemia, as in hypoparathyroidism, tapping the facial nerve (Chvostek's sign) elicits facial muscle twitching. This is caused by enhanced neuromuscular irritability due to low calcium levels. Trousseau's sign or carpopedal spasm is another sign of hypocalcemia. (**Ref. 25,** p. 291)

2. **(A)** See explanation and reference above.

3. **(C)** Permanent hypoparathyroidism is a rare complication of thyroidectomy occurring especially when the thyroid is removed for malignancy. Transient hypoparathyroidism may result from ischemic insult to the parathyroid glands during thyroid surgery, but recovery should be expected. (**Ref. 25,** p. 290)

4. **(B)** The early features of acute appendicitis, including the point where maximal tenderness may occur, were described by McBurney. He described this point as being "located exactly between 1½–2 in. from the anterior spinous process of the ileum on a straight line drawn from that process to the umbilicus." The incision used in this operation was also named after him. (**Ref. 21,** p. 10)

5. **(B)** The highest incidence of appendicitis follows closely the peak of lymphoid tissue in the organ. This peak occurs at adolescence. In older patients, the obstruction that causes the problem is

usually due to something other than lymphoid hyperplasia (fecalith, seeds, etc.). (**Ref. 14,** p. 191)

6. **(C)** All answers except ruptured corpus luteum cyst have a high likelihood that surgical repair is necessary. A ruptured corpus luteum cyst may mimic appendicitis, but operation is not required if this can be determined with relative certainty. (**Ref. 25,** pp. 450–451)

7. **(D)** Keloids are true tumors arising from connective tissue elements of the dermis. They grow beyond the limits of the original incision. Overactive proliferation of fibroblasts is fundamental in their pathogenesis. (**Ref. 25,** p. 1141)

8. **(B)** Carcinoma of the glans is almost completely eliminated by circumcision in infancy; it is markedly decreased by circumcision later in life. It is a slow-growing neoplasm. Poor hygiene, over time, appears to have a role in development of this lesion. (**Ref. 23,** p. 1765)

9. **(D)** The tall peaked T waves strongly suggest hyperkalemia, which is a frequent concomitant of renal insufficiency. This peaking of the T waves is the earliest EKG manifestation of elevated potassium levels. (**Ref. 25,** p. 133)

10. **(A)** In hyperkalemic patients prolongation of the P-R interval may occur, as well as the other changes noted. Early therapy is mandatory to prevent ventricular fibrillation. (**Ref. 25,** p. 133)

11. **(D)** All treatments mentioned except Spironolactone lower serum potassium either by displacing it into cells or excreting it. Spironolactone is a potassium-retaining diuretic that is not useful in cases of hyperkalemia. (**Ref. 25,** p. 134)

12. **(D)** The patient does not have enough renal function to excrete the potassium load. He is also developing signs of congestive heart failure and volume overload. A diuretic will not help, but dialysis and ultrafiltration will. (**Ref. 25,** p. 134)

13. **(B)** Superior sulcus or Pancoast tumors arise in the lung apex. The vast majority are of the squamous cell type. Apical lordotic

views or tomograms may be helpful in identifying early lesions. (**Ref. 21**, pp. 1750–1751)

14. **(C)** Pancoast tumors can metastasize early to surrounding structures. They may also invade the cervical sympathetic plexus. Early metastasis to the pancreas would be unlikely. (**Ref. 21**, pp. 1750–1751)

15. **(C)** In Horner's syndrome patients develop miosis. Severe pain may be present in this syndrome. Anhidrosis may develop on the same side of the lesion. (**Ref.25**, p. 351)

16. **(C)** Ototoxicity can result from ethacrynic acid alone or, more commonly, when used in combination with aminoglycosides. Care should, therefore, be exercised in prescribing such a combination. (**Ref. 23**, p. 163)

17. **(B)** Aminoglycosides can produce renal damage in patients with preexisting renal disease. Such subjects are more likely to develop ototoxicity. Pharmacologically dosed aminoglycoside therapy based on creatinine clearance and measured antibiotic levels is recommended. (**Ref. 23**, p. 1479)

18. **(C)** Pain, pallor, paralysis, paresthesias, and pulselessness (the 5 Ps) are hallmarks of acute arterial insufficiency. A pink extremity is not. (**Ref. 25**, p. 747)

19. **(E)** The heart is the most frequent site of origin of arterial emboli. The embolus most frequently originates as a clot in the left atrium as a consequence of atrial fibrillation, or in the left ventricle following myocardial infarction. Other arterial sources include septic heart valve vegetations and mural thrombi from ventricular aneurysms. (**Ref. 25**, p. 747)

20. **(A)** Secondary erythrocytosis is common in smokers who are also at increased risk of developing bronchogenic carcinoma. Bony metastases may cause considerable pain and result in fractures, as well as pressure on adjacent nerves. (**Ref. 27**, pp. 439–444)

21. **(B)** In patients with bronchogenic carcinoma with painful bony metastases radiotherapy may offer palliation. It may also be useful in some patients with bronchial obstruction, involvement of

nerve roots, as well as those with active hemoptysis or mediastinal involvement. (**Ref. 27,** p. 444)

22. (**B**) Bronchogenic carcinoma is associated with hypercalcemia due to bone reabsorption at sites of metastasis. Likewise, peripheral neuropathy, weakness, and inappropriate ADH syndrome are common. (**Ref. 25,** p. 1302)

23. (**C**) According to the Rule of Nines, burns involving the upper extremity would comprise 9.0% of the total body surface (4.5% for the anterior aspect and 4.5% for the posterior aspect). Burns of a lower extremity are considered to involve twice as much body surface as for upper extremity burn. (**Ref. 25,** p. 243)

24. (**A**) Fine needle aspiration of this mass would be the most direct method to gain diagnosis. If the mass is a cyst, fluid may be removed and the mass should disappear. If solid, cytologic material may be obtained for analysis. CT and ultrasound are more expensive than fine needle aspiration and do not fully address the problem. Biopsy is reserved. (**Ref. 25,** pp. 298–300)

25. (**E**) Needle direction for the biopsy is necessary because the mass is not palpable and therefore inaccessible to nondirected fine needle cytology. Excisional biopsy should be performed, but will require needle direction. (*Note:* Initial diagnosis may also be accomplished by stereotactic core biopsy, but this is not an answer option.) (**Ref. 25,** pp. 296–301)

26. (**C**) Excisional biopsy is indicated because the mass is palpable; needle direction is unnecessary. (**Ref. 25,** p. 298)

27. (**B**) The ability of ultrasound to determine the cystic nature of breast lesions is very reliable. Nonpalpable mammographic densities, which appear to be cystic because of their shape, may have cystic character confirmed by ultrasound. (**Ref. 25,** p. 294)

28. (**B**) DPL is rapid, easy to perform, and does not require moving a hemodynamically unstable patient to other areas of the hospital. These qualities, plus its sensitivity for detecting an intraperitoneal source of bleeding, make it the test of choice in evaluating unstable trauma patients for the possibility of intraperitoneal hemorrhage. (**Ref. 21,** p. 266)

29. **(A)** CT scanning allows evaluation of solid organs that are injured as well as an estimate of the extent of injury and likelihood of success of nonoperative management. (**Ref. 21,** pp. 266–267)

30. **(D)** While CT scanning of the chest is developing some favor in excluding traumatic aortic disruption, arteriography remains the definitive test. Patients with a deceleration mechanism of injury and a wide or indistinct mediastinum, as seen on chest x-ray, should be evaluated for traumatic aortic disruption. (**Ref. 21,** p. 264)

31. **(E)** While a chest radiograph, DPL, or CT scan may suggest a traumatic diaphragm injury, none has a high degree of accuracy. Exploratory laparotomy or laparoscopy may be necessary. (**Ref. 21,** p. 265)

32. **(B)** DPL confirms the presence of intraperitoneal hemorrhage. This is a nonspecific finding that may result in laparotomy. At operation, a liver laceration that is no longer bleeding, or a similar problem not requiring operative repair, may be found as the source of the small amount of blood (20–30 ml) necessary to produce a positive DPL. (**Ref. 21,** p. 266)

33. **(C)** The patient is unable to extend his fourth finger because the extensor tendon to this finger has been eroded and weakened by tenosynovitis with resultant rupture. (**Ref. 25,** p. 1172)

34. **(D)** Treatment requires repair of the dorsal hood of the middle extensor tendon so that it becomes effective in its action. Immobilization and NSAIDs may be part of the treatment, but will not fully address the problem without operative repair. (**Ref. 25,** p. 1172)

35. **(D)** After thoracotomy, atrial arrhythmias are not uncommon. The patient has a ventricular response of 150 as determined by dividing the number of large blocks encompassed by two successive QRS complexes, i.e., 2 into 300. (**Ref. 17,** p. 142)

36. **(C)** The patient has atrial flutter with a 2:1 block. A classic "sawtooth pattern" characteristic of flutter waves is easily discernible in several leads. (**Ref. 17,** p. 142)

37. **(E)** Depending on the exact cause of the tachyarrhythmia and its resistance to therapy, all the treatments mentioned are reasonable except a beta-agonist, which would likely make the arrhythmia worse. (**Ref. 25,** p. 381)

38. **(C)** Lymphogranuloma venereum may develop from 5 days to 3 weeks after sexual exposure. The patient has developed secondary lesions because of regional lymph node infection. The enlarged lymph nodes became adherent and suppurative. Eventually buboes may develop. (**Ref. 27,** pp. 1648–1649)

39. **(B)** Infection with *C. trachomatis* can result in lymphogranuloma venerum (LGV). Patients with LGV should be tested for other sexually transmitted illnesses. (**Ref. 25,** p. 119)

40. **(B)** Doxycycline is frequently used in treatment. Erythromycin is also used. The other medications are either ineffective or not initially indicated. (**Ref. 25,** p. 119)

41. **(C)** In patients with hallux valgus, the first toe is angulated away from the body's midline toward the other toes. In some patients with this condition, the great toe may ride over or under the other toes. (**Ref. 25,** p. 1105)

42. **(B)** The first metatarsal head is quite prominent medially. The subject has rheumatoid arthritis, a condition that is frequently associated with bunions with bursal formation and lateral deviation of the toes. (**Ref. 25,** pp. 1105–1106)

43. **(B)** The chest x-ray shows rib fractures. The patient is a poor historian and may not remember the fall or other trauma that caused it. The other choices are either not suggested by the chest x-ray or not able to be diagnosed by the study. (**Ref. 25,** pp. 225–229)

44. **(D)** Fractured ribs may result in a tear in the lung. A limited pneumothorax with spontaneous absorption, or even tension pneumothorax, may develop. Hemorrhage can result from injury to an intercostal vessel. Retained secretions and atelectasis may develop, as may a flail chest, especially if there are bilateral multiple rib fractures, or fracture of the sternum. (**Ref. 25,** pp. 225–229)

45. **(A)** The diagram is that of a sliding hiatal hernia showing herniation of the stomach along the axis of the esophagus. (**Ref. 25**, p. 422)

46. **(B)** A paraesophageal hernia is pictured. This hernia is distinguished by paraaxial herniation of a portion of the stomach. (**Ref. 25**, p. 421)

47. **(A)** Sliding hiatal hernias may be accompanied by gastroesophageal reflux. In these cases, medical management should be attempted first. If unsuccessful, operation is indicated. In the case of a paraesophageal hernia, surgical repair is recommended even if symptoms are few. Paraesophageal hernias have a higher incidence of complications; most worrisome is strangulation. (**Ref. 25**, pp. 421–426)

48. **(D)** All the other answers are usually associated with these cysts. The cysts do not undergo malignant change. (**Ref. 21**, p. 1165)

49. **(D)** The development of polycythemia is associated with a higher incidence of cerebral and pulmonary thrombosis. Patients with this disorder are also at risk from paradoxical emboli and endocarditis. (**Ref. 21**, p. 1911)

50. **(D)** Empyema, purulent material in the pleural space, does not usually cause hemoptysis. Pneumonias, bronchiectasis, and cancer may lead to empyema. (**Ref. 21**, pp. 1723–1724)

51. **(B)** Ultrasound is reliable, noninvasive, and the preferred initial test in cases of asymptomatic AAA. A CT scan may be useful in cases where leakage is suspected. Arteriography is reserved for selected cases where operation is planned in the near future. Doppler indices do not diagnose aneurysmal disease. MRI is presently more costly and without distinct advantage. (**Ref. 21**, p. 1567)

52. **(A)** Aneurysms may rupture, fistulize to veins or parts of the gut, thrombose, and embolize. Dyspepsia is not a usual complication of AAA. (**Ref. 21**, p. 1567)

53. **(A)** 4% of patients with untreated AAA die of unrelated causes. An AAA usually indicates the presence of widespread vascular disease. (**Ref 21**, p. 1567)

54. **(B)** This pain pattern is most suggestive of a renal stone passing down the ureter. Characteristics are abrupt onset, radiation as described, and lack of increase in pain with palpation early in the course of the illness. Patients do not seem to be able to remain still due to waves of ureteral colic. (**Ref. 25,** p. 937)

55. **(C)** This is most suggestive of ruptured diverticulitis, although a ruptured ectopic pregnancy (not a choice) may present like this with accompanying hypotension. The acute onset and spreading peritonitis is characteristic of a ruptured viscus. (**Ref. 25,** p. 668)

56. **(A)** Classic presentation of appendicitis with initial pain of obstruction of the appendiceal lumen mediated via the foregut nerves giving rise to poor localization of pain. When inflammation of the appendiceal surface finally causes pain in the parietal peritoneum of the abdominal cavity, better somatic localization results. (**Ref. 25,** p. 443)

57. **(E)** Pain resulting from early pancreatitis is described in this question. If the process becomes more severe, diffuse abdominal pain and tenderness occur. This may mimic a ruptured viscus or ruptured abdominal aortic aneurysm. (**Ref. 25,** p. 443)

58. **(D)** Gallbladder pain frequently awakens patients at night and radiates as described. The pain also characteristically lasts for hours and may be relieved by vomiting. (**Ref. 25,** p. 444)

59. **(C)** A second organ from the same donor (not usually possible) would also undergo hyperacute rejection. Pretransplant cross-match testing between donor and recipient should identify patients with preformed antibodies. All the other statements are true. (**Ref. 21,** p. 368)

60. **(A)** Cholelithiasis and alcohol abuse together account for about 80% of pancreatitis. All the other choices are lesser causes. (**Ref. 25,** pp. 569–570)

61. **(B)** Although serum amylase is useful in diagnosis of acute pancreatitis, the actual level does not correlate with the severity of the disease. Eleven criteria (Ranson's criteria) that predict

the severity of the episode can be obtained within 48 hours of admission. (**Ref. 25,** p. 574)

62. **(D)** The description is that of a typical indirect inguinal hernia. As the hernia enlarges, it follows the course of the spermatic cord into the scrotum. LGV and other causes of inguinal adenopathy do not disappear and reappear as easily. The same is true of a femoral artery aneurysm. An incarcerated inguinal hernia does not readily reduce with changes in position. (**Ref. 21,** p. 1139)

63. **(B)** The hernia has become incarcerated, i.e., intestine or other abdominal contents have become trapped within the hernia sac at the fascial opening. While an incarcerated inguinal hernia is sometimes difficult to clinically distinguish from painful groin adenopathy, the recent previous exam makes the diagnosis of the latter less likely. (**Ref. 21,** p. 1139)

64. **(C)** Attempt at manual reduction can be made using sedation and Trendelenburg position providing no signs of bowel infarction (fever, leukocytosis, peritonitis) are present. If reduction is successful, the hernia should be repaired on an urgent basis. If it cannot be reduced, the repair should be performed emergently to relieve the incarceration before strangulation occurs. Further observation and needle biopsy have no place. (**Ref. 21,** p. 1139)

65. **(B)** Venous stasis ulcers are usually associated with incompetent perforating veins, which connect the superficial and deep venous systems. Prior DVT contributes to the development of this phenomena. (**Ref. 21,** p. 1496)

66. **(B)** Initial treatment is aimed at decreasing venous hypertension (elevating the legs) and by increasing flow through the deep venous system via elastic stockings or other compressive dressings. (**Ref. 21,** p. 1497)

67. **(A)** Rest pain is ischemic pain at rest. It is usually improved by hanging the extremities over the edge of a bed. Its presence heralds amputation if blood flow to the extremity is not improved. Ischemic ulcers are frequently also present in this population. (**Ref. 25,** p. 742)

68. **(C)** These are usually the result of pressure applied to an area of decreased sensation (spinal cord lesion, coma, diabetic neuropathy). **(Ref. 25,** p. 90)

69. **(D)** Tetanus prophylaxis should always be checked for currency with puncture wounds. These wounds are so-called "tetanus-prone." **(Ref. 25,** p. 110)

70. **(E)** Antibiotic therapy is the primary therapy for cellulitis. It may be adjunctive with other lesions noted, but used alone will not be curative. **(Ref. 25,** pp. 741–746, 803–805)

71. **(C)** The patient is in critical condition from a left-sided tension pneumothorax. He requires immediate needle decompression of the left chest followed by chest tube insertion. Intravenous access is important, but not as much as correction of the tension pneumothorax. All other choices would likely prove to be fatal errors. **(Ref. 1,** pp. 113–125)

72. **(D)** The patient is suffering from pericardial tamponade. X-rays and negative peritoneal lavage have excluded source of continuing hemorrhage. Distended neck veins and muffled heart tones suggest the diagnosis. **(Ref. 1,** pp. 113–125)

73. **(D)** A pericardiocentesis is necessary to remove blood from the pericardium and allow the heart to again become an effective pump. This should be followed by a thoracotomy to repair the site of bleeding or the condition will recur. **(Ref. 1,** pp. 113–125)

74. **(B)** This patient has a ruptured diaphragm suggested by chest x-ray and nasogastric tube identifying the stomach as being in the left chest. **(Ref. 1,** pp. 113–125)

75. **(D)** The bleeding time measures platelet function. Adequate plate numbers must be present for correct interpretation of the test. **(Ref. 21,** p. 91)

76. **(E)** Euglobulin lysis times, as well as fibrin plate lysis tests, are used to measure fibrinolytic activity. Patients with accelerated fibrinolysis bleed related to clot destruction rather than inadequate clot formation. **(Ref. 21,** p. 92)

77. **(C)** The platelet count is usually less than 100,000 in cases of DIC. **(Ref. 24,** p. 92)

78. **(B)** The activated PTT test is used to monitor anticoagulation with heparin. **(Ref. 21,** p. 92)

79. **(A)** The PT is used for monitoring the dose of coumarin. High-dose, long-term heparin may affect the PT. If this occurs, the pro-thrombin-proconvertin test may be used. **(Ref. 21,** p. 92)

80. **(D)** Aspirin interferes with thromboxane synthesis necessary for adequate platelet function. Other drugs may also impair platelet function despite the presence of an adequate platelet count. **(Ref. 21,** p. 90)

81. **(C)** To prevent nonmechanical bleeding, greater than 80% of normal factor VIII levels are necessary in patients with classical hemophilia A when these individuals are being prepared for operation. **(Ref. 21,** p. 93)

82. **(D)** Prothrombin complex is high in the factor IX needed to treat hemophilia B. **(Ref. 21,** p. 93)

83. **(E)** DDAVP may be useful as the sole therapy in minor to moderate hemostatic challenges in some patients with von Willebrand's disease. **(Ref. 21,** p. 93)

84. **(A)** FFP contains therapeutic amounts of all coagulation factors except platelets. It is frequently used for rapid replenishment of vitamin K–related factors when hemorrhage due to deficiency occurs. Vitamin K , given orally or parenterally, will also be effective, but may take 24 hours or more. **(Ref. 21,** p. 93)

85. **(B)** Cryoprecipitate is high in fibrinogen (factor I) and von Willebrand's factor. **(Ref. 21,** p. 93)

86. **(C)** Patients with gastric outlet obstruction of long duration lose (via nasogastric suction or vomiting) large amounts of gastric acid rich in hydrogen ion. If they also become dehydrated, their kidneys will attempt to conserve sodium and excrete hydrogen ion.

This produces a "paradoxical" acid urine from a patient with metabolic alkalosis. (**Ref. 21,** pp. 65–70)

87. (**A**) Normal saline would be the choice to rapidly restore intravascular volume and chloride deficit. (**Ref. 25,** p. 139)

88. (**B**) Loss of intrinsic factor from removal of large portions of the stomach result in poor vitamin B12 absorption in the terminal ileum. Blood cell maturation is affected, as well as peripheral nerve metabolism. The other choices are much less likely. (**Ref. 25,** p. 474)

89. (**C**) Parenteral vitamin B12 obviates the absorption problem caused by loss of intrinsic factor. Oral therapy may be inadequate. Iron therapy alone would not address the vitamin deficiency; other choices have no bearing on the problem. (**Ref. 25,** p. 52)

90. (**B**) Vitamin B12 deficiency may also result from a diseased terminal ileum—the site of B12 absorption. No other answer has a bearing on this issue. (**Ref. 25,** p. 52)

91. (**E**) If hair removal is necessary, it should be done in the operating room as the patient is prepared for operation. (**Ref. 21,** p. 80)

92. (**C**) 72 hours post op is the upper limit of "prophylactic therapy." Many regimens are a single preoperative dose. The infection rate is higher if antibiotics are started post op (as opposed to pre op). Some trauma patients, given an antibiotic prophylactically for possible bowel injury, may not have required it if no bowel injury is found at operation. (**Ref. 21,** p. 225)

93. (**A**) Clean cases are defined as those not entering the alimentary, respiratory, or urinary tract. (**Ref. 21,** p. 222)

94. (**D**) An abscess is considered *infected* and therefore would not be in the *clean-contaminated* class. All other cases are examples of entry into areas of indigenous microflora in a controlled manner. (**Ref. 21,** p. 222)

95. (**B**) Prophylactic antibiotics, in conjunction with mechanical bowel preparation, have significantly decreased colon surgery

infection rates. Prophylactic antibiotics are generally not effective for major burns or pancreatitis. First-generation cephalosporins are not effective for *Pseudomonas;* penicillin is usually used for β-strep infections. (**Ref. 21,** pp. 222–223; **Ref. 25,** pp. 575, 691)

96. **(B)** If the pylorus is obstructed, bile cannot stain the vomitus. This is an important point in the differential diagnosis of infant emesis. (**Ref. 25,** pp. 1212–1213)

97. **(D)** Operative adhesions are a frequent source of intestinal obstruction in adults, but not newborns. Most neonatal adhesions are due to vascular accidents in utero or caused by other choices. (**Ref. 25,** p. 1214)

98. **(A)** Absence of parasympathetic myenteric nerve cells is believed to be the basis of the nonmotility in the affected bowel segment. This produces a functional obstruction. (**Ref. 25,** p. 1218)

99. **(C)** Biopsy of the rectum is the confirmatory diagnosis, although the disorder is suspected upon history and barium enema findings. (**Ref. 25,** p. 1219)

100. **(C)** A colostomy is performed in young children. The colostomy is usually placed in the so-called distal "transition zone" where ganglion cells are present by frozen section examination at the time of operation. (**Ref. 25,** p. 1219)

101. **(C)** The pathology depicted is that of intussusception of the terminal ileum into the colon. Ischemia and hemorrhage arising in the area of the affected bowel may produce the so-called "currant jelly" stool. (**Ref. 25,** p. 1222)

102. **(A)** If the diagnosis is suspected before onset of vascular compromise of the intussuscepted bowel, the ileum may be reduced by careful barium enema. Fever, elevated white cell count, and clinical evidence of peritonitis mitigate against barium enema use. (**Ref. 25,** p. 1223)

103. **(A)** Intussusception frequently occurs in children with apparent normal bowel. In adults, the frequency is less and often there is an

anomaly (lipoma, tumor, etc.) of the intussuscepting segment. (**Ref. 25,** p. 624)

104. **(B)**   Cancer is the leading cause of colonic obstruction in adults. (**Ref. 25,** p. 651)

105. **(C)**   About 50% of colon cancer arises in the rectosigmoid; the right colon is next with 25%. (**Ref. 25,** p. 654)

106. **(D)**   Radiation therapy post op for stage III rectal cancers gives survival rates 30% superior to patients not so treated. (**Ref. 25,** pp. 660–661)

107. **(D)**   A combination of radiation and chemotherapy with fluorouracil and either mitomycin or cisplatin is the preferred treatment. Abdominoperineal resection is reserved for unresponsive tumors. (**Ref. 25,** p. 710)

108. **(E)**   These tumors are rare, with carcinoid being the most common type. About half of adenocarcinomas of the appendix present as appendicitis. Tumors less than 2 cm are generally cured by appendectomy alone. (**Ref. 25,** p. 614)

109. **(A)**   The cecum is the largest part of the colon. Tumors may grow to a fairly large size before producing obstructive symptoms. (**Ref. 25,** p. 654)

110. **(C)**   An obstruction left-sided colon cancer may cause perforation at the cecum because the wall tension is greatest there (LaPlace's law). (**Ref. 25,** p. 652)

111. **(E)**   Sterile anthropometric measurement from the site of intended insertion to the angle of Louis best approximates the appropriate length of CVP catheter insertion. Other arbitrary centimeter measurements do not take into account individual size variability. (**Ref. 6,** videocassette 1)

112. **(A)**   The angle of Louis approximates the appropriate place for CVP tip placement: distal superior vena cava above the pericardium. Catheter tips placed within the heart have increased risk of perforation and arrhythmia production. (**Ref. 6,** videocassette 2)

113. **(C)** Free aspiration of venous blood confirms intravascular position. Chest x-rays are used to confirm intrathoracic position and exclude complication such as pneumothorax. (**Ref. 6,** videocassette 1)

114. **(C)** Due to the small-caliber and high-compliance characteristics, PIC lines do not allow rapid infusion of fluid or accurate hemodynamic monitoring. (**Ref. 6,** videocassette 3)

115. **(A)** Perforation may occur immediately as a result of incorrect catheter placement technique. It may also result from erosion of a catheter (whose tip is against a vessel wall) subjected to cardiorespiratory vibration. (**Ref. 6,** videocassette 2)

116. **(B)** A burst fracture is pictured. These fractures result from a severe axial loading force applied to healthy bone. Unlike osteoporotic bone, healthy bone "bursts" rather than collapses. The risk of neurologic deficit due to cord injury is increased with burst fractures. (**Ref. 25,** p. 1015)

117. **(A)** A compression fracture is pictured. These fractures usually result from trivial trauma to osteoporotic bone, which collapses. This is in contrast to a burst fracture, which may look similar on x-ray, but requires higher suspicion of spinal instability and possible neural injury. (**Ref. 25,** p. 1012)

118. **(B)** The burst nature of the bone during injury is more likely to cause retropulsion of a fragment into the spinal cord. This is much less likely with the collapse of osteoporotic bone as seen in compression fractures. (**Ref. 25,** p. 1015)

119. **(A)** Compression fractures of the thoracic vertebrae are often treated by rest and a corset brace to prevent further hyperflexion. Treatment is about six weeks. (**Ref. 25,** p. 1012)

120. **(A)** Compression fractures represent the most common type of spinal fracture. It is likely this will change as osteoporosis is effectively treated or prevented. (**Ref. 25,** p. 1012)

121. **(C)** The description is characteristic of obstruction (usually kinking) of postprandial secretions in the afferent limb of a

Billroth II gastrojejunostomy. Pain is quickly relieved by emesis, which decompresses the obstructed limb. (**Ref. 14,** pp. 195–197)

122. **(D)** A portion of the intestine excluded from the usual flow of chyme may foster bacterial overgrowth, resulting in the "blind loop" syndrome. (**Ref. 14,** pp. 195–197)

123. **(A)** Early (within 15 minutes of eating) or late (at about 3 hours postprandial) dumping symptoms may occur due to hypertonic gastric contents gaining rapid access to the small bowel, associated hormonal changes, and reactive hypoglycemia. (**Ref. 14,** pp. 195–197)

124. **(B)** Delayed gastric emptying of solids following gastric surgery is probably the most commonly found postgastrectomy syndrome. (**Ref. 14,** pp. 195–197)

125. **(E)** Alkaline reflux gastritis is caused by continuous entrance of bile and duodenal contents into the gastric remnant. Revision to a Roux-en-Y gastrojejunostomy frequently solves this problem. (**Ref. 14,** pp. 195–197)

126. **(A)** The course of "unconsciousness, lucid interval, followed by coma" is characteristic of an epidural hematoma. Initial injury causes the concussion from which the patient recovers. The eye signs and coma are caused by increased intracranial pressure due to hemorrhage from an extradural artery. (**Ref. 25,** p. 822)

127. **(B)** A unilateral dilated pupil and decreasing level of consciousness is very suggestive of elevated intracranial pressure. In this scenario, intracranial hemorrhage is high on the list of differential diagnoses. Either epidural or subdural hemorrhage may produce this problem. Direct eye injury and congenital eye lesion is unlikely due to history. (**Ref. 25,** pp. 817–823)

128. **(D)** Thirty to 50% of severe head injuries correctly managed may not fully recover. Observation only does not deal with the elevated intracranial pressure and is not indicated. All other treatments are useful in limiting secondary brain injury due to swelling. (**Ref. 25,** pp. 817–823)

129. **(A)** Increasing $PaCO_2$ acutely increases cerebral blood flow and thereby elevates intracerebral pressure (ICP). All other noted maneuvers lead to decrease in ICP according to the Monroe-Kellie doctrine. (**Ref. 25,** pp. 810–812)

130. **(B)** The hernia described is a "direct" type and would be independent of cord structures. It is sometimes difficult to distinguish hernia type with confidence preoperatively. (**Ref. 25,** pp. 712–717)

131. **(B)** With extension below the course of the inguinal ligament (a line drawn from the anterior superior iliac spine to the pubic tubercle), it is a femoral hernia. It may also be a sliding or Richter's hernia, but that cannot be told from the examination. (**Ref. 25,** pp. 712–718)

132. **(A)** A fascial defect is mandatory for development of a hernia, and its correction is the fundamental aspect of the surgical repair. All other choices may have a bearing in different hernia types, but not universally. (**Ref. 25,** p. 712)

133. **(C)** The hernia sac (?) in Figure 4-19a is shown to have been dissected from the within spermatic cord and protruding through the internal ring—indirect sac. In Figure 4-19b the sac is shown in the "direct" area behind the spermatic cord. (**Ref. 25,** pp. 714–716)

134. **(B)** Littre's hernia may be umbilical (20%), inguinal (50%), or femoral (20%) in location, but (by definition) it always contains a Meckel's diverticulum within the hernia sac. (**Ref. 25,** p. 721)

135. **(C)** A spigelian hernia most frequently occurs where the semilunar line crosses the semicircular line. There may be some difficulty in palpating the defect if the overlying external oblique fascia is intact. (**Ref. 25,** p. 721)

136. **(A)** The epigastric hernia is a midline hernia through the linea alba above the umbilicus. About 20% are multiple and 80% occur slightly off midline. (**Ref. 25,** p. 719)

137. **(B)** The cephalic stage of gastric secretion is mediated through the vagus nerve. Acetylcholine indicates the receptor where this effect is translated into increased acid production. (**Ref. 25,** p. 476)

138. (A) The presence of protein hydrolysates in the stomach stimulate gastrin secretion from the antrum. The presence of gastric distention also reinforces cephalic phase stimulation. (**Ref. 25, p. 476**)

139. (C) Histamine-2 receptors increase and facilitate acid production. H-2 blockers represent a major therapeutic area for decreasing acid production. (**Ref. 25, p. 479**)

140. (D) Omeprazole inhibits the sodium-potassium-ATP mediated pump, which is the final common pathway for H^+-ion secretion (acid production). (**Ref. 25, p. 479**)

141. (E) Mucous at the luminal surface and throughout the stomach provided a protective effect against cell surface attack in the low pH environment. (**Ref. 25, p. 475**)

142. (A) At a pH below 2.5, gastrin production is inhibited. If the antrum is excluded from acid contact (as in the procedure described), unregulated gastrin production can occur. (**Ref. 25, p. 477**)

143. (B) A truncal vagotomy disconnects vagal innervation, which exerts its major affect through acetylcholine. (**Ref. 25, p. 480**)

144. (A) Gastrinomas produces gastrin in a manner unresponsive to normal regulatory mechanisms. The result is markedly elevated basal acid secretion and peptic ulceration mediated through this receptor. (**Ref. 25, p. 483**)

145. (E) Antacids neutralize HCl after it is produced in the gastric lumen. They do not act to prevent acid production. (**Ref. 25, p. 479**)

146. (A) Glutamine is nonessential under normal conditions of metabolism, but stress markedly increases its use and need. (**Ref. 25, p. 147**)

147. (D) ω-6 fatty acids in balance with ω-3 fatty acids contribute to a normal functioning immune system. Diets high in ω-6 fatty acids depress immune system by decreasing T-cell mitogenesis. (**Ref. 25, p. 149**)

148. **(C)** Cold water fish and fish oils (cod liver oil) are good sources of ω-3 fatty acids. (**Ref. 25,** p. 149)

149. **(D)** Corn, safflower, sunflower, and soy bean oils are good sources of ω-6 fatty acids. (**Ref. 25,** p. 149)

150. **(B)** Arginine enhances T-lymphocyte activation in response to other mitogens. (**Ref. 25,** p. 147)

151. **(A)** Glutamine is the preferred fuel of enterocytes lining the small bowel. It is important in maintaining the gut barrier to bacteria and toxins. (**Ref. 25,** p. 147)

152. **(E)** Vitamins are largely involved as cofactors in energy transfer situations, metabolism, and wound healing. They cannot be synthesized and must be included in the diet. Excess water-soluble vitamins (C, B, etc.) may be excreted in the urine. Fat-soluble vitamins (A, D, E, K) may be stored. (**Ref. 25,** pp. 147–148)

153. **(B)** Secretin infusion will cause a marked increase in the serum gastrin. This is a diagnostic test for Z-E syndrome. All other findings suggest this diagnosis. (**Ref. 14,** p. 194)

154. **(C)** All patients with Sipple's syndrome have medullary thyroid cancer at the time of diagnosis. The other statements are true. (**Ref. 14,** p. 301)

References

1. American College of Surgeons Committee on Trauma: Advanced Trauma Life Support. Chicago, American College of Surgeons, 1993

2. Ayers LN, Whipp BJ, Ziment I: *A Guide to the Interpretation of Pulmonary Function Tests,* 2nd ed. New York, Roerig (a division of Pfizer Pharmaceuticals), 1978.

3. Delp MH, Manning RT (eds): *Major's Physical Diagnosis: An Introduction to the Clinical Process,* 9th ed. Philadelphia, Saunders, 1981.

4. Eastham RD: *A Pocket Guide to Differential Diagnosis.* Bristol, Great Britain, John Wright and Sons, 1980.

5. Frohlich ED (ed): *Rypins' Medical Licensure Examinations,* 14th ed. Philadelphia, Lippincott, 1985.

6. Food and Drug Administration Center for Devices and Radiological Health Office of Training and Assistance Central Catheter Working Group: Central Venous Catheter Complications. Maryland, National Audiovisual Center, 1994.

7. Gottlieb AJ et al.: *The Whole Internist Catalog.* Philadelphia, Saunders, 1980.

8. Hansten PD: *Drug Interactions,* 5th ed. Philadelphia, Lea and Febiger, 1985.

9. Harvey AM, Johns RJ, McKusick VA et al.: *Principles and Practice of Medicine,* 21st ed. New York, Appleton-Century-Crofts, 1984.

10. Henry JB (ed): *Todd-Sanford-Davidsohn: Clinical Diagnosis and Management by Laboratory Methods,* 17th ed. Philadelphia, Saunders, 1984.

11. Heppenstall RB (ed): *Fracture Treatment and Healing.* Philadelphia, Saunders, 1980.

12. Hurst JW (ed): *Medicine for the Practicing Physician.* Boston, Butterworths, 1983.

13. Kelly WN, Harris ED, Ruddy S et al.: *Textbook of Rheumatology.* Philadelphia, Saunders, 1981.

14. Lawrence PF (ed): *Essentials of General Surgery,* 2nd ed. Baltimore, Williams & Wilkins, 1992.

15. Lawrence PF (ed): *Essentials of Surgical Specialties.* Baltimore, Williams & Wilkins, 1993.

16. Marmor L: *Arthritis Surgery.* Philadelphia, Lea & Febiger, 1976.

17. Marriott HJL: *Practical Electrocardiography,* 6th ed. Baltimore, Williams & Wilkins, 1977.

18. Pritchard JA, MacDonald PC (eds): *Williams Obstetrics,* 17th ed. New York, Appleton-Century-Crofts, 1984.

19. Reichel W (ed): *Clinical Aspects of Aging,* 2nd ed. Baltimore, Williams & Wilkins, 1983.

20. Romney SL, Gray MJ, Little AB et al. (eds): *Gynecology and Obstetrics: The Health Care of Women,* 2nd ed. New York, McGraw-Hill, 1981.

21. Sabiston, DC (ed): *Textbook of Surgery,* 14th ed. Philadelphia, W. B. Saunders, 1991.

22. Schwartz LM: *Compendium of Immunology,* 2nd ed. New York, Van Nostrand Reinhold, 1980.

23. Schwartz SI (ed): *Principles of Surgery,* 6th ed. New York, McGraw-Hill, 1994.

24. Stein JH (ed): *Internal Medicine.* Boston, Little, Brown, 1983.

25. Way, LW (ed): *Current Surgical Diagnosis & Treatment,* 10th ed. Norwalk, CT, Appleton & Lange, 1994.

26. Winefield HR, Peay MY: *Behavioral Science in Medicine.* Baltimore, University Park Press, 1980.

27. Wyngaarden JB, Smith LH (eds): *Cecil Textbook of Medicine,* 17th ed. Philadelphia, Saunders, 1985.

5

Pediatrics

William Schwartz, MD
and Esther K. Chung, MD, MPH

DIRECTIONS: Each of the questions or incomplete statements below is followed by a list of suggested answers or completions. Select the **one** that is best in each case.

---

1. The expected time for a baby to triple its birth weight is
   A. 6 months
   B. 9 months
   C. 12 months
   D. 15 months
   E. 18 months

2. A 10-month-old baby has a "large head." On further investigation, the head is in the 50th percentile, while the length is in the 10th percentile and chest circumference is in the 10th percentile. The rest of the physical examination is normal. At this point, which is the **BEST** description of the problem?
   A. A small child with hydrocephalus
   B. Cephalo-somatic disproportion
   C. Modest growth delay with preferential growth of head
   D. Trisomy 13 syndrome
   E. Postmeningitis hydrocephalus

3. A 10-year-old boy is the shortest child in his class. He has had a normal childhood with no serious illness or problems. He has a

good appetite. Both parents are average size. The physical examination is normal. He is at the 3rd percentile for height and weight. The parents are quite anxious. What is the next step in your evaluation?
A. Growth hormone levels
B. CBC
C. Somatomedin level
D. Bone age
E. Give growth hormone

4. Just after birth, an infant's head size will be about what percent of its total adult size?
A. 15%
B. 25%
C. 50%
D. 75%
E. 90%

5. A normal 6-month-old would require about how many calories per kilogram daily?
A. 25
B. 40
C. 75
D. 110
E. 250

6. X-rays of a normal newborn would reveal ossification centers in which of the following?
A. Clavicle
B. Proximal femur
C. Talus
D. Distal tibia
E. None of the above

7. Which one of the following conditions **BEST** describes the growth chart in Figure 5-1?
A. Growth hormone deficiency
B. Genetic short stature
C. Constitutional growth delay
D. Chronic illness
E. Normal variation

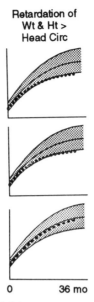

Retardation of
Wt & Ht >
Head Circ

0   36 mo

Figure 5-1 (*Source:* Rudolph.)

8. Which one of the following conditions **BEST** describes the growth chart in Figure 5-2?
   A. Growth hormone deficiency
   B. Genetic short stature
   C. Constitutional growth delay
   D. Chronic illness
   E. Normal variation

9. Characteristics of a infant born to a mother who used crack cocaine extensively during pregnancy include which of the following?
   A. Lip smacking
   B. High-pitched cry
   C. Large tongue
   D. Small head
   E. Easy bruisability

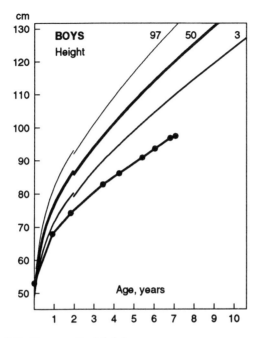

Figure 5-2 (*Source:* Rudolph.)

10. The number of teeth in a normal 2-year-old should be
    A. 10
    B. 16
    C. 20
    D. 24
    E. 28

11. A 5-year-old, previously well male has a fever, headache, irritability, and stiff neck. The rest of the examination is normal. A lumbar puncture reveals clear spinal fluid; 150 WBCs (45 polys, 55 lymphs); protein, 40 mg/dL; glucose, 55 mg/dL; serum glucose, 80 mg/dL. No bacteria are seen on gram stain. The diagnosis of viral meningitis is made. Which of the following statements is **TRUE** about the diagnosis?
    A. The data are consistent with the diagnosis
    B. The percentage of polys is too high
    C. The percentage of lymphs is too low
    D. The glucose should be lower
    E. The protein should be higher

12. A 2-year-old patient has fever and a painful ear. The tympanic membrane is red, dull, and has lost its landmarks. What is the **MOST LIKELY** cause of this infection?
    A. *Listeria*
    B. *Mycoplasma*
    C. *H. influenza*
    D. *S. pneumoniae*
    E. *E. coli*

13. The **MOST LIKELY** cause of osteomyelitis is
    A. *Salmonella*
    B. *Staphylococcus aurea*
    C. *Streptococcus pneumoniae*
    D. *Pseudomonas*
    E. *Escherichia coli*

14. A 3-month-old has fever with rapid respirations and mild retractions. There is good air entry with expiratory wheezes—no rales. Tympanic membranes and abdomen are normal. The **MOST LIKELY** diagnosis is
    A. bronchiolitis
    B. asthma
    C. pneumonia
    D. heart failure
    E. Legionnaire's disease

Questions 15–18: Match the following diagnoses with the five clinical descriptions. Each diagnosis may be used once, more than once, or not at all.

    A. *Listeria monocytes*
    B. Rotavirus infection
    C. *Atypical mycobacteria*
    D. *Salmonella*
    E. *Shigella*
    F. Adenovirus infection
    G. *S. pneumoniae* infection
    H. Kawasaki disease
    I. Tuberculosis
    J. Staphylococcal infection

15. A 9-month-old with a 2-day history of fever and diarrhea; fair urine output; intake of solid foods poor, but good intake of fluids; green stool with more liquid than solid matter

16. A 9-year-old with a 2×3-cm lymph node in the left anterior cervical area that is mobile and tender; weakly positive PPD (5-mm induration)

17. The **MOST LIKELY** organism to cause impetigo in a 6-year-old child

18. The cause of an infection causing bloody diarrhea, foul smelling stools, and seizures

19. Which clinical feature is **LEAST LIKELY** to be present in a 6-year-old girl with a urinary tract infection?
    A. Fever
    B. Flank pain
    C. Dysuria
    D. Frequency
    E. Abdominal pain

20. A 12-year-old has just been cut on his arm by a small piece of glass in his bedroom. The wound is clean but is irrigated with saline. He had full basic immunizations and a tetanus booster three years ago at the time of another injury. When does he need to get a tetanus booster?
    A. Now
    B. In 2 years
    C. In 3 years
    D. In 5 years
    E. In 7 years

21. A 12-year-old girl with acute abdominal pain has a plain film of her abdomen. It shows a normal gas pattern but a calcification in her left lower quadrant that looks like a tooth. The **MOST LIKE-LY** explanation for this is
    A. she swallowed the tooth
    B. an artifact
    C. a fecalith that looks like a tooth
    D. a dermoid cyst
    E. diverticulum

22. Which of the following signs or symptoms is **NOT** usually associated with acute lymphoblastic leukemia?
   A. Joint pain
   B. Fever
   C. Fatigue
   D. Osteomyelitis
   E. Pallor

Questions 23–25: Match the following oncologic diseases with the associated laboratory finding. Each disease may be used once, more than once, or not at all.

   A. Chromosomal anomalies
   B. Destruction of bone in pelvis
   C. Low T cell count
   D. Elevated acid phosphatase
   E. Ecchymosis of eyelid

23. Acute myelogenous leukemia

24. Neuroblastoma

25. Ewing sarcoma

26. A patient with anemia and a low MCV that does not respond to adequate iron treatment will **MOST LIKELY** have
   A. malabsorption of iron from the GI tract
   B. folic acid deficiency
   C. sickle cell anemia
   D. thalassemia
   E. aplastic anemia

27. A patient with a bleeding problem is suspected to have von Willebrand disease. Which of the following tests is compatible with this diagnosis?
   A. Low factor VIII levels
   B. Increased platelet adhesiveness
   C. Platelet antibodies
   D. Low factor IX levels
   E. Prolonged PT

28. The defect in sickle cell anemia has been identified as a
  A. deletion in chromosome 7
  B. substitution of valine for glutamic acid on the beta chain of hemoglobin
  C. inhibitor of fetal hemoglobin synthesis
  D. deficiency of delta heme fraction
  E. substitution of glutamic acid for isoleucine

29. A patient with pallor, frontal and parietal bossing, enlarged maxilla, protrusion of the frontal teeth, and marked malocclusion **MOST LIKELY** has
  A. sickle cell trait
  B. thalassemia
  C. craniostenosis
  D. cleidocranial dysostosis
  E. Pierre Robin syndrome

30. In a 6-year-old with new onset of purpura, which of the following will be compatible with the diagnosis of ITP?
  A. Generalized adenopathy
  B. Prolonged PT
  C. Elevated IgE
  D. Platelet antibodies
  E. Severe abdominal pain

31. Classic hemophilia A is
  A. characterized by absent or low levels of factor IX
  B. characterized by absent or low levels of factor X
  C. a sex-linked recessive disorder
  D. never seen in females
  E. corrected by infusions of PCR coagulant

Questions 32–34: Match the diagnosis with the clinical description. Each diagnosis may be used once, more than once, or not at all.

    A. Trisomy 15
    B. Neiman Pick disease
    C. Lesch Nyhan syndrome
    D. Down syndrome
    E. Autism
    F. Attention deficit–hyperactivity disorder
    G. Post-lyme disease deficit

32. Poor attention span, distractible, normal intelligence, poor school performance

33. Repetitive movements, poor communication skills, low IQ, poor interpersonal relationships

34. Mental retardation, self-destructive behavior, biting

35. A 12-year-old female with staring spells and interrupted speech for several seconds then returns to normal activity. What will the EEG look like in this patient?
    A. Hypsarrythmia
    B. 3/sec spike and dome
    C. Disorganized pattern from temporal lobe area
    D. Seizure spikes from the optic chiasm
    E. None of the above

36. Which feature **BEST** describes cerebral palsy?
    A. Mental retardation
    B. Basal ganglion sclerosis
    C. Generalized spasticity
    D. Choreiform movements
    E. Nonprogressive motor defect

37. Patients with myelomeningocele may have all the following problems **EXCEPT**
    A. hydrocephalus
    B. dislocated hips
    C. cerebellar ataxia

D. urinary tract infections
E. kyphoscoliosis

38. Of the patients with the following diseases, which is **MOST LIKELY** to have a cherry red spot in the macula?
A. Histiocytosis
B. Gaucher disease
C. Optic atrophy
D. Lowe syndrome
E. Tay Sachs disease

39. A patient with cerebellar ataxia **MOST LIKELY** will have had a recent infection with
A. chicken pox
B. strep
C. Lyme disease
D. rubella
E. parvovirus

40. A 1-year-old with a history of jaundice and a total bilirubin of 30 mg/dL as a newborn, now has athetosis, defective vision, spasticity, and poor muscle mass. Where is the lesion in the brain?
A. Hypothalamus
B. Olive
C. Cerebellum
D. Basal ganglia
E. Substantia nigra

41. In the right ventricle of the normal heart, which pressure reading is normal?
A. 40/20
B. 80/60
C. 25/5
D. 120/80
E. 5/2

Questions 42–44: Match the cardiac lesion with the classic associated heart sound. Each answer may be used once, more than once, or not at all.

A. Systolic murmur at upper left sternal border
B. Systolic and diastolic murmur heard at the second intercostal space
C. Systolic murmur at the upper sternal border with radiation to the neck
D. Diastolic murmur heard best at the base
E. Diastolic murmur that disappears with deep breath

42. Atrial septal defect

43. Patent ductus arteriosus

44. Aortic stenosis

45. All the following are associated with acute rheumatic fever **EXCEPT**
   A. changing heart murmur
   B. erythema nodosum
   C. joint pain
   D. fever
   E. elevated sedimentation rate

46. Which change occurs in the newborn's cardiovascular system?
   A. Dilation of the ductus venosus
   B. Left ventricular hypertrophy
   C. Decrease in pulmonary artery pressure
   D. Right atrial dilatation
   E. Biphasic P waves on EKG

47. In a patient with chronic pyelonephritis who develops hypertension, you would expect to find elevated levels of which compound?
   A. 17-OH corticosterone
   B. Leucocidin
   C. Atrial natriuretic factor
   D. Renin
   E. Ergotamine

48. The **MOST COMMON** cardiac cause of cyanosis in the newborn is
    A. teratology of Fallot
    B. patent ductus arteriosus
    C. hypoplastic left heart syndrome
    D. pulmonary hypertension
    E. transposition of the great vessels

49. The cardiovascular lesion **MOST TYPICALLY** associated with Kawasaki disease is
    A. coronary artery aneurysms
    B. myocardiopathy
    C. second-degree heart block
    D. aortitis
    E. pulmonary hypertension

50. The **USUAL** heart rate for a newborn is
    A. 80/min
    B. 100/min
    C. 120/min
    D. 170/min
    E. 195/min

51. Which of the following is **NOT** associated with a functional murmur?
    A. High-pitched murmur at the base
    B. Diastolic murmur —> always pathologic !
    C. Normal EKG
    D. Occurs sometime in more than 25% of children
    E. High-pitched "sea gull"–type murmur at base

52. Which of the following drugs is associated with chest pain?
    A. Heroin
    B. Marijuana
    C. LSD
    D. Cocaine
    E. Angel dust

53. Which of the following features is **NOT** associated with cystic fibrosis?
    A. Nasal polyps
    B. Meconium ileus
    C. Decreased trypsin
    D. Diabetes
    E. Enlarged maxillary glands

Questions 54–55: Match the organism responsible for pneumonia with the clinical situations. Each organism may be used once, more than once, or not at all.

    A. *Adenovirus*
    B. *Staphylococcus*
    C. *Mycobacterium tuberculosis*
    D. *Klebsiella*
    E. *Chlamydia*

54. Six-week-old with conjunctivitis, fever, and cough

55. Six-year-old with fever, cough, and multiple lung abscesses seen on x-ray

56. Which sign or symptom is **NOT** associated with forms of childhood asthma?
    A. Cough
    B. Made worse by exercise
    C. Inspiratory wheeze
    D. Dark circles under eyes
    E. Nasal polyps

57. A 6-week-old male infant has a barky cough with no fever or cyanosis, no rales in lungs, and good air entry. Which of the following is the **MOST LIKELY** diagnosis?
    A. Tracheoesophageal fistula
    B. Croup
    C. Pulmonary sequestration
    D. Bronchiolitis
    E. Vascular ring

58. A premature baby is **MOST LIKELY** to be deficient to a clinically significant degree in which of the following compounds or cells?
   A. Alpha-1 antitrypsin
   B. Surfactant
   C. Eosinophils
   D. Elastin
   E. Mast cells

59. Pulmonary hypertension is associated with which of the following signs or symptoms?
   A. Notched P wave on EKG
   B. Elevated pCO_2
   C. Loud second heart sound at the base of the heart
   D. Increased first heart sound at the apex
   E. Increased breath sounds in sternal area

60. A practical method to monitor pulmonary function at home is
   A. tidal volume
   B. pulse oximetry
   C. inspiratory volume
   D. forced expiratory volume at 1 sec
   E. forced expiratory volume at 1 min

61. An infant with constipation, dry mouth, generalized weakness, decreased sucking and gag reflex **MOST LIKELY** has
   A. polio
   B. Werdnig Hoffman
   C. Guillain-Barré
   D. botulism
   E. none of the above

62. All the following may cause an enlarged tongue **EXCEPT**
   A. hypothyroidism
   B. Hurler disease
   C. arteriovenous malformation
   D. fibroelastosis
   E. lymphangectasia

63. What is the recommended daily dose of vitamin D?
  A. 200 units
  B. 400 units
  C. 600 units
  D. 800 units
  E. 1000 units

64. The caloric needs of a newborn is
  A. 30 kcal/kg/day
  B. 65 kcal/kg/day
  C. 115 kcal/kg/day
  D. 150 kcal/kg/day
  E. 175 kcal/kg/day

65. A 15-year-old will need a diet with how many calories?
  A. 800 kcal/day
  B. 1200 kcal/day
  C. 1500 kcal/day
  D. 1800 kcal/day
  E. 2000 kcal/day

Questions 66–68: Match the description with the diagnosis. Each description may be used once, more than once, or not at all.

  A. Hepatitis A
  B. Hepatitis B
  C. Hepatitis C
  D. Delta hepatitis
  E. Non-A–non-B hepatitis

66. Hepatitis associated with drug users but not transfusion recipients

67. Hepatitis associated with human bites

68. Hepatitis spread by fecal oral route

69. The percent of cases of hepatitis B that become chronic carriers is
    A. 0%
    B. 10%
    C. 25%
    D. 40%
    E. 50%

70. Which of the following conditions is associated with an elevated direct (conjugated) bilirubin?
    A. Sepsis
    B. Spherocytosis
    C. Reye syndrome (hepatic encephalopathy)
    D. Thalassemia
    E. Factor IX deficiency

71. A patient with acute pancreatitis will have which defect?
    A. Elevated trypsin
    B. Elevated amylase
    C. Decreased amylase
    D. Elevated alpha-1 antitripsin
    E. Decreased lipase

72. A large spleen is associated with all the following EXCEPT
    A. Gaucher disease
    B. Epstein-Barr (EB) virus infection
    C. alpha-1 antitrypsin deficiency
    D. chronic myelogenous leukemia
    E. metastatic Wilms tumor

73. Meckel diverticulum
    A. is a remnant of the ductus venosus
    B. is associated with intestinal polyposis
    C. is seen with HIV infection
    D. may lead to anemia
    E. will cause pancreatitis when symptomatic

Questions 74–76: Match the clinical situations of blood in the stools with the following diagnoses. Each diagnosis may be used once, more than once, or not at all.

    A. Inflammatory bowel disease
    B. Milk allergy
    C. Giardia infections
    D. Hookworm infestation
    E. Hemolytic uremic syndrome

74. Bloody diarrhea, *Escherichia coli* infections, and purpura

75. Cough, eosinophilia, intermittent diarrhea, and positive stool guaiac

76. Abdominal pain, blood in stools, lymphoid hyperplasia, narrowing of intestinal lumen

77. A 4-month-old with constipation is found to have the following physical findings: abdominal distension, poor weight gain, no stool in the rectum. Which diagnosis is **MOST CONSISTENT** with this description?
    A. Botulism
    B. Functional megacolon
    C. Rectal fistula
    D. Aganglionic megacolon
    E. Tethered cord

78. The **MOST COMMON** cause of rectal bleeding in a 15-month-old child is
    A. rectal fissure
    B. intestinal polyp
    C. inflammatory bowel disease
    D. arteriovenous malformation
    E. intussusception

79. An infant has severe diarrhea for two days. The physical examination shows an irritable child with no tears. The mouth is dry. The skin is dry but does not tent up when pinched. The diaper is minimally wet. Your estimate of the degree of dehydration is
    A. 2%
    B. 3–5%

C. 5–7%
D. 8–12%
E. cannot estimate from this information

80. What situation **BEST** describes the following electrolyte results: Na = 137; K = 3.0; Cl =91; CO_2 = 32?
    A. Metabolic acidosis
    B. Metabolic alkalosis
    C. Respiratory acidosis
    D. Respiratory alkalosis
    E. Mixed acidosis/alkalosis

81. Which blood gas results are **MOST TYPICAL** of status asthmaticus?
    A. pO_2 = 80, pCO_2 = 40, pH = 7.47
    B. pO_2 = 100, pCO_2 = 42, pH = 7.45
    C. pO_2 = 70, pCO_2 = 58, pH = 7.32
    D. pO_2 = 80, pCO_2 = 38, pH = 7.33
    E. pO_2 = 60, pCO_2 = 42, pH = 7.47

82. Angiotensin is produced in the
    A. kidney
    B. liver
    C. adrenal
    D. right atrium
    E. posterior pituitary

83. Which of the following is the **MOST COMMON** cause of an abdominal mass in a newborn?
    A. Wilms tumor
    B. Neuroblastoma
    C. Uretero pelvic obstruction
    D. Meconium ileus
    E. Hepatoma

84. The newborn can concentrate urine to approximately which level?
    A. 200 mOsm
    B. 300 mOsm
    C. 500 mOsm
    D. 700 mOsm
    E. 1200 mOsm

85. Patients with sickle cell anemia may have all the following renal conditions **EXCEPT**
    A. hematuria
    B. decreased concentrating ability
    C. chronic nephritis
    D. cortical necrosis
    E. papillary necrosis

86. In acute glomerulonephritis secondary to a strep infection, you would expect to see which of the following laboratory results?
    A. Decreased complement
    B. Decreased urinary sodium
    C. Decreased renin
    D. Small kidneys on ultrasound
    E. High cholesterol

87. Nephrotic syndrome in childhood is **MOST LIKELY**
    A. from strep infection
    B. from urinary tract infection
    C. from diabetes
    D. from lupus
    E. idiopathic

88. Which of the following pathological findings is typical of childhood nephrotic syndrome?
    A. Proliferative nephritis
    B. Crescents
    C. Glomerular adhesions
    D. Membranous nephropathy
    E. Normal light microscopy

89. An infant is born with a flat midface, narrow palpebral fissures, low nasal bridge, short upturned nose, and a narrow vermilion border of the upper lip. He is small for gestational age and shows poor growth. Others may have cleft lip, atrial and ventricular septal defects, microphthalmia. These conditions describe
    A. cocaine exposure in utero
    B. HIV infection
    C. fetal alcohol syndrome
    D. heroin exposure
    E. toxoplasmosis

90. Which of the following anatomical findings suggests serious pathology in an otherwise healthy newborn?
   A. Umbilical hernia
   B. Diastasis recti
   C. Single umbilical artery
   D. Cleft lip
   E. None of the above

91. Which of the following diseases is **NOT** associated with jaundice in the newborn?
   A. Galactosemia
   B. Diabetes mellitus in the mother
   C. Breast feeding
   D. Reye's syndrome—hepatic/encephalopathy
   E. Congenital syphilis

92. A 6-hour-old full-term male develops rapid breathing at a rate of 100/min. There are mild substernal retractions and grunting during expiration but no cyanosis. There are clear breath sounds, no rales or rhonchi. Chest x-ray shows prominent pulmonary vascular markings, mild hyperaeration, and mild flattening of the diaphragm. The heart is normal. The **MOST LIKELY** diagnosis is
   A. hyaline membrane disease
   B. transient tachypnea of the newborn
   C. meconium aspiration syndrome
   D. viral pneumonia
   E. congestive heart failure

93. Which one of the following is **NOT** part of the Apgar score?
   A. Blood pressure
   B. Heart rate
   C. Muscle tone
   D. Reflex irritability
   E. Color

94. The scarf sign in the newborn is
   A. a reddening of the neck area from having the umbilical cord wrapped around the neck.
   B. enlargement of the lymphatics in the neck region—cystic hygroma
   C. cyanosis from pulmonary hypertension
   D. accumulation of skin in the chest wall seen in postmature babies
   E. a test to help identify the gestational age of a premature baby

95. Which of the following is **NOT** associated with infants of diabetic mothers?
   A. Spinal agenesis
   B. Hypocalcemia
   C. Transposition of the great vessels
   D. Cataracts
   E. Hyperbilirubinemia

96. A newborn failed the state screening program with values of T_4 of 5.4 and TSH of 448. He is breast-fed and looks well at age 8 days. He is active. He cries with hunger. The physical examination is normal. The repeat findings are $T_4 = 2$, TSH = 476, and TBG = 3.1. Your assessment of these results is
   A. thyroiditis
   B. transient hypothyroidism
   C. immune hypothyroidism
   D. congenital hypothyroidism
   E. normal

97. A patient with anorexia nervosa will have all the following signs or symptoms **EXCEPT**
   A. amenorrhea
   B. fine lanugo hair
   C. bradycardia
   D. constipation
   E. elevated sedimentation rate

98. The accepted treatment of enuresis is
   A. vasopressin analog (DDAVP)
   B. tricyclic antidepressant (Imipramine)
   C. alarm bell set off by moisture

D. counseling parents and child
E. all of the above

99. A 6-year-old does not like school. On further observation, the mother reports these behaviors: increased motor activity, poor sleeping, blurting out answers in class, failure to finish work, and easy distractibility. This condition is **BEST** categorized as
A. autism
B. hyperactivity
C. attention deficit–hyperactivity disorder
D. hyperthyroidism
E. fragile X syndrome

100. A 15-month-old had a first time seizure several hours after the onset of a fever. On physical exam he had an otitis media. The rest of the examination, including the neurological exam, is normal. Which of the following is the **MOST LIKELY** diagnosis?
A. Meningitis
B. Septicemia
C. Pneumococcus
D. Epilepsy
E. Febrile seizure

101. The **USUAL** sequence of sexual maturation in women is
A. breast development, pubic hair, axillary hair
B. axillary hair, pubic hair, breast development
C. breast development, axillary hair, pubic hair
D. pubic hair, breast development, axillary hair
E. pubic hair, axillary hair, breast development

102. A 15-year-old male has large painful breasts. There are no other problems. He has Tanner stage 4 puberty changes. He takes no medications. What is your next step in the assessment or management of him?
A. Estradiol level
B. Testosterone level
C. MR of head
D. Breast biopsy
E. Observation

103. See Figure 5-3. The gram stain of a urethral exudate was obtained in a 16-year-old male. The **MOST LIKELY** diagnosis is
    A. syphilis
    B. gonorrhea
    C. Reiter syndrome
    D. *Herpes genetalis*
    E. chanchroid

104. Which of the following is **TRUE** concerning children's electrocardiograms in comparison with those of adults?
    A. The rate is relatively slower
    B. Variations in the normal are less diverse
    C. The P-R interval is relatively normal
    D. The Q-R-S interval is relatively longer
    E. Sinus arrhythmia is more frequent

105. The majority of children with Down syndrome have _____ chromosomes and are trisomic for number _____ chromosome?
    A. 46, 18
    B. 46, 21
    C. 47, 22

Figure 5-3

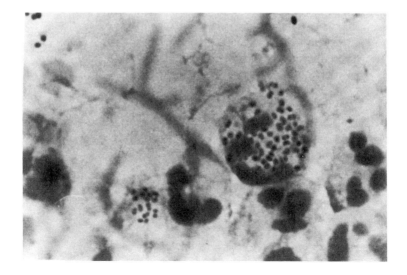

D. 47, 21

E. 38, 20

106. What are the chances that a healthy, term infant will develop clinically evident physiologic jaundice during the first week after birth?
  A. Less than 1%
  B. 5%
  C. 10–15%
  D. 25–50%
  E. Over 80%

107. Specific immune gamma globulin might be used as a prophylaxis in an immunosuppressed subject who is exposed to which of the following?
  A. Mumps
  B. Varicella
  C. Diphtheria
  D. Rabies
  E. Pertussis

108. In prenatal life, which of the following carries oxygenated blood to the inferior vena cava from the umbilical vein?
  A. Foramen ovale
  B. Ductus arteriosis
  C. Umbilical artery
  D. Ductus venosus
  E. None of the above

109. A rash in the inguinal creases and buttocks, which are "beefy red" and macerated with satellite pustules and tiny papules, is **MOST LIKELY**
  A. ringworm
  B. candida albicans diaper rash
  C. contact dermatitis
  D. bullous impetigo
  E. irritant diaper rash

110. A 12-year-old female patient is bothered by "sudden loss of hair." The loss is actually a thinning of the hair rather than total loss. She has been in good health and takes no medication. She was involved in a car accident about three months ago, which was upsetting, but there was no physical injury or trauma to the head. She has a cat and a canary. The **MOST LIKELY** diagnosis is
    A. alopecia areata
    B. alopecia partialis
    C. tinea capitis
    D. telogen effluvium
    E. traction alopecia

111. What type of hemangioma is described **BEST** as "well demarcated, elevated bright red mass composed of numerous coalescing papules or nodules which blanch incompletely with pressure. The deep segment present as ill defined subcutaneous mass often with a bluish hue"?
    A. Nevus flamus
    B. Port wine stain
    C. Strawberry hemangioma
    D. Hemangiosarcoma
    E. Cavernous hemangioma

Questions 112–113: Match the following diagnoses with the appropriate descriptions. Each diagnosis may be used once, more than once, or not at all.

    A. Atopic dermatitis
    B. Contact dermatitis
    C. Seborrheic dermatitis
    D. Histiocytosis X
    E. Lichen planus

112. The **MOST COMMON** childhood disease in which there is a family history of allergies and similar skin lesions; presence of pruritis and lichenification; affected areas include cheeks and extensor surfaces of extremities

113. Begins during the first two months of life; on the head, patches of greasy, yellowish scale which may become worse, progressing to erythematous changes and papules on the forehead; may also be seen on the axillae, neck diaper area, and behind the ears

Questions 114–116: Match the following diagnoses with the appropriate descriptions. Each diagnosis may be used once, more than once, or not at all.

    A. Lyme disease
    B. Juvenile rheumatoid arthritis
    C. Serum sickness
    D. Acute rheumatic fever
    E. Transient synovitis

114. Usually affects children between ages 3 and 6; associated with limp and pain; usually involves the hip, anterior thigh, or knee; temperature is normal or mildly elevated; other symptoms include upper respiratory infection, with limited internal rotation, extension and abduction

115. Starts with a headache, stiff neck myalgia, fatigue, lethargy, and lymphadenopathy; may progress to arthritis of large joints, especially the knees

116. Fever, myalgia, lymphadenopathy, arthralgias, and arthritis following exposure to blood products, drugs, or infectious agents

Questions 117–120: Match the following diseases with the causative agents. Each disease may be used once, more than once, or not at all.

    A. Swimmers' ear
    B. Rocky Mountain spotted fever
    C. Lyme disease
    D. Fitz Hugh Curtis syndrome
    E. Creeping eruption

117. Cutaneous larval migrans

118. Gonococcus

119. *Pseudomonas*

120. *Rickettsia rickettsii*

121. A 16-year-old female has pain in her left hip and knee. She fell on the tennis court yesterday and now cannot walk. The hip is held in external rotation. The **MOST LIKELY** diagnosis is
    A. fracture of the head of the femur
    B. intracapsular hip fracture
    C. contusion of the hip capsule
    D. slipped femoral epiphysis
    E. patellar fracture

Questions 122–123: Match the disease with the site of the genetic defect. Each disease may be used once, more than once, or not at all.

    A. Insulin-dependent diabetes mellitus
    B. Cystic fibrosis
    C. Sickle cell anemia
    D. Maple syrup urine disease
    E. Marfan disease

122. Short arm of chromosome 6

123. Long arm of chromosome 7

124. Siblings of a child with insulin-dependent diabetes mellitus have what percentage probability of developing the disease?
    A. 0%
    B. 5–10%
    C. 25%
    D. 40–50%
    E. 100%

125. Urine that turns purple when ferric chloride is added indicates which situation?
    A. Diabetes
    B. Gaucher disease
    C. Aspirin ingestion
    D. Phenylketonuria
    E. Alkaptonuria

126. Which of the following will cause insulin requirements to **INCREASE** in a child with IDDM?
A. Fever
B. Emotional upset
C. Returning to school after summer camp
D. Addition of corticosteroids
E. All of the above

Questions 127–129: Match the gestational age with the events of the following embryonic developments. Each development may be used once, more than once, or not at all.

A. Limb buds appear
B. Kidneys formed
C. Dermal ridges and creases formed
D. Sex differentiation of internal and external genitalia
E. Return and rotation of intestines into abdominal cavity

127. Day 30 —> limb buds appear

128. Weeks 5–7

129. Week 10

130. A male has mental retardation, high prominent forehead, prominent supraorbital ridges, long narrow face, large ears, prominent mandible, and interstitial fibrosis of the testes. His behavior includes hyperactivity, hand flapping, gaze avoidance, and repetitive behavior. What diagnosis is suggested?
A. Autism
B. William syndrome
C. Burte Sloan syndrome
D. Fragile X syndrome
E. XXY syndrome

Questions 131–135: Match the developmental milestones with the given ages. Each milestone may be used once, more than once, or not at all.

- **A.** Walks alone
- **B.** Stands holding on
- **C.** Waves bye-bye, plays patty cake
- **D.** Says two- to three-word phrases
- **E.** Sits without support, transfers objects

131. 8 months

132. 10 months

133. 12 months

134. 15 months

135. 2 years

136. A 6-month-old has poor growth, hepatomegaly, lymphadenopathy, oral candidiasis, diarrhea, eczema, and low-grade fevers. The **MOST LIKELY** diagnosis is
- **A.** histiocytosis X
- **B.** Gaucher disease
- **C.** IgG deficiency
- **D.** toxoplasmosis
- **E.** HIV infection

Questions 137–141: Match the laboratory findings with the diseases that feature purpura. Each finding may be used once, more than once, or not at all.

- **A.** Normal platelet count, normal megakaryocytes
- **B.** Decreased platelet count, decreased megakaryocytes
- **C.** Decreased platelet count, increased megakaryocytes
- **D.** Decreased platelet count, normal megakaryocytes
- **E.** Normal platelet count, decreased factor VIII

137. Idiopathic thrombocytopenia purpura

138. Aplastic anemia

139. Acute lymphocytic leukemia

140. Von Willebrand disease

141. Anaphylactoid purpura

142. A 1-year-old patient has had a fever as high as 103° F for the past three days. No site of infection was detected. Today there is a rash on both cheeks with circumoral pallor. The **MOST LIKELY** cause of this problem is
    A. unidentifiable viral infection
    B. echoviral infection
    C. parvo viral infection
    D. adenoviral infection
    E. none of the above

143. A 1-year-old has high fevers for four days. Today the fever is gone and a rash appears on the trunk. There is mild redness of the pharynx and mild cervical lymphadenopathy. He is now well except for the rash. The **MOST LIKELY** diagnosis is
    A. scarlet fever
    B. staph scalded skin syndrome
    C. erythema bullosum
    D. roseola
    E. rubeola

144. The baby with a patent ductus arteriosis, cataracts, deafness, and delayed development will **MOST LIKELY** have
    A. toxoplasmosis
    B. rubella
    C. rubeola
    D. cytomegalus
    E. varicella

145. A patient presents with diarrhea associated with abdominal pain, flatus, and nausea. There is no blood in the stool or fever. He lives in a rural area where they have animals, well water, and insecticides. The **MOST LIKELY** cause of his problem is
    A. *shigella*
    B. insecticide poisoning
    C. *salmonella*
    D. ECHO virus
    E. *giardia*

Questions 146–149: Match the toxin with the clinical symptoms. Each toxin may be used once, more than once, or not at all.

    A. Iron
    B. Carbon monoxide
    C. Lead
    D. Insecticide (parathione)
    E. Lidocaine

146. Headache, nausea, confusion, and syncope

147. Nausea and vomiting of blood followed by an asymptomatic period; later abdominal pain, severe bleeding, metabolic acidosis, and shock

148. Cyanotic patient with headache, dizziness, nausea, and dyspnea

149. A patient in "congestive heart failure" with a decreased sensorium

150. Which statement about hydrocarbon ingestion is **NOT TRUE**?
    A. Kerosene absorbed from the GI tract causes CNS and pulmonary symptoms
    B. Hydrocarbons with high volatility will cause CNS damage
    C. The major danger from high-viscosity hydrocarbons is aspiration
    D. Baby oil and motor oils are not toxic unless aspirated in large amounts
    E. Radiographic changes after kerosene ingestion may take 24 hours to develop

Pediatrics

Answer Key

1. C	27. A	53. E	79. C
2. C	28. B	54. A	80. B
3. D	29. B	55. B	81. E
4. D	30. D	56. C	82. B
5. D	31. C	57. E	83. C
6. E	32. F	58. B	84. D
7. C	33. E	59. C	85. D
8. A	34. C	60. D	86. A
9. D	35. B	61. D	87. E
10. C	36. E	62. D	88. E
11. A	37. C	63. B	89. C
12. D	38. E	64. C	90. E
13. B	39. A	65. C	91. D
14. A	40. D	66. D	92. B
15. B	41. C	67. B	93. A
16. C	42. A	68. A	94. E
17. J	43. B	69. B	95. D
18. E	44. C	70. A	96. D
19. B	45. B	71. B	97. E
20. E	46. C	72. E	98. E
21. D	47. D	73. D	99. C
22. D	48. E	74. E	100. E
23. A	49. A	75. D	101. A
24. E	50. C	76. A	102. E
25. B	51. B	77. D	103. B
26. D	52. D	78. B	104. E

105. D	117. E	129. E	141. A
106. D	118. D	130. D	142. C
107. B	119. A	131. E	143. D
108. D	120. B	132. C	144. B
109. B	121. D	133. B	145. E
110. D	122. A	134. A	146. B
111. C	123. B	135. D	147. A
112. A	124. B	136. E	148. E
113. C	125. C	137. C	149. D
114. E	126. E	138. B	150. A
115. A	127. A	139. B	
116. C	128. B	140. E	

Pediatrics

Answers and Comments

1. **(C)** The weight gain of infants averages 20 g/day for the first 6 months and 15 g/day until the first year. They double their birth weight by 4–6 months, and triple the birth weight by a year. They quadruple their weights by two years. (**Ref. 5,** p. 17)

2. **(C)** The head will grow preferentially to the rest of the body when there are inadequate calories. This will cause the head to appear large when the body is small. Caloric deprivation will affect the weight and length before slowing down head growth. (**Ref. 5,** p. 18)

3. **(D)** From the information, this patient is normal. He is within the range of normal size even though he is the shortest in the class. However, many parents want documentation of the diagnosis. This is done with a bone age radiograph, which demonstrates the sequential appearance of ossification of bones in the hands and knee area as the patient ages. This patient will have either a normal or a slightly delayed bone age. If it is slightly delayed, it shows that there is potential for additional growth. The major task is to observe him for determining further growth velocity and the growth achieved in a year. (**Ref. 5,** pp. 130, 133–134, 235)

4. **(D)** The neonate's head size will be about 75% of its total adult size. The rest of its body is only about 25% of its total mature size. (**Ref. 5,** p. 136)

5. **(D)** Daily caloric requirements on a weight basis are highest in infancy and gradually decrease thereafter. By the age of 15, children usually require about 50 cal/kg of body weight. (**Ref. 5,** p. 217)

6. **(E)** The correct answer is the distal femur and proximal tibial epiphyses, cuboid and proximal humeral epiphysis. (**Ref. 5,** p. 133)

7. **(C)** Constitutional growth delay is characterized by normal birth weight and below-average growth velocity in the second year, resulting in short stature in the third year. Then the velocity returns to normal; so the patient grows at a normal rate but is still on the small size. (**Ref. 5,** p. 1573; **Ref. 6,** p. 230)

8. **(A)** Patients with growth hormone deficiency will have satisfactory growth in the first year of life as they react to insulin. Then the grow curve flattens as the failure of the growth hormone takes effect. (**Ref. 5,** p. 1571)

9. **(D)** Cocaine may cause vasoconstriction of placenta and systemic arteries, resulting in premature births in some cases, intracranial bleeding, and seizures. In those infants who are born at term without any major neurologic problem, microcephaly and small size are common findings. Because of poor nutrition in mothers who use cocaine, both problems contribute to the microcephaly and microsomia. (**Ref. 5,** p. 1712)

10. **(C)** Full development of primary dentition occurs from 6 months to 2.5 years. The usual sequence for the primary teeth is central incisor, lateral incisor, first molar, cuspid, and second molar. (**Ref. 5,** pp. 971–975)

11. **(A)** Early in the course of viral meningitis, there may be equal numbers of polys and lymphocytes. In the first six hours, the lymphocytes increase and eventually monocytes predominate. Glucose is normal while protein may be slightly elevated. (**Ref. 5,** p. 1817)

12. **(D)** Studies vary about the percentage of viral and bacterial causes of otitis media. Of the bacterial causes, *Streptococcus pneumoniae* is the most frequent organism. The effect of immu-

nization with *H. influenza* vaccine has decreased this bacterium as a cause otitis media. (**Ref. 5,** p. 940)

13. **(B)** Over 90% of the cases of osteomyelitis are caused by *Staphylococcus aureus* and 5% are from beta hemolytic *Streptococcus*. (**Ref. 5,** p. 563)

14. **(A)** Bronchiolitis, occurring in the winter and spring, is often confused with asthma. It commonly is associated with respiratory syncitial virus. There are edema and inflammation of the small bronchi and bronchioles. (**Ref. 5,** p. 1520)

15. **(B)** Rotavirus is the most important cause of acute gastroenteritis in infants and young children. The incubation period is one to three days. It is spread by the fecal oral route. The peak incidence is in the fall and winter. (**Ref. 5,** p. 670)

16. **(C)** This infection contrasts with tuberculosis infections by involving the cervical nodes, has a PPD-T test that measures 0–15 mm and has a normal chest x-ray. The therapy is the same as for Tb but the mainstay of treatment is excision. (**Ref. 3,** Vol. 14, No. 7, July, 1993; **Ref. 5,** p. 637)

17. **(J)** Impetigo is usually caused by *Staphlococcus* and *Streptococcus pneumoniae* is the second most frequent cause. The order has changed in recent years. Treatment includes careful hand washing, penicillin, dicloxacilin, or erythromycin. (**Ref. 5,** pp. 921–922)

18. **(E)** Shigella diarrhea is associated with high fevers and crampy abdominal pain. Over one-third of patients have a seizure from the neurotoxins, and 40% have blood in the stools. Ampicillin was the major treatment but, as resistance develops, trimethoprim sulfa is more effective. Culture and sensitivity are important guides to the proper treatment. (**Ref. 5,** pp. 605–607)

19. **(B)** Although flank pain can occur in children with urinary tract infections, most UTIs are in the lower tract, producing symptoms of fever and bladder irritability, such as dysuria and frequency. Upper tract infections more frequently occur as part of ureteral reflux and congenital anomalies. The upper tract infections may

be serious, leading to renal failure, while lower tract infections do not affect renal function. (**Ref. 5,** p. 1289)

20. **(E)** Once the patient is immunized with tetanus toxoid, the booster should occur every 10 years. With clean minor wounds, the 10-year schedule is satisfactory. If the wound is dirty, neglected, or had poor circulation in the area, dT should be given if the last toxoid were given 5 years ago. (**Ref. 4,** p. 462; **Ref. 5,** p. 624)

21. **(D)** Dermoid cysts or cystic teratomas in adolescent girls are the most common ovarian tumor in children or adolescents. These tumors contain tissue from all three germ layers, including skin, hair, and sebaceous glands. They may enlarge and produce symptoms of torsion or peritonitis. (**Ref. 6,** pp. 153–154)

22. **(D)** Some patients will have hemorrhage or sepsis as the presenting signs, but most have slow onset of symptoms such as pallor, easy bruisability, lethargy, anorexia, malaise, intermittent fever bone pain, arthralgia, abdominal pain. Joint pain is often diagnosed as rheumatoid arthritis or traumatic injury when it is the first sign of acute lymphoblastic leukemia with involvement of the bone marrow in the area. Bone marrow examination will provide the information for diagnosis. Sometimes bone marrow aspiration is difficult because of the tightly packed marrow or fibrosis of the marrow. (**Ref. 5,** p. 1187)

23. **(A)** Chromosome abnormalities are found in almost 100% of AML cases. In the adult form of chronic myelogenous leukemia, the Philadelphia chromosome is present in 90% of the cases. These genetic characteristics correlate with the treatment success of some subtypes of these forms of leukemia. Most of the cases of leukemia in children are acute lymphoblastic leukemia. (**Ref. 5,** pp. 1192–1193)

24. **(E)** When periorbital metastasis occurs, proptosis and periorbital ecchymosis ("black eyes") occurs. Neuroblastoma, arising from the neural crest tissue, is the most common extracranial solid tumor in childhood. It commonly arises in either the adrenal gland or in the paraspinal area. The other common abdominal tumor, Wilms tumor, arises in the kidney. Neuroblastoma metastasizes to lymph nodes, bone marrow, liver, skin, the orbits, and bone. It pro-

duces catecholamines such as vanillylmandellic acid (VMA) and homovanillic acid (HVA). (**Ref. 6,** pp. 577, 1201–1203)

25. **(B)** Ewing sarcoma, the second most common bone tumor in children, accounts for about 30% of primary bone tumors. Osteogenic sarcoma, or osteosarcoma, is the most common bone tumor. The most common sites of involvement in Ewing sarcoma is the pelvis proximal extremities, upper tibia, and rib. The patients present with pain and soft tissue mass. If the lesions are in the vertebrae, there may be neurologic defects. The classic radiographic finding is a lytic, destructive bone lesion with laminar perisoteal reaction, which results in the classic onion skin appearance. (**Ref. 5,** pp. 1205–1206)

26. **(D)** The MCV (mean corpuscular volume) is a good way to start the investigation of a patient with anemia. The causes of anemia with low MCV are iron deficiency, chronic disease, lead poisoning, thalassemia, and thalassemia trait, spherocytosis. Malabsorption of iron from the GI tract is uncommon. Folic acid deficiency will cause a high MCV. Sickle cell anemia has many sized cells as well as reticulocytes that contribute to the high MCV. Aplastic anemia is usually associated with normal MCV. (**Ref. 5,** p. 1097)

27. **(A)** Von Willebrand disease has platelet dysfunction and decreased level of factor VIII. The von Willebrand factor promotes platelet adhesion to exposed vascular collagen and transports factor VIII. Patients typically have nosebleeds and easy bruisability. Menorrhagia is often a problem in affected females. (**Ref. 5,** p. 1164)

28. **(B)** Sickle cell anemia occurs when valine replaces glutamic acid on the 6th position on the beta globulin chain of hemoglobin. The molecule then leads to polymerization of the sickle hemoglobin. Sickling leads to chronic hemolysis with an increased risk of infection and painful crises. Sickle cell anemia occurs in 1 in 600 African-Americans, and the trait appears in 1 in 12. Other forms include sickle thalassemia and sickle hemoglobin C. (**Ref. 5,** p. 1122; **Ref. 6,** pp. 447–457)

29. **(B)** Thalassemia stems from the abnormal synthesis of one of the globulin polypeptide chains. Alpha thalassemia is usually

caused by deletion of one or more globulin genes, while beta thalassemia may also be due to gene deletion. The chronic hemolysis causes the bone marrow to produce more red cells. This increase in production leads to hypertrophy of the bone marrow and cosmetic changes of prominent forehead and maxillary bones as well as malocclusion problems. As the hemolysis progresses, the spleen enlarges, causing abdominal pain, lumbar lordosis, and anorexia. The chronic anemia will strain the heart, producing cardiac dilatation. (**Ref. 5,** p. 1129)

30. **(D)** Idiopathic (immune) thrombocytopenia is an acquired platelet disorder of childhood. Platelets from patients with ITP typically show increased amounts of IgG associated with the platelet membrane in vitro. In some, antiplatelet antibodies can be detected by Western Blot techniques. The PT and PTT are normal. Bleeding and mucosal bleeding are the most prominent symptoms. Severe abdominal pain and generalized adenopathy are not likely to be seen in patients with ITP. (**Ref 2,** p. 1689)

31. **(C)** Hemophilia A, classic hemophilia, or factor VIII deficiency involves males with some female carriers having decreased levels of factor VIII. Severe cases have less than 1% of factor VIII, while moderate cases have from 1 to 5% factor VIII. The PTT level is elevated; clotting time is prolonged only in severe cases. (**Ref. 5,** pp. 1162–1163)

32. **(F)** Attention deficit–hyperactivity disorder involves a series of behaviors including restlessness, distractibility, impulsive behavior, excessive talking, interruptions, and engaging in dangerous activities. The children with ADHD present problems in schools when they are expected to follow classroom routine. Ideally the children need a team evaluation to rule out other medical problems and develop a treatment plan. There are no major neurological problems, although minor or soft signs may be present, but have no significance. Routine CT or EEG are not necessary for diagnosis. Treatment includes educational programs, family counseling, and, in many cases, drugs such as methyphenidate (Ritalin). (**Ref. 6,** pp. 718–723)

33. **(E)** Autism consists of three primary characteristics: social indifference or failure to develop normal social responses; absent

or abnormal speech and language development; and restricted, stereotyped responses to objects. Most autistic children have IQs of less than 70. The cause is unknown. (**Ref. 6,** pp. 710–714)

34. (**C**)   Lesch-Nyhan syndrome, a disorder of purine metabolism, is characterized by mental retardation, cerebral palsy, choreoathetosis, and self-destructive behavior. They classically bite themselves and can destroy lips or amputate fingers. The X-linked disease is produced by abnormal activity of HGPRT-hypoxanthine guanine phosphoribosyl transferase enzyme, which results in high levels of uric acid in the blood and in the urine, gouty arthritis, hematuria, and renal calculi. (**Ref. 5,** p. 318)

35. (**B**)   This generalized seizure disorder also known as absence seizures appears as momentary lapses in awareness with amnesia. There is no warning or postictal state. (**Ref. 5,** p. 1771)

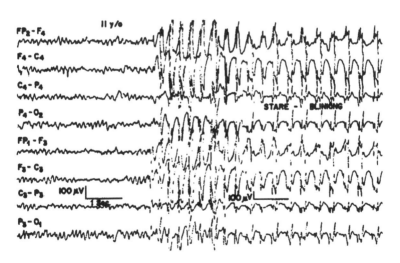

Figure 5-4 (*Source:* Rudolph.)

36. (**E**)   The definition of cerebral palsy (CP) concentrates on the nonprogressive motor defects, not intelligence. While many children have no known cause, some will have a history notable for events such as meningitis, maternal drug use, head trauma, and asphyxia. Two main groups, spastic and nonspastic CP, correlate

somewhat with the location of the brain defects: Spastic CP involves the motor cortex, nonspastic in the other areas. Associated disabilities include strabismus, feeding and speech disorders, motor disabilities, constipation, orthopedic deformities, and behavior difficulties. (**Ref. 6,** pp. 672–682)

37. **(C)** The degree of central nervous system difficulties is related to the spinal level of the myelomeningocele; the lower the lesion, the less disruption of function. There is an associated hydrocephalus, which may be congenital, acquired, or not present. The dislocated hips arise from muscle paralysis and imbalance of opposing muscle groups around the hips. Neurogenic bladder dysfunctions lead to urinary retention and infection. (**Ref. 6,** pp. 660–671)

38. **(E)** Ganglioside G_{m2} buildup in the neurons secondary to hexosaminidase A deficiency will cause the neurologic problems seen in Tay Sachs disease. After four to five months of normal development, the patient will have a startle reaction to loud noises. The head becomes enlarged and a cherry red spot is seen in the macula. This is followed by seizures and hyperactive reflexes, and later by blindness and deafness. Death occurs before the fourth year. (**Ref. 5,** p. 357)

39. **(A)** Acute cerebellar ataxia and acute cerebritis often follow varicella, mycoplasma, and other viral infections such as enterovirus, influenza virus, myxovirus. It may also be secondary to acute labyrinthitis and drug intoxication. Brain tumors and hydrocephalus—rare causes—must be considered in the differential diagnosis. Patients with these later conditions will have papilledema and headaches. In those problems associated with varicella and other viruses, the duration of ataxia is limited in time. There is no evidence of papilledema and no characteristic laboratory abnormalities. (**Ref. 5,** p. 1821)

40. **(D)** Bilirubin levels greater than 25–30 mg/dL are associated with kernicterus or bilirubin encephalopathy. The basal ganglia are particularly susceptible to the toxic effects of bilirubin. Damage results in choreoathetosis, tremors, oculomotor paralysis, and spasticity. (**Ref. 2,** pp. 449, 2120)

41. (C)   Normal pressures in the infant's heart are: right atrium mean pressure, 2–6; right ventricle, 15–25/2–5; left atrium mean pressure, 5–10; left ventricle, 8–130/5–10. (**Ref. 5**, p. 1337)

42. (A)   Usually asymptomatic, this lesion is characterized by a systolic ejection murmur best heard at the left mid- and upper sternal borders. The murmur is preceded by a loud S1. It is followed by a widely split, fixed S2, which is due to increased right ventricular diastolic volume and prolonged ejection time. (**Ref. 1**, p. 1170; **Ref. 5**, p. 1369)

43. (B)   Patent ductus arteriosus is often associated with a machinery-like murmur which begins in early systole and ends in late diastole. It may radiate to the left clavicle or down the left sternal border. Additionally, this lesion is associated with a wide pulse pressure and bounding arterial pulsations. (**Ref. 1**, p. 1173; **Ref. 5**, p. 1361)

44. (C)   Most children with this lesion will be asymptomatic. On routine physical examination, there is usually a systolic ejection murmur at the upper left sternal border, which radiates to the neck and down the sternal border. It is usually accompanied by a thrill over the suprasternal notch. (**Ref. 1**, p. 1180; **Ref. 5**, p. 1379)

45. (B)   Clinical manifestations of rheumatic fever include carditis, polyarthritis, subcutaneous nodules, chorea, and a rash referred to as erythema marginatum. The diagnosis is typically made with the guidance of Jones criteria, which include the manifestations above, as well as arthralgia, fever, and elevated sedimentation rate. Evidence of recent streptococcal infection, along with specified Jones criteria, indicates a high probability of acute rheumatic fever. (**Ref. 5**, p. 493)

Erythema nodosum is the appearance of painful, erythematous, subcutaneous nodules usually found on the extensor surfaces of the arms and legs. In the United States, the most common cause of this disease is streptococcal infection; however, it has been associated with a wide variety of drugs and diseases, including penicillin and sulfonamides, syphilis, tuberculosis, and sarcoidosis. (**Ref. 5**, pp. 425, 827)

46. (C) At birth, there is a transition from fetal circulation to adult-type circulation in the normal newborn. Many changes occur, including a decrease in pulmonary artery pressure, closure of the ductus arteriosus, obliteration of the ductus venosus, and closure of the foramen ovale. Following closure of the ductus arteriosus and a decrease in pulmonary vascular resistance, the pressure in the right ventricle decreases. Pressure in the left atrium and the left ventricle increase as a result of increased pulmonary blood flow and pulmonary venous return. The increase in the left atrial pressure is believed to facilitate the closure of the foramen ovale. (**Ref. 1,** pp. 1144–1145)

47. (D) Chronic pyelonephritis may cause inflammation in the parenchyma of the kidney with local obliteration of blood vessels. Ischemia, which results from decreased renal perfusion, stimulates increased renin secretion. Renin causes an increase in angiotensin II production, which leads to subsequent vasoconstriction and hypertension. 17-hydroxycorticosteroids are excreted in the urine, and are useful in the measurement of daily glucocorticoid production. They are elevated in a form of congenital adrenal hyperplasia, called 11-hydroxylase deficiency. Leucocidin is a substance produced by some bacteria that destroys leukocytes. Atrial natriuretic factor is produced in response to an increase in extracellular volume. It causes a marked natriuresis, decreases blood pressure, and inhibits secretion of renin and vasopressin. Ergotamine is a substance that is most often used to treat migraine headaches. (**Ref. 2,** pp. 1830–1831, 2004)

48. (E) Though tetralogy of Fallot is the most common cyanotic heart lesion in patients with congenital heart disease who survive beyond infancy, transposition of the great arteries is the most common cause of cyanosis in the neonate. In this lesion, the aortic root arises from the right ventricle and the main pulmonary artery arises from the left ventricle. Patent ductus arteriosus is considered a left-to-right shunt, and blood flows from the aorta to the pulmonary artery. It is not a cyanotic heart lesion. In hypoplastic left heart syndrome, there is underdevelopment of the entire left heart. Affected patients present with varying degrees of cyanosis and heart failure. Pulmonary hypertension of the newborn describes the persistence of fetal circulation and is characterized by cyanosis and respiratory distress. It is often associated with infection, central nervous system abnormalities, polycythemia, and pulmonary parenchymal disorders. (**Ref. 5,** pp. 1270, 1306, 1314, 1322, 1393)

49. **(A)** Kawasaki disease is characterized by fever for at least five days, conjunctivitis, changes of the oropharyngeal mucosa, cervical adenopathy, and rash. Within the first two weeks of illness, 10 to 40% of affected children will have evidence of coronary vasculitis. The cardiovascular lesions most typically associated with this disease are coronary artery aneurysms. Second-degree heart block is very uncommon in children; however, arrhythmias are seen in Kawasaki disease, as are pericarditis, myocarditis, endocarditis, and heart failure.

The term *myocardiopathy* or *cardiomyopathy* refers to heart muscle disease that exists in the absence of congenital heart disease, abnormal coronary arteries, valvular disease, and hypertension. It may be either primary or secondary to a variety of systemic diseases. Pulmonary venous hypertension may result from lesions, including congenital mitral stenosis and mitral insufficiency; primary pulmonary hypertension is of unknown etiology. Aortitis, which typically involves the thoracic aorta, is a common manifestation of tertiary syphilis. (**Ref. 1,** pp. 629, 1183, 1210)

50. **(C)** The newborn heart rate has a normal range of 90–160 bpm, with an average awake heart rate of 120–130 bpm. At rest, the heart rate may drop as low as 100 bpm, and may occasionally drop to 80 bpm. Newborns with heart rates greater than 160 bpm are considered to be tachycardic. Persistent tachycardia and bradycardia require further investigation since they may be early signs of heart disease, sepsis, or other conditions. (**Ref. 5,** p. 119)

51. **(B)** Murmurs not associated with significant hemodynamic abnormalities are referred to as functional or innocent murmurs. On routine examination they are present in over 30% of children. The most common is a medium-pitched, vibratory systolic ejection murmur. Others include innocent pulmonic murmurs that are high-pitched and early-systolic, and venous hums caused by turbulence of blood in the jugular system. A high-pitched "sea gull"–type murmur is an example of an innocent murmur. Diastolic murmurs are not considered to be innocent murmurs, and are found in a number of cardiac lesions. Examples include pulmonary valve insufficiency (associated

with a high-pitched blowing diastolic murmur along the left sternal border), mitral stenosis (associated with a long diastolic rumbling murmur at the apex), and mitral insufficiency (often associated with a rumbling mid-diastolic murmur at the apex). (**Ref. 1,** p. 1132; **Ref. 5,** p. 1321)

52. **(D)** Cocaine and its free base form, crack, cause vasoconstriction and coronary spasm. Crack has been associated with angina, cardiac arrhythmias, and sudden death. Heroin has minimal effects on the cardiovascular system. Marijuana causes tachycardia in new and experienced users; it also causes mild elevations in systolic and diastolic blood pressures. Acute ingestions of hallucinogens, such as LSD and PCP ("angel dust") are associated with cardiac arrhythmias and hypertension. (**Ref. 5,** pp. 747, 753, 756)

53. **(E)** Cystic fibrosis is a genetic disease associated with dysfunction of the exocrine glands. There is failure to clear mucous secretions, a paucity of water in mucous secretions, elevated salt content of sweat and other secretions, and chronic respiratory infection. Clinical manifestations include nasal polyposis, sinusitis, pneumonia, reactive airway disease, pancreatitis associated with decreased trypsin production and diabetes, meconium ileus, intussusception, and failure to thrive. (**Ref. 1,** p. 1106; **Ref. 2,** p. 1491)

54. **(A)** Adenovirus may cause cough, coryza, pharyngitis, conjunctivitis, pneumonia, and fever in infants and children. Chlamydial pneumonia occurs during the first six months of life, and presents with cough, tachypnea, but no fever. (**Ref. 5,** p. 577)

55. **(B)** *Staphylococcus aureus* causes a necrotizing pneumonitis, complicated by empyema, pneumatoceles, bronchopleural fistulas, and pyopneumothorax. In children, mycobacterium tuberculosis may cause asymptomatic illness. Reactivation tuberculosis is uncommon in children, and is referred to as adult pulmonary tuberculosis. It is associated with low-grade fever, cavitation, productive cough, and at times mild hemoptysis.
    Klebsiella pneumoniae causes pneumonia in debilitated or immunosuppressed patients, and is unusual in otherwise healthy infants and children. It may have a fulminant course, associated with purulent secretions, cavitations, and pulmonary abscesses. (**Ref. 1,** pp. 704, 765, 1081)

56. **(C)** Asthma is characterized by recurrent episodes of wheezing, coughing, and dyspnea. The wheezing is classically expiratory since there is difficulty expelling air from the bronchioles. Those who develop asthma in the first two decades of life are more likely to have associated atopic diseases, such as allergic rhinitis. Allergic rhinitis is associated with dark circles under the eyes.

Exposure to air pollutants, allergens, and tobacco smoke may increase airway hyperreactivity in patients with asthma. Some may have asthma that is induced only by exercise. During an acute exacerbation, expiratory wheezes are prominent, but inspiratory wheezes may also be present. Nasal polyps are associated with immotile cilia syndrome and cystic fibrosis, aspirin sensitivity, and allergies. (**Ref. 5**, pp. 436–437)

57. **(E)** A barky cough in a 6-week-old male is concerning for the diagnosis of a congenital disorder, such as a vascular ring. Vascular rings around the trachea and esophagus occur and produce varying degrees of compression. Other associated symptoms include wheezing and vomiting.

Viral croup is usually seen in infants and children, ages 3 months to 5 years. Classically, the patient presents with barky cough and stridor. The diagnosis of tracheoesophageal fistula is typically made in the newborn period when the infant has choking, cyanosis, or coughing with an attempted feed. Of the five major forms, esophageal atresia with distal tracheoesophageal fistula occurs most commonly (seen in 87% of patients with tracheoesophageal fistula). Pulmonary sequestration refers to a nonfunctioning embryonic and cystic pulmonary tissue that receives its entire blood supply from the systemic circulation. On physical exam, patients with this lesion may have dullness to percussion and decreased breath sounds in the area of the sequestration. Bronchiolitis occurs during the first two years of life and is characterized by a paroxysmal wheezy cough, dyspnea, and irritability. (**Ref. 1**, pp. 941–942, 1063, 1065, 1075, 1183)

58. **(B)** Surfactant is a mixture of phospholipids and proteins, and appears in the amniotic fluid at approximately 30 weeks gestation. It reduces surface tension in the airspaces of the lung. When there is a deficiency, as in premature infants, surface tension is high at the interface between alveolar gas and the alveolar wall. This results in progressive atelectasis and the development of hyaline membrane disease. Alpha-1 antitrypsin deficiency is an inherited autosomal recessive condition that involves the lungs and liver of affected patients. Peripheral eosinophils are low in all newborns. Mast cells are specialized cells that play a role in atopic diseases. Elastin is a yellow, elastic fibrous mucoprotein that is found in the connective tissue of elastic structures. It may be overproduced in patients with Hurler syndrome. (**Ref. 1**, p. 1036; **Ref. 5**, pp. 431, 1069, 1382, 1438)

59. **(C)** The main causes of pulmonary hypertension are left ventricular failure and increased pulmonary resistance with or without increased pulmonary blood flow. Clinically these patients will have a loud pulmonary component of the second heart sound. Often a systolic ejection click is present. As the hypertension continues, there will be tricuspid regurgitation. The EKG will show peaked P waves, contrasted with the notched P wave seen in left atrial hypertrophy. (**Ref. 5**, pp. 1325, 1388–1389)

60. **(D)** The forced expiratory volume at 1 sec FEV_1 detects the abnormality in air flow measurements in patients with asthma. There are inexpensive peak flow meters that can be used at home to detect early changes from asthma. (**Ref. 5**, p. 507)

61. **(D)** *Clostridium botulinum* will interfere with the cholinergic transmission of nerves by interfering with the release of acetylcholine in response to nerve stimulation. Epidemics have been associated with ingestion of honey and with breast feeding. The usual incubation period for food-borne botulism is 12–36 hours (range 6 hours to 8 days). A toxin neutralization bioassay in mice is used to identify *botulinum* toxin in serum stool or foods. In infants *C. botulinum* or toxin can be detected in stools. Toxin is found in only 10% of cases. Electromyography can also be used to demonstrate a characteristic pattern of brief, small, abundant motor action potentials. (**Ref. 4**, p. 161)
    Treatment requires admission to the intensive care for observation and possible ventilatory support. Although boulinum antitoxin is available, it is not usually given to infants since it might induce lifelong sensitivity to equine antigens and there is no evidence that it is effective for infants. Antibiotics do not improve the paralysis. (**Ref. 4**, pp. 160–162)

62. (D) Macroglossia is seen in hypothyroidism, glycogen storage disease, Beckwith-Wiedemann syndrome (macrosomia, macroglossia omphalocele, facial hemangioma, and mental retardation). Anatomical changes secondary to abnormalities of the lymphatic or arteriovenous malformations will cause large tongues. Endocardial fibroelastosis is a rare cardiac problem where the ventricles or atria are lined with a thick white tissue. (**Ref. 5,** pp. 1416, 1470)

63. (B) The supply of vitamins is usually adequate in infant formula or breast milk. Breast-fed infants not exposed to sunlight will need vitamin D. Fluoride does not pass through breast milk; so all breast-fed babies need supplemental fluoride. Iron is needed by 4–6 months in the form of iron drops or iron-fortified cereal. (**Ref. 5,** pp. 237, 1644)

64. (C) The recommendation from the Academy of Pediatrics is 115 kcal/kg/d from 0 to 6 months and 105 kcal/kg/d from 7 to 12 months. For premature infants the requirement is 120 kcal/kg/d. (**Ref. 5,** p. 241)

65. (C) A good rule of thumb for estimating calorie needs is 1000 kcal plus 100 for each year. (**Ref. 5,** p. 341)

66. (D) Delta hepatitis is coinfective with hepatitis B. Chronic carriers of hepatitis B are at risk of chronic liver disease caused by hepatitis delta virus. (**Ref. 5,** p. 673)

67. (B) Hepatitis B infection was first documented by blood transfusions but later by sexual transmission, oral routes such as human bites, and during delivery. Because the carrier rate is high, especially in Asia and Africa (10–15%), hepatitis B is a major health problem. The recent recommendation to start immunization against hepatitis B is an attempt to protect infants from hepatitis B and its chronic carrier state, which can cause liver cancer. (**Ref. 5,** pp. 672–673)

68. (A) Hepatitis A is spread by the fecal oral route. Epidemics are found in areas with infected shellfish and in countries with poor sanitation. (**Ref. 5,** p. 672)

69. **(B)** Ninety percent of patients infected with hepatitis B recover; the remaining 10% develop persistent antigenemia. The presence of HBsAg for more than 6 months is indicative of the chronic carrier state. In chronic active hepatitis cases, most are HBsAg-negative. These cases are mainly females who respond to corticosteroids, have high titers to smooth muscle antibodies, and negative HBs antigen and antibody. Cases of chronic active hepatitis that are HBsAg-positive are typically males, do not respond to corticosteroids, and are often positive to the HBs antibody. **(Ref. 5,** p. 1077)

70. **(A)** With more sophisticated and specific tests available, the type of bilirubin—conjugated or unconjugated—provides clues, not diagnoses of the cause of jaundice. In general, the hemolytic anemias cause elevation of the indirect or unconjugated bilirubin. Finding a direct bilirubin would make one think of biliary obstruction or sepsis. Reye syndrome is not associated with jaundice. **(Ref. 5,** pp. 1054–1059)

71. **(B)** Unfortunately, the laboratory tests are not specific for acute pancreatitis. The classic changes are early elevation of amylase and then elevated lipase. There are many cases of acute pancreatitis, as seen on ultrasound with a large pancreas and decreased density, with normal amylase levels. Most cases of pancreatitis are idiopathic, related to infection, trauma, and congenital anomalies. **(Ref. 5,** pp. 1044–1045)

72. **(E)** The causes of splenomegaly include hemolytic disease (thalassemia, spherocytosis), inflammatory and infectious diseases (malaria, SBE, TB, lupus), and malignancy (leukemia, lymphoma, Hodgkin disease). Except for neuroblastoma, few solid malignancies metastasize to the spleen. **(Ref. 5,** p. 1153)

73. **(D)** This anomaly occurs in about 2% of people. It stems from the residual omphalomesenteric or vitelline duct, which connects the yolk sac to the midintestinal area. About 50% are asymptomatic but gastric mucosa (seen in 35% of patients) in the diverticulum can produce gastrointestinal bleeding and anemia. Technetium pertechnetate nuclear scans are diagnostic in 85 to 90% of the cases. **(Ref. 5,** p. 1033)

74. **(E)** Hemolytic uremic syndrome (HUS), characterized by hemolytic anemia, thrombocytopenia, and renal insufficiency, usually starts with a mild illness with cough, vomiting, and mild diarrhea. When the child becomes markedly ill with hemolysis, bleeding, and decreased platelets, three systems are involved: the kidney, gastrointestinal tract, and brain. The symptoms include anemia, purpura, and bleeding in the kidneys, intestines, and brain. The peripheral smear shows burr and helmet cells, along with schistocytes. The urine will show red cells, protein, and red cell casts. The patient may be anuric for several days to many weeks. Usually, the anuria lasts about two weeks. Many cases are associated with an *E. coli* infection. Some patients will be confused with ulcerative colitis. (**Ref. 5**, pp. 1028, 1264)

75. **(D)** Hookworm infection is caused by either *Necator americanus* or *Ancylostoma duodenale,* which are found most commonly in the southern United States. The initial infection is characterized by a skin rash, followed by a cough, low-grade fever, acute abdominal disturbance, intermittent diarrhea, and eosinophilia. Symptoms depend on the nutritional status of the patient and the number of reinfections. The diagnosis is made by finding ova in the stool. Most infections are not significant clinically unless the number of ova is high when the patient develops anemia. (**Ref. 5**, p. 722)

76. **(A)** Inflammatory bowel disease includes both Crohn disease and ulcerative colitis. Crohn disease frequently involves the ileocecal area. It typically presents with diarrhea and weight loss. Patients may have periumbilical pain, which is increased with meals. They may also have abscesses or bowel perforation. Ulcerative colitis usually presents with rectal bleeding and a change in bowel consistency. Abdominal pain, fever, weight loss, and anemia are other symptoms or signs. Many clinical and laboratory features are similar in the two conditions. Endoscopy and radiologic studies help differentiate the two problems. (**Ref. 5**, pp. 1022–1025)

77. **(D)** Congenital aganglionic megacolon (Hirschsprung disease) may present in the newborn period with bowel obstruction but is usually diagnosed in childhood because of failure to thrive, irri-

tability, poor feeding, and constipation. The rectal examination will show an empty rectum. Barium enema will show a narrowed area where there are no ganglion cells. Biopsy of the involved area will help establish the diagnosis. (**Ref. 5,** p. 1039)

78. **(B)**   In children, juvenile intestinal polyps are the most frequent cause of intestinal bleeding in the 2 to 5-year-old age group. In the first year of life, the leading cause of rectal bleeding is anal fissures, usually associated with passage of large stools. GI infections at any age may cause bleeding. (**Ref. 6,** pp. 333–336)

79. **(C)**   Minimal dehydration (3–5%) is characterized by dry mucous membranes and thirst. Moderate dehydration 5–7% includes loss of fluid around the eyes and dry skin, which may tent. The patient with severe dehydration will have tachycardia, oliguria, and marked decrease in skin turgor. (**Ref. 5,** p. 231)

80. **(B)**   In a patient with vomiting, there is a loss of hydrogen and chloride in addition to dehydration. The decreased intravascular volume will stimulate the renin-angiotensin-aldosterone secretion, which conserves sodium and increases the excretion of potassium. The sodium is conserved as sodium bicarbonate. This results in an increase in the bicarbonate level and a metabolic alkalosis. (**Ref. 5,** p. 229)

81. **(E)**   Status asthmaticus indicates that a person with asthma is unresponsive to initial therapy or is at risk for respiratory failure. There is airway narrowing and varying degrees of airway obstruction, resulting in ventilation-perfusion mismatch and subsequent hypoxemia. In moderate case, hyperventilation leads to respiratory alkalosis and hypocapnia. The blood gas in answer B is a normal blood gas. Answer C represents combined respiratory and metabolic acidosis as well as hypoxemia. This is a blood gas one might see in a burn victim, who suffers from volume loss and smoke inhalation. In answer D there is evidence of hypoxemia and a metabolic acidosis, as may be seen in a patient with sepsis. (**Ref. 5,** p. 509–510)

82. **(B)**   The renin-angiotensin system starts in the kidney where renin is made in the juxtaglomerular apparatus. Renin acts on angiotensin, which is made in the liver to produce angiotensin I,

which, in turn, is converted to angiotensin II in the lung. Angiotensin II is a vasoconstrictor. (**Ref. 5,** p. 1231)

83. **(C)** The most common causes of abdominal masses in the newborn are both renal, ureteropelvic obstruction (UPJ) and multicystic kidneys. Other renal causes are renal vein thrombosis and tumors. Both Wilms tumor and neuroblastoma are rare in the newborn and more common in older infants. UPJ can occur at any age either as a mass or as hematuria. Multicystic kidneys are dysplastic kidneys with few functional glomeruli and no significant function. (**Ref. 5,** p. 174)

84. **(D)** The infant's kidney can perform many of the complicated functions needed for the maintenance of body water and electrolytes. It cannot match the adult kidney's ability to concentrate. While the adult can produce concentrated urine of 1200 mOsm, the infant can concentrate only to 700–800 mOsm. When the infant has a fever or has gastrointestinal losses, this limitation becomes clinically significant. (**Ref. 5,** p. 1233)

85. **(D)** Recurrent microvascular thromboses secondary to sickling of the red blood cells in the renal arterioles will cause hematuria, reduced concentrating ability, and proteinuria. With repeated episodes, chronic nephritis may develop in older patients. Classically, papillary necrosis, with sloughing of the renal papilla and massive hematuria, will develop. Fortunately, this a rare occurrence, although hematuria is quite common. (**Ref. 5,** p. 1276)

86. **(A)** In acute poststreptococcal glomerulonephritis, complement binds to the immune complexes consisting of the antigen and antibody. This will depress the complement levels about two weeks after the streptococcal infection. The serum complement returns to normal four to six weeks after the drop in complement. In acute nephritis, the urinary sodium may be elevated, the renin may be increased, the kidneys may be large, and the cholesterol is normal. (**Ref. 5,** pp. 1260–1262)

87. **(E)** Childhood nephrotic syndrome has no known cause in most cases. In adults, there are few idiopathic cases, while most are associated with systemic diseases such as diabetes, drugs, hepati-

tis, and collagen disease. The few cases in children with known causes include hemolytic uremic syndrome, anaphylactoid purpura, drugs, lymphomas, and hepatitis. Most have a poor prognosis, while the idiopathic cases have a good prognosis, eventually. (**Ref. 6,** p. 580)

88. **(E)** Childhood nephrotic syndrome (minimal change nephrosis, nil disease) is characterized by proteinuria, edema, low serum albumin, and high serum cholesterol. It is most frequently seen in children 1 to 3 years of age. In contrast to adults, most cases in children are idiopathic. They usually respond to corticosteroids and most cases eventually will be cured. Renal biopsies will show normal glomeruli on routine light microscopy studies. On electron microscopy, the basement membrane will lose the foot processes. (**Ref. 5,** p. 1276; **Ref. 6,** p. 583)

89. **(C)** As little as two drinks of alcohol a day may produce these defects. All pregnant women should avoid alcohol. These patients with fetal alcohol syndrome also may have developmental delay, mental retardation, and hyperactivity. (**Ref. 5,** p. 438)

90. **(E)** In an otherwise healthy infant, any one of these findings alone would not suggest serious pathology. An umbilical hernia is related to the underdeveloped periumbilical musculature of the anterior abdominal wall. It usually closes before age 5. Diastasis recti is a gap between the abdominal rectus muscles in the midline, and it closes with increased use of the abdominal muscles. A single umbilical artery occurs in 1% of newborns. Of these newborns, 15% have other anomalies that are obvious to the examiner. Isolated cleft lip is not associated with other serious lesions. In cases such as in this question, other defects are rarely encountered. (**Ref. 5,** p. 173)

91. **(D)** Metabolic diseases such as galactosemia and diabetes, as well as congenital infections such as syphilis, cause jaundice as the liver becomes affected by the primary disease. Breast feeding is associated with prolonged jaundice in infants in 1 of 200 births, starting gradually and peaking in the second or third week. It is not associated with kernicterus. In Reye syndrome, hepatic failure and encephalopathy occur in older children. The liver loses its many functions but there is no jaundice. (**Ref. 5,** pp. 1054–1057)

92. **(B)** This description of the newborn with rapid respirations and no other major findings suggests transient tachypnea of the newborn (TTN) or persistent postnatal pulmonary edema. Not all infants have tachypnea, and some may have the fluid enter the lungs postnatally. There may be cyanosis, which clears with supplemental oxygen. TTN usually resolves by day 3 or 4. Abnormal breath sounds and radiographs will help diagnose the other conditions. **(Ref. 5,** pp. 1483–1485)

93. **(A)** Virginia Apgar devised this rating scale to measure the degree of intrapartum stress at birth. Most normal infants have a score of 8–10 at 5 min. Commonly there is a deduction in the score for cyanotic extremities. Most developmentalists rely on the 5-min score to help identify infants who may be at risk for neurological problems. **(Ref. 5,** p. 193, note the error on p. 193 under Apgar score, line 5)

94. **(E)** This sign is elicited by pulling the hand across the chest wall to the opposite shoulder. In a 28-week-old newborn, the elbow can reach the other shoulder. At 32 weeks there is some resistance. At 36 weeks, the elbow just passes the midline, and in full-term babies, the elbow does not reach the midline. The other features of the Dubowitz tests are: posture, heel-to-ear maneuver, popliteal angle, dorsiflexion angle of the foot, and return to flexion of the forearm. **(Ref. 5,** p. 176)

95. **(D)** Infants of mothers who have diabetes are prone to many problems including congenital anomalies, macrosomia, respiratory distress, low serum glucose and calcium, hyperbilirubinemia, polycythemia, persistent pulmonary hypertension syndrome, and cardiomyopathy. The congenital anomalies more frequently involve the heart (VSD and transposition of the great vessels) and the spinal agenesis–caudal regression syndrome. **(Ref. 5,** pp. 203–205)

96. **(D)** The signs of hypothyroidism in the newborn are absent or subtle. Some may have prolonged jaundice, transient hypothermia, enlarged posterior fontanel, or respiratory distress. (The normal values are $T_4 > 6 \, \mu/dL$ and $TSH = 20\mu U/mL$.) In this case, the high TSH indicates that the thyroid is not responding to the stimulus of TSH. The state programs select out the lower 10% of the babies for further study so that they can detect the rare case before brain damage occurs. (**Ref. 5,** p. 1634)

97. (**E**)   Anorexia nervosa, commonly occurring among young women, affects many of the body functions as a result of severe malnutrition. These include metabolic disturbances of the liver, hypothalamic-pituitary axis, and electrolyte disorders. The body functions slow down. The patients have a decreased sedimentation rate. (**Ref. 5,** pp. 108–109)

98. (**E**)   Enuresis is diagnosed after age 5 when most children are toilet trained. There are many studies supporting a variety of causes of this problem, but in general enuresis has no apparent cause. The treatments are mainly empirical since they are not directly interfering with a pathologic malfunction. The variety of approaches needs to match the wishes of the patients with the treatment style of the physician. (**Ref. 5,** pp. 110–111)

99. (**C**)   These behaviors are characteristics of ADHD, a problem that involves about 10% of the population. While it may result from underlying problems such as Tourette syndrome, Reye syndrome, or fetal alcohol syndrome, it usually occurs in otherwise healthy children. Treatment requires a skillful team to help the child overcome some behaviors, increase self-esteem, and help the family restructure its relationships. (**Ref. 5,** pp. 115–116; **Ref. 6,** p. 718)

100. (**E**)   Febrile seizures occur after the onset of a fever in susceptible infants. It classically lasts a few minutes with no abnormality of the neurologic exam when the patient awakens. If the patient looks well, there is no need to investigate the cause of the seizure—this time. Observation is required to assure that the patient remains well. Treatment and laboratory testing are dependent on the philosophy of the doctors. (**Ref. 5,** p. 1792)

101. (**A**)   The usual sequence of appearance of secondary sexual characteristics is breast buds, pubic hair, and axillary hair. The Tanner scale outlines the five stages of appearance of pubic hair and breast size in females and testicular size and penis size in males. (**Ref. 3,** Vol. 8, No. 2, August 1986)

102. (**E**)   This pubertal gynecomastia occurs in males most commonly during Tanner 2–4, with peak incidence at 14 years. Spontane-

ous regression usually occurs in several months but it may persist for several years. The exact mechanism is unclear. Drugs (estrogen, testosterone, tricyclic antidepression medication, marijuana) and endocrine disorders cause this problem in rare situations. (**Ref. 5,** p. 61)

103. **(B)** Typical bean-shaped gram-negative diplococci are clearly seen within polymorphonuclear leukocytes in a gram stain of the urethral exudate. This finding is consistent with a diagnosis of gonorrhea. (**Ref. 3,** p. 195)

104. **(E)** Sinus arrhythmia is often related to respiratory phases, with speeding of the heart during inspiration and slowing during expiration. Both phasic and nonphasic forms of sinus arrhythmia are especially common in children and require no treatment. (**Ref. 1,** p. 1191)

105. **(D)** Down syndrome (trisomy 21) is the most frequently occurring chromosomal abnormality in humans. One in 600–800 live births are affected by this disorder. (**Ref. 5,** p. 296)

106. **(D)** Jaundice usually becomes clinically apparent during the second or third day of life. Indirect bilirubin levels are usually below 12 mg/dl, with peak levels occurring on days 5–7. With hemolytic jaundice, which is usually from ABO incompatibility or Rh sensitization, a bilirubin level of 20 is felt to be harmful while, in nonhemolytic states, a bilirubin level may rise higher before active treatment. (**Ref. 5,** p. 1055)

107. **(B)** VZIG (varicella zoster immune gamma) globulin should be given to immunocompromised individuals within 48 hours of exposure to varicella and to immunosuppressed patients with progressive varicella. In most cases, the disease is uncomfortable to the patient but not dangerous. Few children will get encephalitis, pneumonia, or superimposed bacterial (*S. pneumoniae*) infections. In special circumstances, the use of VZIG will prevent the disease or modify it. (**Ref. 4,** pp. 515–516)

108. **(D)** After birth, the ductus venosus is obliterated and becomes the ligamentum venosum. The foramen ovale connects the right and left atria. The ductus arteriosus connects the aorta to the pulmonary artery. (**Ref. 1,** p. 1145)

109. **(B)** This red rash with satellite lesions in the intertrigenous regions is most likely a candida albicans infection, which favors warm moist areas such as those between fingers, neck folds, corners of the mouth, and axillae. Ringworm usually has a circular appearance. Contact dermatitis may be red but does not have satellite lesions outside the contact area. Irritant diaper rash usually spares the intertrigenous areas. (**Ref. 5,** p. 926)

110. **(D)** This thinning of the hair after a severe stress affects hair follicles in the growing phase and shifts the follicles into the resting phase. Hairs are shed when the growing phase resumes 2–3 months after the stress. The hair will return to a normal pattern of growth. (**Ref. 5,** p. 917)

111. **(C)** This hemangioma sits on the skin as if a lump of putty were put there. It typically becomes larger, gets a grayish blue frosting, and then involutes. Size and location do not affect prognosis. Port wine stains are lesions with dilated capillaries in the dermis. Cavernous hemangiomas are soft subcutaneous, often bluish, ill defined masses, often referred to as "a bag of worms." (**Ref. 5,** pp. 913–915)

112. **(A)** Eczema is a generic term that denotes edema within the epidermis. In acute eczema, vesicles and blisters are formed. Atopic dermatitis is caused by dry skin, heat infection, specific allergens, topical irritants, or psychological factors. There may be an allergic component where certain foods may cause flare-ups of the skin lesions. The skin is dry. The middle of the face is usually spared. Chronic scratching will cause lichenification, increased markings of the skin. (**Ref. 5,** pp. 884–886)

113. **(C)** Seborrheic dermatitis may present as a cradle cap with greasy yellow scale in the newborn period. In older children, it presents as dandruff. Other locations include the forehead, cheeks, axillae, neck, behind the ears, and diaper area. (**Ref. 5,** p. 883)

114. **(E)** Transient synovitis is a nonspecific, self-limited inflammation of the hip joint of unknown etiology. It is usually associated with an upper respiratory infection. There is a normal temperature or low-grade fever. Laboratory tests are normal. If persistent,

Legg-Calve-Perthes disease (aseptic necrosis of the femoral head) needs to be ruled out. (**Ref. 5,** p. 1947)

115. **(A)** A multiple system disease, Lyme disease, may include headache, stiff neck myalgia, arthralgias, malaise, fatigue, lethargy, and lymphadenopathy. Ten percent have cardiac manifestations, which include myocarditis, pancarditis, and conduction disturbances. One-third of the patients will remember having a tick bite. The organism is *Borrelia burdorferi.* (**Ref. 5,** p. 592)

116. **(C)** Serum sickness follows drug reactions, such as penicillin, insect bites, and more recently transplantation. Formerly, injections of antisera made from horses were the major culprits. It is a delayed type of immediate hypersensitivity. The illness may last 7–10 days. In the late stages, eosinophilia is present. (**Ref. 5,** p. 519)

117. **(E)** Nematode larvae produce pruritic reddish papules at the site of skin entry. As the larvae migrate through the skin, they leave an irregular wavy track, which is also pruritic. Two drugs, thiabendazole or albendazole (not yet approved by the FDA), are suggested. The disease is self-limited and can be treated with ethyl chloride spray at the area ahead of the visible track. (**Ref. 4,** pp. 172–173)

118. **(D)** Fitz Hugh Curtis, a perihepatitis, causes right upper quadrant tenderness or an audible friction rub. It may cause right shoulder pain. Liver function is normal. It is associated with both gonococcal and chlamydia infections. It enters into the differential diagnosis of abdominal pain in a sexually active female. (**Ref. 6,** p. 524)

119. **(A)** External otitis media, a common infection found in swimmers, will cause pain when the external ear is touched or pulled. Other causes are local trauma. It is frequently caused by *Pseudomonas aeruginosa* and *Staphylococcus aureus.* Human schistosome will cause a papular pruritic rash called swimmer itch. (**Ref. 5,** pp. 732, 942)

120. **(B)** Rocky Mountain spotted fever is caused by *Rickettsia ricketsii.* It is transmitted to humans by tick bites. Although named for the Rocky Mountain area, it is widespread in the United States. Many cases are reported in the East Coast area, as well as in Southeastern and South Central United States. The disease is char-

acterized by fever, rash, headache, muscle pain, nausea, and vomiting. The rash occurs on the palms of the hand and soles of the feet. It is seen also in drug sensitivities and syphilis. The patients may have low sodium levels from the loss of sodium into the extravascular space. Treatment is chloromycetin in children less than 9 and tetracycline for older children. Tetracycline is contraindicated in young children because it will interfere with the enamel formation of teeth. (**Ref. 4,** pp. 402–403; **Ref. 5,** p. 696)

121. (**D**) This condition of teenagers is bilateral in 30% of cases. The epiphysis falls posteriorally and medially, and there is proximal and anterior migration of the femoral metaphysis. The cause is unknown. This may represent a local manifestation of a more general disorder of endochondrial ossification. Radiographs of AP and lateral views confirm the diagnosis with the characteristic "ice cream falling off the cone" appearance. Treatment is with spica cast and careful rehabilitation. Some cases may require surgery. (**Ref. 5,** pp. 1941–1942)

122. (**A**) The HLA region, the major histocompatibility complex, is located on the short arm of chromosome 6. This complex contains loci of genes involved in the immune response and cell-cell interactions. Each child has one HLA region, with haplotypes inherited from each parent. Siblings with IDDM share common haplotypes 55 to 60% of the time, compared with 25% in siblings without IDDM. (**Ref. 5,** pp. 348–350)

123. (**B**) CF is transmitted as a recessive disorder. The gene is located on the long arm of chromosome 7. Seventy percent of the patients have a deletion of three base pairs that code for the amino acid, phenylalanine. The other 30% include over 100 different mutations. Sickle cell disease involves the substitutions of valine for glutamic acid on the 6th position from the N-terminal end of the beta globulin chain. Maple syrup urine disease is a branched chain ketoaciduria with a characteristic odor in the urine of maple syrup. (**Ref. 5,** pp. 1123, 1526)

124. (**B**) Siblings of a child with IDDM have a 5–10% risk of developing diabetes. (**Ref. 5,** p. 352)

125. (**C**) Aspirin and phenothiazides will turn urine purple when ferric chloride is added. PKU turns urine blue-green, which

fades. Alkaptonuria turns urine green, which fades rapidly. Urine from patients with Gaucher disease does not react to ferric chloride. (**Ref. 5**, p. 287)

126. **(E)** Stress from these conditions will require additional insulin doses. Infections are short-term stresses, which will raise blood sugar levels. Since physical activity will decrease the insulin requirements, returning to school where there is more sedentary time will require additional insulin doses. (**Ref. 5**, p. 345)

127. **(A)** Activities around the fourth week of gestation include neural tube closure at day 27; limb bud appearance at day 30; branchial arches, clefts, and pouches formation in weeks 4 to 5. (**Ref. 5**, p. 425)

128. **(B)** The kidneys and mature heart are also formed. (**Ref. 5**, p. 425)

129. **(E)** Sex differentiation of internal and external genitalia occur from week 7 to week 10. At the tenth week, the intestinal contents, which have previously moved from outside the abdomen, now return to the abdominal cavity. At this time, when the return is not correctly performed, conditions such as intestinal malrotation occur. The cecum will not reach the right lower quadrant but will locate to another quadrant. The dermal ridges form in weeks 13 to 19. (**Ref. 5**, p. 425)

130. **(D)** This form of mental retardation accounts for 40% of X-linked mental retardation involving 4–5 per 10,000 males. About one-third of female carriers are reported as slow. These patients may exhibit signs of autism. Reports state that a significant percent of males with autism have fragile X syndrome. Patients with William syndrome have growth delay, mental retardation, stellate iris, hypoplastic nails, supravalvular aortic stenosis, and characteristic facies. XXY syndrome, or Klinefelter syndrome (seminiferous tubule dysgenesis), is associated with mental retardation in some cases. These patients are tall males with small firm testes and poorly developed secondary sexual characteristics. (**Ref. 5**, pp. 418, 446–447, 1662)

131. **(E)**; 132. **(C)**; 133. **(B)**; 134. **(A)**; 135. **(D)** These answers reflect the upper limits of the normal range by which the milestones should be reached. Most children will achieve these mile-

stones earlier. These answers reflect the time after which the child may be demonstrating a developmental delay. (**Ref. 5,** p. 1683)

136. **(E)** These symptoms reflect the immunodeficiency problems of children with HIV infection: abnormal B cell function, relative hypogammaglobulinemia, decrease in CD4 cell count, and an abnormality in antibody-mediated immunity. (**Ref. 5,** pp. 471–472)

137. **(C)** In this form of purpura, the platelets are coated with increased amounts of IgG or IgM resulting in rapid destruction of platelets. The bone marrow responds to this low platelet count with increased young megakaryocytes. ITP follows viral infections in 80% of the cases. (**Ref. 5,** p. 1159)

138. **(B)** Bone marrow suppression may occur after radiation and cytotoxic drugs, as well as following exposure to insecticides (DDT or Lindane), solvents such as benzene, and other drugs such as chloramphenicol, tridione, mesantoin, and sulfonamides. (**Ref. 5,** p. 1107)

139. **(B)** In patients with acute lymphocytic leukemia (ALL), the bone marrow becomes infiltrated with leukemic cells, decreasing the megakaryocytes and peripheral platelets. (**Ref. 5,** p. 1187)

140. **(E)** This autosomal dominant disease causes mild to moderate bleeding. The platelets are normal, but there is a defect in the adhesion to exposed vascular collagen. Decreased factor VIII is secondary to decreased amount of von Willebrand factor, which transports the factor VIII. The most common symptoms are nosebleeds and easy bruising. (**Ref. 5,** pp. 1164–1165)

141. **(A)** Since this is a vasculitis with leaking of the red cells into the tissue rather than a problem with platelets or clotting factors, the bone marrow and platelet count will be normal. The purpura typically occur on the buttocks and flexor surfaces of the legs. Renal and intestinal lesions are common. (**Ref. 5,** p. 490)

142. **(C)** Erythema infectiosum, or Fifth's disease, is caused by parvovirus. The rash may spread to the trunk and may be pruritic. (**Ref. 5,** p. 683)

143. **(D)**   This classic pattern of fever followed by a rash is exanthem subitum or roseola infantum, caused by human herpesvirus-6. **(Ref. 4,** p. 272)

144. **(B)**   Rubella infection early in pregnancy produces a spectrum of defects resulting in either stillborns, abortions, or live births with a panoply of problems, including red-purple macular "blueberry muffin" lesions, hepatitis, hemolytic anemia, patent ductus arteriosus, hearing loss, cataracts, glaucoma, retinopathy, encephalitis. In childhood, they may develop diabetes. Fortunately, immunizations will prevent this infection and the resultant problems. **(Ref. 5,** p. 690)

145. **(E)**   The hint about the well water should make you investigate the stools for *giardia*. *Giardia* is the most frequent identifiable agent of waterborne diarrhea. Cysts may be seen in the stool, although it may take three stool examinations to find the cysts. The most effective treatment is quinacrine hydrochloride (Atabrine) or metronidazole (Flagyl) in younger children. **(Ref 3,** Vol. 14, No. 7, July 1993; **Ref. 4,** p. 194)

146. **(B)**   These patients are usually exposed to carbon monoxide in cars, poorly ventilated houses with house heaters, or house fires. Symptoms may progress from mild headache to coma with hypotension, encephalitis, and cardiac arrhythmias. Few people will exhibit the cherry red lips that are so widely described. **(Ref. 5,** pp. 793–794)

147. **(A)**   Iron poisoning will cause early changes of hemorrhagic gastroenteritis followed by a quiet period of up to 12 hours. Then, in ingestions of large amounts, the third phase will develop with circulatory collapse, hepatic and renal failure, bleeding, and coma. The iron pills can be seen on radiographs as radiodense particles in the gastrointestinal tract. Serum iron levels will confirm the diagnosis. Treatment with desferoxamine, if used early, will help reverse the poisoning. **(Ref. 5,** p. 806)

148. **(E)**   Methemoglobinemia, the oxidized form of hemoglobin that is incapable of carrying oxygen, may result from local anesthetics, sulfa drugs, nitrites, and aniline dyes. The cyanotic appearance stems from the dark brown color of the blood containing methemoglobin. A drop of blood from the patient placed on filter paper next to a normal patient's blood will demonstrate the brown color. Treatment is with methylene blue. (**Ref. 5,** p. 809)

149. **(D)**   Insecticides containing organophosphates (anticholinesterases) will cause excessive salivation and sweating, mimicking some symptoms of heart failure. They also produce diarrhea, urination, and muscle fasciculations. The problems may be reversed with atropine, 2-PAM, or protopam. (**Ref. 5,** pp. 814–815)

150. **(A)**   Kerosene is a high-viscosity, low-volatility liquid. It causes pulmonary damage from aspiration, not absorption from the stomach. In general, there are two components to hydrocarbon toxicity: volatility and viscosity. Agents such as benzene and carbon tetrachloride have high volatility, causing CNS dysfunction. Kerosene and turpentine have high viscosity, which will lead to aspiration and pulmonary damage. (**Ref. 1,** p. 1779)

References

1. Behrman R (ed): *Nelson Textbook of Pediatrics,* 14th ed. Philadelphia, W. B. Saunders, 1991.

2. Oski FA (ed): *Principles and Practice of Pediatrics,* 2nd ed. Philadelphia, Lippencott, 1994.

3. *Pediatrics in Review,* Vol. 14, No. 7 (July 1993).

4. *Red Book Report of the Committee on Infectious Disease American Academy of Pediatrics 1994.*

5. Rudolph A (ed): *Rudolph's Pediatrics,* 19th ed. Norwalk, CT, Appleton & Lange, 1991.

6. Schwartz MW (ed): *Pediatric Primary Care,* 2nd ed. Chicago, Yearbook, 1987.

6

Gynecology and Obstetrics

Samuel L. Jacobs, MD, FACOG

GYNECOLOGY

DIRECTIONS: Each of the questions or incomplete statements below is followed by a list of suggested answers or completions. Select the **one** that is best in each case. If more than one answer is correct, the question will state the number of responses to select. Choose exactly this number.

1. A 24-year-old white female G_0 presents in moderate distress to the ER, complaining of sudden onset of a temperature of 39.5° C, watery diarrhea and vomiting, and a diffuse macular sunburn-like rash over her body. Vaginal exam reveals a superabsorbent tampon in place. Vaginal culture is done, and the **MOST PROBABLE** causative organism is

    A. *Yersinia enterocolitica*
    B. *Clostridium deficile*
    C. *Escherichia coli*
    D. *Staphylococcus aureus*
    E. *Neisseria gonorrhoea*

2. In the preceding patient, the **MOST APPROPRIATE** antibiotic would be
   A. penicillin
   B. nafcillin
   C. metronidazole
   D. doxycycline
   E. ampicillin

3. All the following are epidemiologic risk factors for cervical cancer **EXCEPT**
   A. family history
   B. cigarette smoking
   C. young age at first intercourse
   D. multiple male partners
   E. HPV infection

4. An 18-year-old sexually active white female has a history of abnormal cytology on her most recent Pap smear. She undergoes colposcopy in the clinic, at which time a biopsy is performed. The biopsy is negative, and the endocervical curettage is positive. The **MOST APPROPRIATE** next step would be
   A. reassurance
   B. repeat Pap in 6–8 weeks
   C. cone biopsy
   D. repeat colposcopy in 6–8 weeks
   E. cervical canal cryotherapy

5. A patient has squamous cell cancer of the cervix involving the upper one-third of the vagina. There is neither parametrial involvement nor extension to the pelvic wall, but there is unilateral hydronephrosis on IVP. She would be staged as
   A. IIIB
   B. IIIA
   C. IIB
   D. IIA
   E. IVA

6. All the following are risk factors for the development of ovarian epithelial carcinoma **EXCEPT**
   A. nulliparity
   B. oral contraceptives
   C. obesity
   D. talcum powder
   E. positive family history

7. Ovarian cancer spreads by all of the following routes **EXCEPT**
   A. lymphogenous
   B. hematogenous
   C. celomic metaplasia
   D. adjacent spread (transcelomic)

8. A 64-year-old woman with epithelial ovarian cancer goes to the operating room for staging and treatment. She has tumor on her left ovary and obvious implants on abdominal peritoneal surfaces. These implants are all <2 cm in diameter. Nodes are negative. The treatment of choice for this stage is
   A. cytoreductive surgery
   B. radiation therapy
   C. chemotherapy
   D. A & B
   E. A & C

9. The five-year survival rate for this stage is best quoted to be
   A. 10%
   B. 30%
   C. 50%
   D. 85%
   E. 99%

10. The **MOST COMMON** presentation of vulvar neoplasia is
    A. dysuria
    B. perineal pain
    C. vaginal discharge
    D. pruritus
    E. asymptomatic

11. The **MOST COMMON** histologic type of vulvar cancer is
    A. squamous cell
    B. basal cell
    C. melanoma
    D. adenocarcinoma
    E. sarcoma

12. The following are risk factors for the development of vulvar neoplasia (select **THREE**)
    A. yeast infections
    B. ulcerative colitis
    C. endometrial cancer
    D. vulvar dystrophy
    E. previous cervical dysplasia
    F. trichomoniasis
    G. history of HPV infection

Questions 13–14: Match the **APPROPRIATE** treatment with the appropriate stage of vulvar cancer (an option may be used only once or not at all):

    A. Stage 0
    B. Stage I
    C. Stage II
    D. Stage III
    E. Stage IV

13. Wide local resection

14. Chemotherapy

15. The **MOST FREQUENTLY** occurring type of degeneration that a uterine fibroid undergoes is
    A. sarcomatous
    B. cystic
    C. myxomatous
    D. carneous
    E. hyaline

Questions 16–19: Refer to Figure 6-1. Select the **MOST LIKELY** location of the fibroid. Use each letter in the figure only once.

16. Menometrorrhagia _____

17. Confusion with an ovarian mass on pelvic exam _____

18. Dystocia _____

19. Asymptomatic _____

20. All the following are risk factors for endometrial adenocarcinoma (select **FOUR**).
    A. IUD usage
    B. Nulliparity
    C. Obesity
    D. Strenuous exercise
    E. HPV infection
    F. Late menarche
    G. Chronic anovulation
    H. Late menopause

21. In a 56-year-old woman with post-menopausal bleeding, the **MOST HELPFUL** diagnostic test would be
    A. pelvic ultrasound
    B. histologic sampling of the endometrium
    C. Pap smear
    D. CBC/diff
    E. progestin challenge

22. The **MOST APPROPRIATE** treatment for Stage I adenocarcinoma of the endometrium is
    A. total abdominal hysterectomy with bilateral salpingo-oophorectomy
    B. total abdominal hysterectomy without bilateral salpingo-oophorectomy
    C. radical hysterectomy with bilateral salpingo-oophorectomy and pelvic lymphadenectomy
    D. total vaginal hysterectomy without bilateral salpingo-oophorectomy
    E. primary external radiation therapy followed by total abdominal hysterectomy and bilateral salpingo-oophorectomy

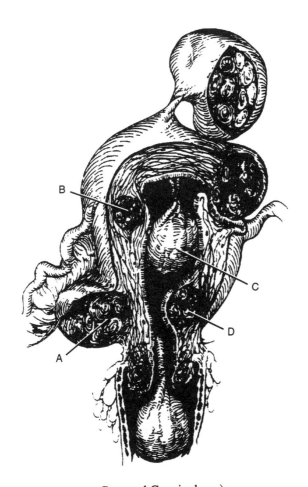

Figure 6-1 (*Source:* Gant and Cunningham.)

Questions 23–25: A 52-year-old white female in good health with irregular menses comes to your office for a routine annual check-up. She has been somewhat depressed lately and is concerned that she may be going through menopause.

23. You would tell her that the age of onset of menopause **IS** related to
    A. height
    B. race
    C. oral contraceptive use
    D. cigarette smoking
    E. age of menarche

24. You also counsel her about **FOUR** risk factors of osteoporosis, which are
    A. uterine fibroids
    B. low calcium diet
    C. caffeine
    D. diabetes mellitus
    E. IUD usage
    F. sedentary lifestyle
    G. estrogen usage
    H. cigarette smoking

25. Your treatment recommendations may include all the following **EXCEPT**
    A. estrogens
    B. calcium
    C. GnRH agonists
    D. progestogens
    E. exercise

Questions 26–29: In Figure 6-2, a basal body temperature graph (where X = menses), select the appropriate time in the menstrual cycle for the following tests. Use each letter only once or not at all.

26. Post-coital test _____

27. Endometrial biopsy _____

28. Peak progesterone level _____

29. Hysterosalpingogram _____

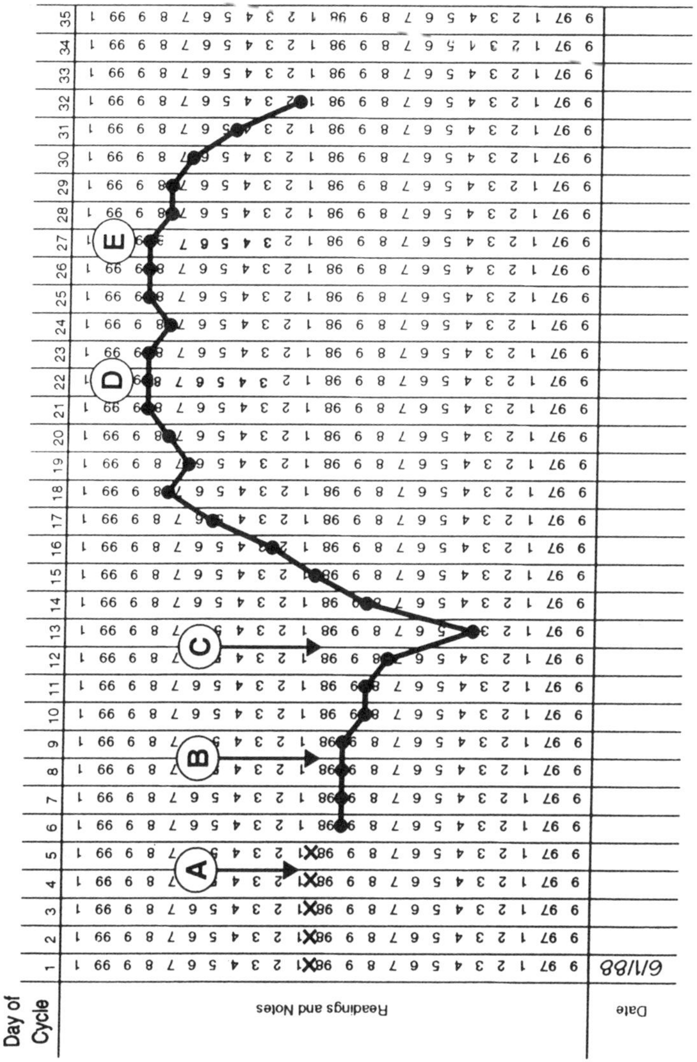

Figure 6-2

Questions 30–34: Refer to Figure 6-3. Select the appropriate graph for each of the following hormones. Use each letter once.

30. Estradiol _____

31. LH _____

32. Progesterone _____

Figure 6-3 (*Source:* DeCherney and Pernoll.)

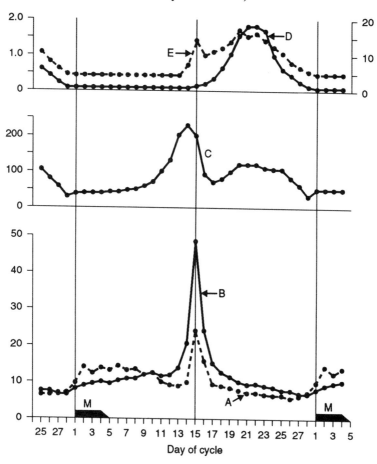

33. FSH _____

34. 17-OH progesterone _____

35. You deliver a full-term infant with ambiguous genitalia. A uterus is found to be present, and the karyotype turns out to be 46 XX. The *next* step in the work-up would include which **THREE** of the following?
   A. 17-OH progesterone level
   B. Chest x-ray
   C. History of excessive androgens in mother
   D. Serum electrolytes
   E. IVP
   F. Laparotomy for gonadectomy

36. A 22-year-old white woman presents to your office with a history of mildly increasing facial hair and irregular menstrual cycles. She is sexually active, but not interested in becoming pregnant at this time. Her DHEA-S is normal, her testosterone level is minimally elevated, and she is most interested in cosmetic results. The treatment of choice would be
   A. bilateral oophorectomy
   B. oral contraceptives
   C. long-term GnRH agonist therapy
   D. expectant management
   E. dexamethasone

37. The incidence of male factor infertility is approximately
   A. 40%
   B. 20%
   C. 10%
   D. <5%
   E. 75%

38. A 27-year-old African-American female with regular 28-day cycles has a two-year history of primary infertility. Her partner's semen analysis is WNL, as is the post-coital testing. Endometrial biopsy is in phase and the peak progesterone level is appropriate. The hysterosalpingogram shows bilateral fill of tubes, but no spill from either side. The next step in the work-up would be

   A. two cycles of documented basal body temperature charting
   B. referral to an IVF center
   C. ovulation induction agents (e.g., clomiphene citrate)
   D. anti-sperm antibody testing
   E. surgery to open the tubes

39. The physiologic function of hCG appears to be to

   A. initiate menstruation
   B. maintain the corpus luteum
   C. maintain the placenta
   D. inhibit the pituitary
   E. stimulate estrogen release

40. All the following are **ABSOLUTE** contraindications to oral contraceptive use **EXCEPT**

   A. migraines
   B. thromboembolic disease
   C. breast cancer
   D. cerebrovascular disease
   E. active liver disease

41. All the following are considered local **BARRIER** methods of contraception **EXCEPT**

   A. condom
   B. IUD
   C. sponge
   D. foam
   E. diaphragm

42. An 11th-grader who has never been pregnant comes into your office for contraceptive counseling. She has been sexually active for over one year and has had one episode of gonorrhea from one of her previous partners. The **MOST APPROPRIATE** method for her would be

   A. abstinence
   B. condoms

C. oral contraceptives
D. IUD
E. condoms and oral contraceptives

43. All the following theories have been proposed to explain endometriosis. The **MOST COMMONLY** accepted explanation of them is
A. hematogenous dissemination
B. lymphogenous dissemination
C. hyperprolactinemia
D. celomic metaplasia
E. retrograde menstruation

44. Endometriosis is **MOST COMMONLY** found on/in the
A. uterosacral ligaments
B. appendix
C. vagina
D. ovary
E. tube

45. The diagnosis of endometriosis can be definitively made on the basis of
A. history
B. physical exam
C. Pap smear
D. ultrasound
E. laparoscopy

46. The **BEST** medical treatment of choice for endometriosis is
A. oral contraceptives
B. GnRH agonists
C. danazol
D. spironolactone
E. dexamethasone

47. On biopsy, histologically, endometriotic lesions **MOST COM-MONLY** consist of which **THREE** of the following?
A. Glandular cells
B. Stromal cells
C. Target cells
D. Germ cells
E. Psammoma bodies
F. Hemosiderin-laden marrophages

48. In the United States, about how many women will develop breast cancer in their lifetime?

 A. 1/10
 B. 1/100
 C. 1/1000
 D. 1/10,000
 E. 1/100,000

49. Routine mammography should be obtained with what frequency (select **THREE**)?

 A. Yearly after age 40
 B. Initially between 35–40
 C. Yearly after age 50
 D. Every other year after age 40
 E. Initially at age 50
 F. Every other year after age 50

50. All the following are associated with demonstrable increased risk for breast cancer **EXCEPT**

 A. menopause after age 55
 B. menarche before age 12
 C. nulliparity
 D. lactation
 E. positive family history

51. All the following statements are **TRUE** about PMS **EXCEPT**

 A. symptoms include bloatedness, irritability, food cravings
 B. symptoms must occur in the second half of the cycle
 C. there must be a symptom-free period of at least 7 days in the first half of the cycle
 D. progesterone is the definitive therapy
 E. the highest incidence is in women in their late twenties to early thirties

52. A young woman who is being worked up for infertility has been measuring her basal body temperature, which has just risen. About how many days should her basal temperature remain elevated until the next menses?

 A. 2–4 days
 B. 6–8 days
 C. 9–10 days

  D. 14–15 days
  E. 24–28 days

53. Two separate FSH levels exceeding how many milli-international units/mL may objectively confirm the presence of menopause?
  A. 1–5
  B. 10–20
  C. 25
  D. 40
  E. 100

54. The **USUAL** duration of a menstrual flow is
  A. 1–2 days
  B. 3 days
  C. 4–6 days
  D. 7 days
  E. 8–10 days

55. A 15-year-old girl is brought to the emergency room by her mother, who states that the girl's appetite has been extremely poor and she has lost 20 lb in the past three months. Menarche was at age 13, but the patient has not had her period for several months. The **MOST LIKELY** diagnosis is
  A. hyperthyroidism
  B. Addison's disease
  C. anorexia nervosa
  D. juvenile diabetes
  E. Turner's syndrome

56. How often do ectopic pregnancies occur in the United States?
  A. 1/50
  B. 1/100
  C. 1/200
  D. 1/400
  E. 1/2000

Questions 57–58: Refer to Figure 6-4.

57. All the following statements are **TRUE** about Figure 6-4 **EXCEPT**
    A. it is more common before age 20 or after age 40
    B. it affects one in every 2000 pregnancies in the United States
    C. the "complete" type is entirely of maternal origin
    D. it is rarely associated with clinical hyperthyroidism
    E. it may be associated with pregnancy-induced hypertension during the second trimester

58. Usually, the **BEST** treatment for this condition is which of the following?
    A. Immediate evacuation upon diagnosis
    B. Expectant management until 28 weeks, then delivery by c-section
    C. Propylthiouracil and supportive therapy
    D. Immediate methotrexate chemotherapy for all cases
    E. Immediate hysterectomy for all cases

59. A 32-year-old woman is diagnosed as having an ectopic pregnancy. All the following have been implicated in the etiology of this disorder **EXCEPT**
    A. adhesions
    B. IUD

Figure 6-4 (*Source:* Gant and Cunningham.)

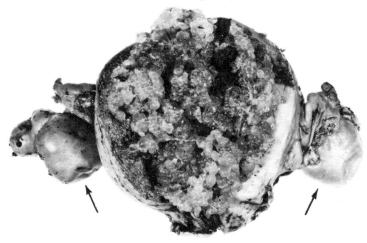

C. salpingitis
D. previous abdominal surgery
E. oral contraceptives

60. Pelvic relaxation associated with estrogen deficiency is associated with development of all the following **EXCEPT**
   A. cystoceles
   B. urethroceles
   C. enteroceles
   D. rectoceles
   E. uterine prolapse

61. All the following statements are **TRUE** of the girl pictured in Figure 6-5 **EXCEPT**
   A. she has Turner's syndrome
   B. her serum gonadotropins are increased
   C. she will probably suffer from primary amenorrhea
   D. she is tall for her age
   E. her karyotype is 45 XO

Figure 6-5 (*Source:* Jones HW Jr, Scott WW: Hermaphroditism, *Genital Anomalies and Related Endocrine Disorders*, 2nd ed. Williams & Wilkins, 1971.)

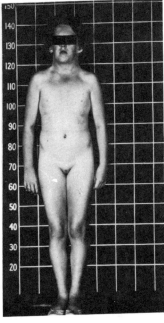

62. All the following may cause galactorrhea **EXCEPT**
   A. bromocryptine
   B. Cushing's syndrome
   C. phenothiazines
   D. oral contraceptives
   E. hyperprolactinemia

63. The pelvic diaphragm consists of all the following structures **EXCEPT**
   A. coccygeus muscles
   B. mons pubis
   C. inner surface of the ischial spines
   D. levator ani muscles
   E. peritoneum

64. A 24-year-old sexually active woman presents with lower abdominal pain, seven weeks of amenorrhea, and vaginal bleeding. A palpable mass is noted in the adnexal area of the uterus. She is tachycardic and hypotensive. The **MOST LIKELY** diagnosis is
   A. adnexal torsion
   B. Mittelschmerz
   C. ectopic pregnancy
   D. gram-negative sepsis
   E. degenerating fibroid

65. All the following may cause dyspareunia **EXCEPT**
   A. decreased lubrication
   B. anorgasmia
   C. vaginismus
   D. endometriosis
   E. pelvic adhesions

66. In dysfunctional uterine bleeding, all the following are **TRUE EXCEPT**
   A. patients may show irregular spotting with or without heavy menses
   B. D&C is the treatment of choice
   C. sonogram may aid in the diagnosis
   D. pregnancy must be ruled out
   E. one of the most common causes is anovulation

Questions 67–69: Match the **BEST** treatment for the type of vaginal discharge listed. Use each answer once or not at all.

A. Acyclovir
B. Doxycycline
C. Metronidazole
D. Clotrimazole

67. Frothy yellow-green discharge _____

68. Cottage cheese-like white exudate _____

69. Mucopurulent discharge _____

Questions 70–75: For women aged 15 to 44 years, match the first-year contraceptive failure rate seen in Figure 6-6 with the corresponding form of contraception used. Use each answer once.

70. Rhythm method _____

71. Oral contraceptives _____

72. Condoms _____

73. Foam, cream, and jelly _____

74. IUDs _____

75. Diaphragms _____

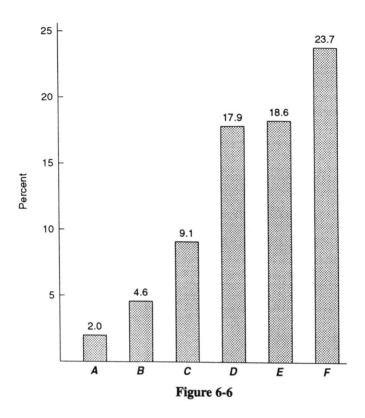

Figure 6-6

OBSTETRICS

76. Three weeks after giving birth, a nursing 31-year-old woman developed chills, fever, and marked engorgement of her left breast, which became painful, hard, and erythematous. The **MOST LIKELY** offending organism is
   A. *Streptococcus faecalis*
   B. *Streptococcus viridans*
   C. *Staphylococcus epidermidis*
   D. *Staphylococcus aureus*
   E. *Escherichia coli*

Questions 77–79: Refer to Figure 6-7. Match the correct letter to each case scenario. Each letter is used only once.

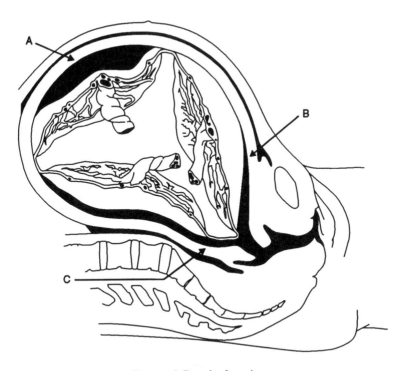

Figure 6-7 (*Source:* Gant and Cunningham.)

77. A 21-year-old G_1 P_0 presents at 34 weeks with painless spotting
_____

78. A 36-year-old G_4 P_3 presents at term with painful bleeding
_____

79. A 27-year-old G_2 P_1 presents at term with hypertonic contractions and fetal distress _____

80. If amniocentesis were to be performed on a pregnant woman after 34 weeks of gestation, the ratio of lecithin to sphingomyelin would **NORMALLY** be about
   A. 4:1
   B. 2:1
   C. 1:1
   D. 1:2
   E. 1:4

81. Coagulation factors were measured in a 25-year-old pregnant woman. Which of the following coagulation factors would be expected to **DECREASE** during a normal pregnancy?
    A. Factor I
    B. Factor VII
    C. Factor VIII
    D. Factor IX
    E. None of the above

82. On the assumption that labor occurs 280 days from the beginning of the last menstrual period, the date of confinement is estimated by adding 7 days to the first day of the last menstrual period and subtracting 3 months. This is referred to as
    A. Naegele's rule
    B. William's rule
    C. Friedman's rule
    D. Kelly's rule
    E. Marshall's rule

83. Which of the following tests is **MOST COMMONLY** used to help diagnose rupture of the membranes?
    A. Phenylpropanolamine
    B. Nitrazine
    C. Clinitest
    D. Ketostix
    E. None of the above

84. How much is the recommended total weight gain for pregnancy?
    A. 5–8 lb
    B. 10–12 lb
    C. 14–18 lb
    D. 18–22 lb
    E. 22–27 lb

85. Approximately how many grams of elemental iron should be given daily throughout the latter half of pregnancy and throughout lactation?
    A. 30 mg
    B. 60 mg
    C. 90 mg
    D. 160 mg
    E. 325 mg

86. A 24-year-old woman is in her last month of pregnancy. Her utero-placental blood flow would be **APPROXIMATELY**
   A. 100 mL/min
   B. 250 mL/min
   C. 500 mL/min
   D. 750 mL/min
   E. 1000 mL/min

87. Compared to the nonpregnant state, a pregnant woman's resting heart rate would be expected to
   A. decrease about 10–15 bpm
   B. decrease about 25–30 bpm
   C. increase about 10–15 bpm
   D. increase about 25–30 bpm
   E. remain about the same as before pregnancy

88. What is the reported prevalence of asymptomatic bacteriunia in pregnant women?
   A. Less than 1%
   B. 2–12%
   C. 15–20%
   D. 30%
   E. Over 40%

89. All the following are widely accepted criteria used to confirm the diagnosis of heart disease in pregnancy **EXCEPT**
   A. cardiac enlargement
   B. continuous heart murmur
   C. diastolic murmur
   D. systolic murmur
   E. bradycardia

90. Postpartum hemorrhage has **USUALLY** been defined as the loss of about how much blood during the first 24 hours after delivery?
   A. >50 mL
   B. >250 mL
   C. >500 mL
   D. >750 mL
   E. >1000 mL

91. All the following are **TRUE** of the use of magnesium sulfate in preeclampsia **EXCEPT** that it
  A. reduces cerebral irritability
  B. controls and prevents seizures
  C. is easily regulated
  D. causes general CNS depression
  E. does not usually seriously affect the fetus

92. All the following are **TRUE** of placenta previa **EXCEPT**
  A. it may be total, partial, or marginal
  B. bleeding usually occurs in the third trimester
  C. bleeding is usually painless
  D. the usual treatment is caesarean section
  E. digital exam of the cervix is the best way to confirm the diagnosis

93. The contraction stress test is contraindicated in all the following situations **EXCEPT**
  A. a previous classical caesarean section
  B. hydramnios
  C. presence of multiple fetuses
  D. placenta previa
  E. suspected oligohydraminos

94. Respiratory function tests were determined in a 24-year-old pregnant woman. A **DECREASE** would be expected for which of the following?
  A. Minute ventilation
  B. Tidal volume
  C. Minute oxygen uptake
  D. Residual volume
  E. Respiratory rate

95. In instructing an expectant mother about potential danger signals during pregnancy, all the following should be reported **IMMEDIATELY EXCEPT**
  A. ankle swelling
  B. blurred vision
  C. facial swelling
  D. abdominal pain
  E. escape of fluids from the vagina

96. A pregnant woman is diagnosed as having abruptio placentae. Which of the following findings might be consistent with **SEVERE** abruptio placentae?
    A. Vaginal bleeding
    B. Disseminated intravascular coagulation
    C. Tenderness of the uterus
    D. Evidence of hypervolemia
    E. Preterm labor

97. Abdominal ultrasonography should be able to detect an intrauterine pregnancy when the βHCG is greater than or equal to
    A. 6 mIU/mL
    B. 60 mIU/mL
    C. 600 mIU/mL
    D. 6000 mIU/mL
    E. none of the above

98. The usual presumptive signs and symptoms in a patient with early pregnancy include all the following **EXCEPT**
    A. amenorrhea
    B. breast tenderness and enlargement
    C. generalized fatigue
    D. infrequency of urination
    E. morning sickness

99. General contraindications for oxytocin induction of labor include all the following conditions **EXCEPT**
    A. previous classical c-section with rupture of membranes
    B. grand multiparity
    C. fetal distress
    D. post-dates
    E. multiple fetuses

Questions 100–107: Refer to Figure 6-8. Match the values for the PO$_2$, hemoglobin, PCO$_2$, and bicarbonate that would **NORMALLY** be expected to be found in the maternal and fetal blood. Each value may be used only once.

100. 32 mm Hg _____

101. 95 mm Hg _____

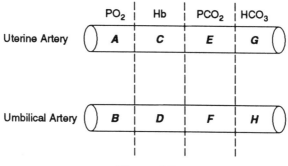

Figure 6-8

102. 15 mm Hg _____

103. 48 mm Hg _____

104. 25 mM/L _____

105. 18.8 mM/L _____

106. 16 g/dL _____

107. 12 g/dL _____

Questions 108–112: Match the appropriate letter to the question. The answers may be used once, more than once, or not at all.

    A. Median episiotomy
    B. Mediolateral episiotomy
    C. Both
    D. Neither

108. Loss of blood is greater _____

109. Dyspareunia more likely to occur _____

110. Easier of the two to repair _____

111. Improper healing is more frequent _____

112. Extension through the anal sphincter is more frequent _____

113. All the following are **TRUE** about twin pregnancies **EXCEPT**
    A. they occur in 1/88 births
    B. they may be monozygotic or dizygotic
    C. twin-to-twin transfusion may result from A-V anastomoses
    D. they should always be delivered by caesarean section
    E. they have a higher risk of preterm labor

114. A 23-year-old woman is Rh negative and 22 weeks pregnant. All the following statements are **CORRECT EXCEPT**
    A. if her child is Rh positive, there is a 16% likelihood of isoimmunization
    B. severe isoimmunization may result in hydrops fetalis
    C. Rh incompatibility accounts for almost 98% of hemolytic disease of the newborn
    D. administration of D-immune globulin (Rhogam®) is administered to all non-sensitized women at 28 weeks gestation
    E. immediate intrauterine exchange transfusion is mandatory in all cases

Questions 115–119: Refer to Figure 6-9. Match the milestones of pregnancy with the **APPROXIMATE** times at which they appear.

115. Morning sickness _____

116. Fetal activity _____

117. First missed menses _____

118. Uterus palpable above pubic symphysis _____

119. Conception _____

Questions 120–122: Refer to Figure 6-10. Match the likelihood of having a Down syndrome child with respect to maternal age.

120. Mother is 45 years old _____

121. Mothers of all ages _____

122. Mother is 40 years old _____

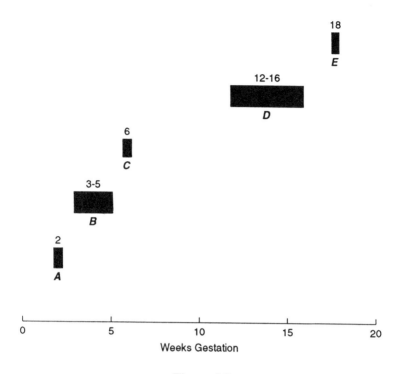

Figure 6-9

Questions 123–125: Match the appropriate letter to the question. Each answer may be used only once.

    A. Highest in protein
    B. Highest in lactose
    C. Lowest in fat
    D. None of the above

123. Human colostrum

124. Human mature milk

125. Cow's milk

126. Late deceleration patterns (type II dips) on a fetal monitoring strip represent
    A. cord compression
    B. pulmonary immaturity

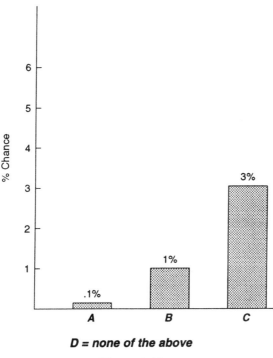

D = none of the above

Figure 6-10

    C. pulmonary hypoxia secondary to decreased perfusion of the intervillous spaces
    D. congenital cardiac conduction defects
    E. entry of the fetal head into the pelvic brim

127. The seven cardinal movements of labor (**IN ORDER**) are
    A. engagement, descent, flexion, internal rotation, extension, external rotation, expulsion
    B. engagement, extension, flexion, internal rotation, external rotation, descent, expulsion
    C. engagement, internal rotation, external rotation, extension, flexion, descent, expulsion
    D. engagement, flexion, external rotation, internal rotation, descent, extension, expulsion
    E. engagement, external rotation, descent, internal rotation, flexion, extension, expulsion

128. Which of the following is the **TOP** cause of maternal mortality?
- **A.** Anesthesia-related death
- **B.** Embolism
- **C.** Hemorrhage
- **D.** Infection
- **E.** Hypertensive disease

129. The hemostatic mechanism **MOST IMPORTANT** in combating postpartum hemorrhage is
- **A.** increased blood clotting factors in pregnancy
- **B.** intramyometrial vascular coagulation due to vasoconstriction
- **C.** contraction of the myometrium to compress vessels and obliterate their lumina
- **D.** markedly decreased blood pressure in the uterine venules
- **E.** fibrolysis inhibition

130. After a normal vaginal delivery, the non-nursing mother will **USUALLY** have her first menstrual period
- **A.** 2 weeks after delivery
- **B.** 6 to 8 weeks after delivery
- **C.** 4 to 6 weeks after delivery
- **D.** 10 to 14 weeks after delivery
- **E.** all of the above

131. The smallest anteroposterior diameter of the pelvic inlet is called
- **A.** interspinous diameter
- **B.** true conjugate
- **C.** diagonal conjugate
- **D.** obstetric conjugate
- **E.** none of the above

132. Routine pelvic examination is contraindicated in which of the following situations during pregnancy?
- **A.** Carcinoma of the cervix
- **B.** Gonorrhea
- **C.** Prolapsed cord
- **D.** Placenta previa
- **E.** Active labor

133. A newborn who at 1 minute of age has a heart rate of 90, an irregular respiratory rate, a grimace, and is pale, limp, and blue has an APGAR rating of

A. 1
B. 3
C. 5
D. 7
E. 9

134. Oxytocin is an nonapeptide and is chemically very similar to

A. ACTH
B. LH
C. FSH
D. vasopressin (ADH)
E. insulin

135. All the following are components of the biophysical profile **EXCEPT**

A. fetal breathing movements
B. non-stress test
C. membrane status
D. adequate amniotic fluid volume
E. adequate fetal tone

136. Effective uterine contractions have all the following characteristics **EXCEPT** they

A. occur every 3 to 4 min
B. exert 50 to 60 mm Hg pressure
C. are palpable only in true labor
D. have a duration of 30 to 90 sec
E. have periods of relaxation between contractions

137. Postpartum hemorrhage that is unresponsive to oxytocin and uterine massage is **MOST LIKELY** due to

A. vaginal lacerations
B. placenta accreta
C. uterine atony
D. ruptured uterus
E. coagulopathy

138. The third stage of labor comprises
  A. from delivery of the infant to separation and expulsion of the placenta
  B. delivery of the infant
  C. surgical repair of the episiotomy
  D. complete dilation of the cervix and expulsion of the fetal head
  E. adequate documentation of the delivery

139. Refer to Figure 6-11. A 21-year-old primigravida is admitted in labor with a double footling breech presentation, ruptured membranes, and cervix 6 cm dilated. An electronic fetal monitor is put in place. During the course of the labor, the pattern displayed in Figure 6-11 was noted. The **MOST LIKELY** cause of the pattern is
  A. fetal head compression
  B. abruptio placentae
  C. uteroplacental insufficiency
  D. cord prolapse
  E. maternal expulsive efforts

140. Arrest of labor in active phase is **BEST** illustrated by which of the following curves shown in Figure 6-12? Choose the correct letter.

Figure 6-11

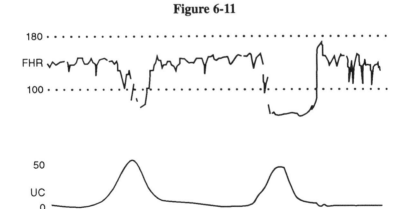

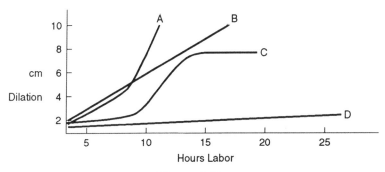

Figure 6-12

141. The type of drug **MOST EFFECTIVE** in the treatment of preterm labor is
   A. alpha adrenergic agonists
   B. beta adrenergic agonists
   C. alpha adrenergic blockers
   D. beta adrenergic blockers
   E. parasympathomimetics

142. In the 38th week of pregnancy, vaginal bleeding associated with a live fetus in the breech presentation suggests
   A. imminent preterm labor
   B. premature separation of a normally implanted placenta
   C. a short umbilical cord
   D. multiple gestation
   E. placenta previa

143. A patient is seen in the early third trimester of pregnancy with acute onset of chills, fever, nausea, and backache. Her temperature is 102° F. The urinary sediment reveals many bacteria and white blood cells. Which of the following is the **MOST LIKELY** diagnosis?
   A. Acute appendicitis
   B. Ruptured uterus
   C. Pyelonephritis
   D. Abruptio placentae
   E. Labor

144. The latent phase of labor
    A. follows the phase of maximum slope and precedes the second stage
    B. follows the acceleration phase and precedes the phase of maximum slope
    C. follows the active phase
    D. precedes the active phase
    E. follows the deceleration phase

145. Premature rupture of the membranes is **MOST STRICTLY** defined as rupture at any time prior to
    A. a stage of fetal viability
    B. the second stage of labor
    C. the 32nd week of gestation
    D. the onset of labor
    E. the 38th week of gestation

146. Severe preeclampsia is defined as being "severe" by all the following **EXCEPT**
    A. a persistent blood pressure of 160 mm Hg or more systolic or 110 mm Hg or more diastolic
    B. the development of convulsions in the absence of neurological disease
    C. proteinuria of 5 g or more in 24 hours
    D. oliguria (500 ml or less in 24 hours) and a rising plasma creatinine level
    E. severe thrombocytopenia or overt intravascular hemolysis

147. The leading cause of neonatal death is
    A. congenital anomalies
    B. prematurity
    C. birth trauma
    D. maternal sepsis
    E. pregnancy-induced hypertension

Questions 148–150: Match the appropriate letter to the question. Each letter may be used once, more than once, or not at all.

    A. True labor
    B. False labor
    C. Both
    D. Neither

148. Uterine contractions palpable

149. Cervix does not dilate

150. Cannot be stopped by sedation

Gynecology and Obstetrics

Answer Key

GYNECOLOGY

1. D	20. B, C, G, H	39. B	58. A
2. B	21. B	40. A	59. E
3. A	22. A	41. B	60. E
4. C	23. D	42. E	61. D
5. A	24. B, C, F, H	43. E	62. A
6. B	25. C	44. D	63. B
7. C	26. C	45. E	64. C
8. E	27. E	46. B	65. B
9. B	28. D	47. A, B, F	66. B
10. D	29. B	48. A	67. C
11. A	30. C	49. B, C, D	68. D
12. D, E, G	31. B	50. D	69. B
13. A	32. D	51. D	70. F
14. E	33. A	52. D	71. A
15. E	34. E	53. D	72. C
16. C	35. A, C, D	54. C	73. D
17. A	36. B	55. C	74. B
18. D	37. A	56. B	75. E
19. B	38. E	57. C	

OBSTETRICS

76. D	95. A	114. E	133. B
77. B	96. B	115. C	134. D
78. C	97. D	116. E	135. C
79. A	98. D	117. B	136. C
80. B	99. D	118. D	137. A
81. E	100. E	119. A	138. A
82. A	101. A	120. C	139. D
83. B	102. B	121. A	140. C
84. E	103. F	122. B	141. B
85. A	104. H	123. C	142. E
86. C	105. G	124. B	143. C
87. C	106. D	125. A	144. D
88. B	107. C	126. C	145. E
89. D	108. B	127. A	146. B
90. C	109. B	128. B	147. B
91. D	110. A	129. C	148. C
92. E	111. B	130. B	149. B
93. E	112. A	131. D	150. A
94. D	113. D	132. D	

Gynecology and Obstetrics

Answers and Comments

GYNECOLOGY

1. **(D)** *Key Words:* sudden temperature, sunburn-like rash, superabsorbent tampons
   This is a case of toxic shock syndrome. It is associated with the use of superabsorbent tampons. The causative organism is *Staphylococcus aureus.* (**Ref. 2,** p. 781)

2. **(B)** *Key Words:* sudden temperature, sunburn-like rash, superabsorbent tampons
   The drug of choice to treat *Staphylococcus aureus,* a penicillinase-producing bacteria, would be nafcillin, a beta-lactamase-resistant antibiotic. (**Ref. 2,** p. 782)

3. **(A)** *Key Words:* epidemiologic risk factors, cervical cancer
   Cervical cancer seems to be associated with the same risk factors for sexually transmitted diseases, such as young age at first intercourse, multiple partners, smoking, etc. There is no relationship to family history. (**Ref. 3,** p. 222)

344

4. **(C)** *Key Words:* sexually active, abnormal cytology, colposcopy, negative biopsy, positive endocervical curettage (ECC)
The management here is quite clear. In light of her previously abnormal Pap, she underwent colposcopy, which resulted in a discrepancy between the biopsy and the ECC. In such cases, a cone biopsy must be performed to resolve this discrepancy. Repeating a Pap or a colposcopy will only delay making a definitive diagnosis. (**Ref. 3**, p. 223)

5. **(A)** *Key Words:* cervical cancer, upper third of vagina, hydronephrosis
The staging here is consistent with IIIB cervical cancer. Even though there is no parametrial involvement, all cases of hydronephrosis are included. (**Ref. 3**, p. 226)

6. **(B)** *Key Words:* risk factors, ovarian cancer
One of the current theories on the pathogenesis of epithelial ovarian cancer may be related to the monthly break and repair of the ovarian capsule associated with ovulation. The oral contraceptive may actually be protective against ovarian cancer because of its inhibition of ovulation. The other factors listed are considered risk factors. (**Ref. 3**, p. 240)

7. **(C)** *Key Words:* ovarian cancer, spread
Ovarian cancer most commonly spreads by direct extension, but may also spread via the lymphatics or the blood vessels. Coelomic metaplasia is one of the hypotheses on the pathogenesis of endometriosis, not ovarian cancer. (**Ref. 3**, p. 241)

8. **(E)** *Key Words:* ovarian cancer, obvious abdominal implants < 2 cm, negative nodes
This is a case of Stage IIIB ovarian cancer, the primary objective for which is to surgically remove as much tumor as possible, followed by chemotherapy. Radiation therapy is very limited, and is not the treatment of choice for IIIB ovarian cancer. (**Ref. 3**, p. 242)

9. **(B)** *Key Words:* ovarian cancer, obvious abdominal implants < 2 cm, negative nodes
Five-year survival is about 30% in Stage III ovarian cancer. (**Ref. 2**, p. 965)

10. **(D)** *Key Words:* common presentation, vulvar neoplasia
About two-thirds of patients with vulvar neoplasia present with a history of longstanding pruritis or a small vulvar lesion. The remainder are asymptomatic. (**Ref. 3,** p. 214)

11. **(A)** *Key Words:* most common histology, vulvar cancer
About 90% of vulvar cancer is squamous cell in origin. Less commonly are melanomas, sarcomas, adenocarcinomas, and basal cell cancers. (**Ref. 3,** p. 214)

12. **(D, E, G)** *Key Words:* risk factors, vulvar cancer
Vulvar cancer is associated with many of the same risk factors as for cervical disease, such as HPV infection, vulvar intraepithelial neoplasia, and certain vulvar dystrophies. (**Ref. 3,** p. 214)

13. **(A)** *Key Words:* vulvar cancer, wide local resection
Stage 0 vulvar cancer refers to carcinoma in situ, and is adequately treated by wide local resection. (**Ref. 3,** p. 216)

14. **(E)** *Key Words:* vulvar cancer, chemotherapy
Chemotherapy is usually indicated in the most advanced cases of vulvar cancer, often with distant metastases. Most involve platinum-based combination therapy. (**Ref. 3,** p. 218)

15. **(E)** *Key Words:* degeneration, fibroid
Fibroids can undergo different types of degenerative change, the most common being hyaline degeneration. Sarcomatous degeneration refers to malignant change, and occurs most rarely—less than 0.5% of all cases. (**Ref. 3,** p. 25)

16. **(C)** *Figure 6-1:* pedunculated fundal fibroid
Of all the fibroids pictured, this is the one most likely to cause abnormal uterine bleeding. (**Ref. 3,** p. 24)

17. **(A)** *Figure 6-1:* intraligamentous fibroid
By virtue of its anatomic location, it may be confused for an ovarian mass on pelvic examination. These tumors actually may arise in the broad ligament without uterine attachment. (**Ref. 3,** p. 23)

18. **(D)** *Figure 6-1:* cervical submucous fibroid
Myomas in the cervix or lower uterine segment may obstruct labor and may be confused with the fetal head. (**Ref. 3,** p. 374)

19. **(B)** *Figure 6-1:* intramural fibroid
Subserous or intramural uterine fibroids may be totally asymptomatic, even though they may attain great size. (**Ref. 3**, p. 24)

20. **(B, C, G, H)** *Key Words:* risk factors, endometrial cancer
Any condition that leads to unopposed or prolonged estrogen exposure to the endometrium may be a risk factor for endometrial cancer. Thus chronic anovulation, late menopause, early menarche, nulliparity, and obesity are implicated. Other risk factors include diabetes, estrogen replacement therapy, and estrogen-producing ovarian tumors. (**Ref. 3**, p. 231)

21. **(B)** *Key Words:* post-menopausal bleeding
Post-menopausal bleeding is abnormal, and must be thought of as a malignancy until proven otherwise. Thus, a histologic specimen of the endometrial cavity is required for diagnosis by either office endometrial biopsy or a D&C in the operating room. (**Ref. 3**, p. 233)

22. **(A)** *Key Words:* treatment, Stage I adenocarcinoma endometrium
Total abdominal hysterectomy with bilateral salpingo-oophorectomy is the treatment of choice for Stage I endometrial adenocarcinoma. *Post*operative external radiation therapy is indicated in cases of documented lymph node involvement. (**Ref. 3**, p. 235)

23. **(D)** *Key Words:* age of onset, menopause, related factors
The age of onset of menopause is *not* related to height, weight, race, oral contraceptive use, age at menarche, parity, or socioeconomic conditions. However, smoking *is* related to the age of onset of menopause. (**Ref. 3**, p. 192)

24. **(B, C, F, H)** *Key Words:* risk factors, osteoporosis
The classic presentation of the patient at risk for osteoporosis is a thin, fair-haired, smoker of Northern European origin. Other risk factors include a low-calcium diet, hypoestrogenism, early menopause, caffeine intake, alcohol, and a sedentary lifestyle. (**Ref. 3**, p. 193)

25. **(C)** *Key Words:* treatment, osteoporosis
Estrogen, progestins, calcium, and exercise are all part of the treatment regimen for menopause and osteoporosis. GnRH agonists would be contraindicated in women with osteoporosis, because

they can potentially worsen the condition via their hypoestrogenic action. (**Ref. 3,** p. 195)

26. **(C)** *Figure 6-2:* days 12–13
The post-coital (Sims-Huhner) test is a reflection of the interaction between the sperm and the cervical mucus. It is done prior to ovulation, when there is maximal estrogenic mucus effect. (**Ref. 3,** p. 187)

27. **(E)** *Figure 6-2:* days 26–28
Biopsy of the endometrium is taken about 2–3 prior to the onset of the next expected menses, and is histologically "dated" as a reflection of the progesterone-related changes in the endometrium. (**Ref. 3,** p. 187)

28. **(D)** *Figure 6-2:* day 21
Progesterone is produced by the corpus luteum from ovulation through the next menses. It is responsible for the $1°$ F rise in the basal body temperature. Peak secretion occurs in the mid-luteal phase around day 21 of a 28-day cycle, where ovulation has occurred on day 14. (**Ref. 3,** p. 187)

29. **(B)** *Figure 6-2:* day 8
A hysterosalpingogram (HSG) is performed 2–7 days after cessation of menses in order to evaluate the uterine cavity and tubal patency. It should not be done after ovulation (day 14) because of the risk of interrupting an early pregnancy, nor during menses because of the chance of intravasation of dye, and the possibility of retrograde menstruation leading to endometriosis. (**Ref. 3,** p. 187)

30. **(C)** *Figure 6-3:* estradiol
(**Ref. 2,** p. 132)

31. **(B)** *Figure 6-3:* LH
(**Ref. 2,** p. 132)

32. **(D)** *Figure 6-3:* progesterone
(**Ref. 2,** p. 132)

33. **(A)** *Figure 6-3:* FSH
(**Ref. 2,** p. 132)

34. (E) *Figure 6-3:* 17-OH progesterone
(Ref. 2, p. 132)

35. (A, C, D) *Key Words:* ambiguous genitalia, uterus present, 46 XX karyotype
In this case of female pseudohermaphrodism, it is most important to get a 17-OH progesterone and electrolytes, to rule out congenital adrenal hyperplasia, most commonly associated with a 21-hydroxylase deficiency. One must also rule out a history of maternal androgen ingestion. **(Ref. 3,** pp. 156–157)

36. (B) *Key Words:* mild facial hair, irregular cycles, sexually active, normal DHEAS, minimally elevated testosterone, not interested in pregnancy
This is a classic case presentation of mild hirsutism associated with chronic oligo-ovulation secondary to polycystic ovarian disease (PCOD). There is mild excess ovarian androgen production (testosterone), which is best controlled by oral contraceptives. Since she is sexually active and not interest in pregnancy, these will also be good for contraception. Dexamethasone would be appropriate in cases of adrenal hyperandrogenism (i.e., DHEAS elevation). **(Ref. 3,** p. 178)

37. (A) *Key Words:* male factor infertility
About 40 to 45% of all infertile couples have male factor infertility, while 40 to 45% have female-factor infertility. Ten percent of couples have unexplained infertility. **(Ref. 3,** p. 186)

38. (E) *Key Words:* regular cycles, normal work-up, HSG-no spill
This is a case of distal tubal obstruction, which is amenable to surgical therapy, resulting in a 10–15% chance for conception. If surgery is unsuccessful, IVF would be the next step. Ovulation induction is useless, since she is probably ovulatory already. BBT charting will only prolong the treatment. **(Ref. 3,** p. 189)

39. (B) *Key Words:* physiologic function, hCG
The most apparent function of hCG is to maintain the function of the corpus luteum in early pregnancy. HCG does not initiate menstruation, nor does it maintain the placenta. HCG does stimulate progesterone release, not estrogen release. **(Ref. 3,** pp. 272–273)

40. **(A)** *Key Words:* absolute contraindications, oral contraceptives
    Migraine headaches are a relative contraindication to the oral
    contraceptive. All the others are absolute contraindications. (**Ref.
    1**, p. 232)

41. **(B)** *Key Words:* local barrier methods
    Condoms, sponges, spermicidal foams, and diaphragms are all
    locally acting barriers to conception, i.e., they prevent the sperm
    and the egg from getting together. The IUD does not prevent con-
    ception, and therefore is not a barrier method of contraception. Its
    true mechanism of action is unknown. (**Ref. 3**, p. 201)

42. **(E)** *Key Words:* never pregnant, gonorrhea, previous partners
    In light of this young woman's STD history, she should be coun-
    seled to use the oral contraceptive for pregnancy prevention *and*
    the condom for disease prevention. Abstinence is unrealistic, and
    an IUD would be a poor choice in a sexually active nulligravida
    with a history of STDs. (**Ref. 3**, p. 201)

43. **(E)** *Key Words:* most commonly accepted theory, endometriosis
    All the theories listed are possible explanations for the pathogen-
    esis of endometriosis, but the most commonly accepted theory is
    Sampson's theory of retrograde menstruation. (**Ref. 3**, p. 180)

44. **(D)** *Key Words:* endometriosis, most commonly found
    If retrograde menstruation is the most commonly accepted expla-
    nation for endometriosis, then logically the ovary, being the first
    site in contact with the distal end of the tube, is the most common
    site for the disease. All the other answers are possible but less
    common. (**Ref. 3**, p. 181)

45. **(E)** *Key Words:* definitive diagnosis, endometriosis
    Although a good history and physical examination may lead us to
    suspect endometriosis, it can be definitively diagnosed only by
    means of laparoscopy or laparotomy, with a biopsy of the sus-
    pected implants, if possible. It cannot be diagnosed by Pap smear
    or ultrasound. (**Ref. 3**, p. 180)

46. **(B)** *Key Words:* best medical treatment, endometriosis
    GnRH agonists and danazol work equally well in the medical
    treatment of endometriosis, but danazol has potent androgenic
    side effects, and therefore is not as good. The oral contraceptive

contains estrogen and may not work as well. Neither spironolactone nor dexamethasone is appropriate for the treatment of endometriosis. (**Ref. 3,** p. 181)

47. (**A, B, F**) *Key Words:* histology, endometriosis
The most common histologic picture is that of endometrium itself, i.e., glands and stroma. Often there are also hemosiderin-laden macrophages present. (**Ref. 3,** p. 180)

48. (**A**) *Key Words:* epidemiology, breast cancer
One out of every ten women will develop breast cancer in her lifetime. (**Ref. 3,** p. 102)

49. (**B, C, D**) *Key Words:* routine mammography, frequency
Opinion differs, but the ob/gyn literature recommends routine mammography initially between ages 35 and 40, every other year from 40 to 50, then yearly after age 50. (**Ref. 3,** p. 104)

50. (**D**) *Key Words:* increased risk, breast cancer
Epidemiologic factors that increase risk for breast cancer include irradiation, white race, menarche <12, menopause >55, first baby >30, alcohol, and a positive family history. Lactation and breast feeding do not appear to influence breast cancer risk. (**Ref. 3,** pp. 102–103)

51. (**D**) *Key Words:* PMS
Since the cause of PMS is unknown, there is no specific definitive treatment that works in all cases. The other statements are all true. (**Ref. 2,** p. 662)

52. (**D**) *Key Words:* basal body temperature, elevation
The basal body temperature rises approximately $1°$ F after ovulation, and remains elevated for the duration of the luteal phase until the onset of the next menses, when the temperature drops back down to baseline. (**Ref. 3,** p. 186)

53. (**D**) *Key Words:* FSH level, menopause
Two separate FSH levels >40 mIU/mL are consistent with menopause. (**Ref. 4,** p. 321)

54. (**C**) *Key Words:* duration, menstrual flow
The duration of the menstrual flow varies from 4 to 6 days. (**Ref. 3,** p. 10)

55. **(C)** *Key Words:* ER, poor appetite, 20-lb weight loss, 2° amenorrhea
Anorexia nervosa is the most logical diagnosis. Addison's disease may also present similarly, but is much less common. Hyperthyroidism and juvenile diabetes are usually associated with weight loss despite *increased* appetite. Turner's syndrome usually presents as primary amenorrhea, without the other weight changes. (**Ref. 3,** p. 168)

56. **(B)** *Key Words:* frequency, ectopic pregnancy
More than one in 100 pregnancies in the United States are ectopic. (**Ref. 3,** p. 60)

57. **(C)** *Figure 6-4:* hydatidiform mole
Complete moles have a 46 XX karyotype and are entirely of paternal origin. The other statements are true. (**Ref. 3,** pp. 246–247)

58. **(A)** *Figure 6-4:* hydatidiform mole
The treatment of choice for uncomplicated molar disease is immediate evacuation upon diagnosis. This is usually accomplished by suction curettage, although hysterotomy may be necessary. (**Ref. 3,** pp. 247–249)

59. **(E)** *Key Words:* ectopic, etiology
Combination oral contraceptives are not considered a cause of ectopics. (**Ref. 3,** p. 60)

60. **(E)** *Key Words:* pelvic relaxation, estrogen deficiency
Uterine prolapse, unlike other conditions, is usually associated with trauma secondary to childbirth. (**Ref 3,** p. 112)

61. **(D)** *Figure 6-5:* Turner's syndrome
Turner's syndrome females are usually very short, with an average adult height less than 60 in. (**Ref. 2,** pp. 110–111)

62. **(A)** *Key Words:* galactorrhea
All are associated with galactorrhea except for bromocryptine, a dopamine agonist that is the treatment for galactorrhea. (**Ref. 2,** p. 1120)

63. **(B)** *Key Words:* pelvic diaphragm
The mons pubis is not part of the pelvic diaphragm. (**Ref. 3,** p. 4)

64. **(C)** *Key Words:* sexually active, pain, amenorrhea for 7 weeks, bleeding, adnexal mass, hypotension, tachycardia
This is a ruptured ectopic pregnancy complicated by hemoperitoneum and impending hypovolemic shock. Sepsis would present with a fever, and the other diagnoses listed do not at all fit the severity of this picture. **(Ref. 3, p. 63)**

65. **(B)** *Key Words:* dyspareunia
Dyspareunia may cause anorgasmia, rather than vice versa. **(Ref. 3, p. 86)**

66. **(B)** *Key Words:* dysfunctional uterine bleeding (DUB)
DUB appears commonly at both ends of a woman's reproductive lifespan, and is most commonly associated with anovulatory cycles. D&C, although palliative, is rarely curative. Ultrasound of the endometrial lining may help to rule out endometrial hyperplasia. **(Ref. 3, p. 97)**

67. **(C)** *Key Words:* frothy, yellow-green, discharge
This is the discharge from trichomoniasis. Metronidazole is the drug of choice. **(Ref. 3, p. 44)**

68. **(D)** *Key Words:* cottage cheese, exudate
This is the discharge from candidiasis. Clotrimazole is the drug of choice. **(Ref. 3, p. 44)**

69. **(B)** *Key Words:* mucopurulent, discharge
This is the discharge from chlamydia cervicitis. Doxycycline is the drug of choice. **(Ref. 3, p. 44)**

70. **(F)** *Figure 6-6:* 23.7%
The first-year failure rate in typical users of rhythm is about 24%. **(Ref. 3, p. 198)**

71. **(A)** *Figure 6-6:* 2.0%
The first-year failure rate in typical users of oral contraceptives is 2%. **(Ref. 3, p. 198)**

72. **(C)** *Figure 6-6:* 9.1%
The first-year failure rate in typical users of condoms is 10%. **(Ref. 3, p. 198)**

73. **(D)** *Figure 6-6:* 17.9%
The first-year failure rate in typical users of spermicides is 18%.
(**Ref. 3**, p. 198)

74. **(B)** *Figure 6-6:* 4.6%
The first-year failure rate in typical users of IUDs is 5%. (**Ref. 3**, p. 198)

75. **(E)** *Figure 6-6:* 18.6%
The first-year failure rate in typical users of diaphragms is 19%.
(**Ref. 3**, p. 198)

OBSTETRICS

76. **(D)** *Key Words:* 3 weeks post-partum, nursing, fever, breast engorgement
The symptoms of suppurative mastitis appear about the third or fourth week post-partum. The most common offending organism is *Staphylococcus aureus* from the infant's nose and throat. (**Ref. 3**, p. 386)

77. **(B)** *Figure 6-7:* partial placenta previa
A partial placenta previa is so named because it partially covers the internal os. As the uterus grows larger, some separation and painless bleeding may occur. (**Ref. 3**, p. 435)

78. **(C)** *Figure 6-7:* abruptio placenta with external hemorrhage
This reflects separation of the placenta from its site of implantation in the uterus, before delivery of the fetus, and is associated with painful bleeding. (**Ref. 3**, p. 433)

79. **(A)** *Figure 6-7:* abruptio placenta with concealed hemorrhage
This is a very dangerous form of abruption because there is no external bleeding. This may result in uterine hypertonus and even fetal demise before it is diagnosed. (**Ref. 3**, p. 433)

80. **(B)** *Key Words:* lecithin to sphingomyelin (L-S) ratio, after 34 weeks

The L-S ratio, a sign of fetal lung maturity reaches 2:1 or more after 34 weeks gestation, when the risk of respiratory distress is slight. (**Ref. 3,** p. 328)

81. **(E)** *Key Words:* coagulation factors decrease, pregnancy
Factors I, VII, VIII, IX, and X all increase during pregnancy, while factors XI and XIII decrease somewhat. (**Ref. 3,** p. 284)

82. **(A)** *Key Words:* add 7 days, subtract 3 months, last menstrual period
Naegele's rule is used to calculate the estimated date of delivery. (**Ref. 3,** p. 322)

83. **(B)** *Key Words:* diagnosis, rupture of membranes
Nitrazine paper is used as a colorimetric pH assay. The pH of normal vaginal secretions range in pH between 4.5 and 5.5, while amniotic fluid is 7.0 to 7.5, resulting in a characteristic color change in the nitrazine paper. (**Ref. 3,** p. 341)

84. **(E)** *Key Words:* total weight gain, pregnancy
It is generally recommended that women gain 22–27 lb during pregnancy. (**Ref. 3,** p. 324)

85. **(A)** *Key Words:* elemental iron, latter half pregnancy
Every pregnant woman should be given at least 30 mg of elemental iron, supplied as a simple iron salt, such as ferrous gluconate or sulfate. (**Ref. 3,** p. 325)

86. **(C)** *Key Words:* last month pregnancy, uteroplacental blood flow
Uteroplacental blood flow increases to more than 500 mL/min in late pregnancy. (**Ref. 3,** p. 278)

87. **(C)** *Key Words:* resting heart rate, pregnancy
Resting pulse increases about 10–15 bpm in pregnancy, with a 10% increase in cardiac volume (**Ref. 3,** p. 285)

88. **(B)** *Key Words:* asymptomatic bacteriuria, pregnancy
The reported prevalence of asymptomatic bacteriuria during pregnancy varies between 2 and 12%, depending on parity, race, and socioeconomic status. (**Ref. 3,** p. 448)

89. (D) *Key Words:* heart disease criteria, pregnancy
In normal pregnancy, functional systolic heart murmurs are quite common. The other criteria would be consistent with heart disease. (**Ref. 3,** p. 446)

90. (C) *Key Words:* post-partum hemorrhage
Post-partum hemorrhage is defined as >500 mL blood loss within the first 24 hours post-partum. It is the cause of 25% of deaths from obstetrical hemorrhage. (**Ref. 3,** p. 383)

91. (D) *Key Words:* magnesium sulfate, pre-eclampsia
Magnesium sulfate is used to treat pre-eclampsia and eclamptic seizures, without causing generalized CNS depression in either the mother or the fetus. (**Ref. 3,** p. 430)

92. (E) *Key Words:* placenta previa
A digital examination of the cervix is contraindicated if the diagnosis of placenta previa is suspect. Ultrasound would be the best way to make the diagnosis. (**Ref. 3,** pp. 434–436)

93. (E) *Key Words:* contraction stress test (CST), contraindications
Oligohydramnios is an indication, rather than a contraindication, for CST. (**Ref. 3,** p. 332)

94. (D) *Key Words:* respiratory function, pregnancy
The residual volume and functional residual capacity are decreased in pregnancy. The respiratory rate changes little, but the tidal volume, minute ventilation, and minute oxygen uptake are increased in pregnancy. (**Ref. 3,** p. 286)

95. (A) *Key Words:* danger signals, pregnancy
Ankle swelling can be normal depending on the patient's weight, gestational age, and level of activity. All the other items listed are potential danger signals. (**Ref. 3,** p. 323)

96. (B) *Key Words:* severe abruption
Disseminated intravascular coagulation is a sign of severe abruption, leading to possible fatal hemorrhage and fetal demise. This is associated with hypofibrinogenemia <150 mg/dL, along with elevated fibrin-degradation products. (**Ref. 3,** p. 434)

97. **(D)** *Key Words:* abdominal ultrasound, β-hCG levels
When the β-hCG level is greater than or equal to 6000 mIU/mL, evidence of an intrauterine gestational sac should be seen using abdominal ultrasonography, and above 2000 mIU/mL with vaginal sonography. (**Ref. 3,** p. 64)

98. **(D)** *Key Words:* early pregnancy symptoms
Amenorrhea, breast tenderness, fatigue, and morning sickness are all early symptoms of pregnancy. Urinary frequency is also common. (**Ref. 3,** p. 257)

99. **(D)** *Key Words:* oxytocin contraindications, induction of labor
Post-dates would be a definite indication for oxytocin induction of labor. The other items are all relative or absolute contraindications and would necessitate caesarean section. (**Ref. 3,** p. 359)

100. **(E); 101. (A); 102. (B); 103. (F); 104. (H); 105. (G); 106. (D); 107. (C)** *Figure 6-8*
The uterine artery carries oxygenated blood from the heart to the uterus in the maternal circulation. Therefore uterine arterial values for pO_2, hemoglobin, pCO_2, and HCO_3, respectively, are 95 mm Hg, 12 g/dL, 32 mm Hg, and 18.8 mM/L. The umbilical artery carries deoxygenated fetal blood away from the fetus toward the placenta. Therefore umbilical arterial values for pO_2, hemoglobin, pCO_2, and HCO_3, respectively, are 15 mm Hg, 16 g/dL, 48 mm Hg, and 25 mM/L. (**Ref. 5,** p. 174)

108. **(B)** *Key Words:* blood loss greater
Mediolateral episiotomy results in greater blood loss than midline episiotomy. (**Ref. 3,** p. 347)

109. **(B)** *Key Words:* dyspareunia
Dyspareunia is more common after a mediolateral episiotomy due to faulty healing. (**Ref. 3,** p. 347)

110. **(A)** *Key Words:* easy repair
Midline episiotomy is much easier to repair because of the natural apposition of the tissue in the midline of the perineum. (**Ref. 3,** p. 347)

111. **(B)** *Key Words:* improper healing
Improper healing occurs more frequently after mediolateral episiotomy because of the difficulty of the repair compared to a midline repair. (**Ref. 3,** p. 347)

112. **(A)** *Key Words:* anal sphincter extension
Unfortunately, this is the only "down" side of doing a midline episiotomy. Otherwise the advantages of a median episiotomy far outweigh the disadvantages. (**Ref. 3,** p. 347)

113. **(D)** *Key Words:* twin pregnancies
Twins do not have to be delivered by caesarean section. In fact, cephalic presentation of the first twin occurs over 75% of the time, and is compatible with vaginal delivery at least for the first twin. The most common indication for c-section is noncephalic presentation for one or both fetuses. All the other statements concerning twin pregnancies are true. (**Ref. 3,** pp. 421–425)

114. **(E)** *Key Words:* Rh negative, 22 weeks pregnant
Intrauterine exchange transfusion for Rh disease may be initiated as early as 22 weeks, but only for severe hemolytic disease as evidenced by an antibody titer no higher than 1:16 as measured by indirect Coombs. The other statements regarding Rh isoimmunization are true. (**Ref. 3,** pp. 415–417)

115. **(C)** *Figure 6-9:* morning sickness
Morning sickness usually occurs about 6 weeks after the onset of the last menstrual period, in response to rising hCG titers. (**Ref. 3,** p. 257)

116. **(E)** *Figure 6-9:* fetal activity
Fetal activity is first recognized by the pregnant woman between 16 and 20 weeks gestation, and is called "quickening." (**Ref. 3,** p. 257)

117. **(B)** *Figure 6-9:* first missed menses
Cessation of menses is highly suggestive of pregnancy. However, other conditions such as anovulation may result in missed menses too. (**Ref. 3,** p. 257)

118. **(D)** *Figure 6-9:* uterus palpable, symphysis pubis
The uterus can be felt through the abdominal wall after 12 weeks gestation above the level of the symphysis pubis. (**Ref. 3,** p. 258)

119. (A) *Figure 6-9:* conception
Conception occurs at ovulation, two weeks after the last menstrual period. **(Ref. 3,** p. 262)

120. (C); 121. (A); 122. (B) *Figure 6-10*
The risk of Down syndrome in mothers of all ages is 1:800 liveborns. At age 40, the risk is 1:100. By age 45, the risk of Down syndrome is 1:32. **(Ref. 3,** pp. 407–408)

123. (C); 124. (B); 125. (A) *Key Words:* milk, protein, lactose, fat
The major components of milk are proteins, lactose, water, and fat. Milk is isotonic with plasma, with lactose accounting for half of the osmotic pressure. Human colostrum is lowest in fat, while human mature mile is highest in lactose and fat. Cow's milk is highest in protein and lowest in lactose. **(Ref. 5,** p. 465)

126. (C) *Key Words:* late decelerations
Late decelerations are usually the consequence of uteroplacental insufficiency leading to pulmonary hypoxia. Entry of the fetal head into the pelvic brim results in early decelerations secondary to head compression. Cord compression is associated with variable decelerations. Neither congenital cardiac conduction defects nor pulmonary immaturity may result in decelerations at all. **(Ref. 3,** pp. 336–338)

127. (A) *Key Words:* cardinal movements, labor
The seven cardinal movements of labor in order are engagement, descent, flexion, internal rotation, extension, external rotation, and expulsion. **(Ref. 3,** pp. 308–309)

128. (B) *Key Words:* top cause, maternal mortality
Embolism, hypertensive disease, and hemorrhage are the top three causes of maternal deaths in the United States, accounting for 20, 17, and 13% of deaths, respectively. Infection accounts for 8% of maternal mortality, while anesthesia-related deaths are about 4%. **(Ref. 3,** pp. 253–254)

129. (C) *Key Words:* hemostasis, post-partum hemorrhage
Obstetric hemorrhage is the consequence of excessive bleeding from the placental implantation site and/or trauma to the genital tract. With placental separation, maternal–fetal vessels are severed abruptly. Thus, contraction of the myometrium, resulting in vessel

compression and obliteration of the lumen, is the most important mechanism in combating post-partum hemorrhage. (**Ref. 3**, p. 432)

130. **(B)** *Key Words:* non-nursing, first menses
If the woman does not nurse, menstrual flow will probably return within 6 to 8 weeks after delivery. (**Ref. 3**, p. 320)

131. **(D)** *Key Words:* smallest A-P diameter, pelvic inlet
The obstetric conjugate is the shortest A-P diameter through which the fetal head must pass in descending through the pelvic inlet. It is normally more than 10 cm longer than the true conjugate and diagonal conjugate. The interspinous diameter is not an A-P diameter, but rather a transverse diameter. (**Ref. 3**, p. 300)

132. **(D)** *Key Words:* routine pelvic exam, contraindicated
Placenta previa is a contraindication to routine pelvic exam; ultrasound is preferable in making the diagnosis. Routine pelvic exam may be performed in all the other situations. (**Ref. 3**, p. 435)

133. **(B)** *Key Words:* heart rate 90, irregular respiration, grimace, pale, limp, blue
APGAR scoring at 1 minute in this case would be heart rate <100 = 1 point, irregular respiration = 1 point, limp muscle tone = 0, grimace reflex activity = 1 point, and blue color, pale = 0. Total points = 3. (**Ref. 3**, p. 312)

134. **(D)** *Key Words:* oxytocin, nonapeptide
Oxytocin and vasopressin are produced in the posterior pituitary gland. Both are chemically very similar. LH, FSH, and ACTH are glycoproteins produced in the anterior pituitary. Insulin is a polypeptide produced in the pancreas. (**Ref. 2**, pp. 138–140)

135. **(C)** *Key Words:* biophysical profile
Membrane status is not part of the biophysical profile. A reactive non-stress test and fetal movements, in addition to the other items listed, *are* part of the biophysical profile. (**Ref. 3**, p. 334)

136. **(C)** *Key Words:* uterine contractions
Uterine contractions may be palpable in false labor as well as true labor. All the other statements are correct. (**Ref. 3**, p. 294)

137. **(A)** *Key Words:* post-partum hemorrhage, unresponsive, most likely cause

Post-partum hemorrhage is most responsive to oxytocin and uterine massage when it is secondary to uterine atony. Although placenta accreta, ruptured uterus, coagulopathy, and vaginal lacerations are unresponsive to oxytocin or uterine massage, vaginal lacerations would be the most common cause of hemorrhage in this situation. All the others are rare. (**Ref. 3,** pp. 432–433)

138. **(A)** *Key Words:* third-stage labor

The first stage of labor ends when the cervix is fully dilated (10 cm). The second stage of labor ends with delivery of the infant. The third stage of labor lasts from delivery of the infant to the separation and expulsion of the placenta. (**Ref. 3,** p. 293)

139. **(D)** *Figure 6-11:* double-footling breech, ruptured membranes, variable decelerations

This is a classic scenario for cord prolapse, especially when membranes are ruptured. Immediate caesarean section should be performed. (**Ref. 3,** pp. 363–364)

140. **(C)** *Figure 6-12*

Curve C represents arrested labor in active phase. Curve A is a normal labor curve, while curve B demonstrates a protracted active phase. (**Ref. 3,** pp. 356–358)

141. **(B)** *Key Words:* drug, preterm labor

Beta agonists are most commonly used in the treatment of preterm labor. The other commonly used agent is magnesium sulfate. (**Ref. 3,** p. 440)

142. **(E)** *Key Words:* third trimester bleeding, breech

This situation is classic for placenta previa. (**Ref. 3,** p. 362)

143. **(C)** *Key Words:* fever, backache, late pregnancy, bacteriuria

This situation is a classic description of pyelonephritis. It is most commonly right-sided and more common after midpregnancy. (**Ref. 3,** p. 448)

144. **(D)** *Key Words:* latent phase, labor

The latent phase of labor precedes the active phase. The active phase consists of the acceleration phase, phase of maximum slope, and deceleration phase. (**Ref. 3**, p. 357)

145. **(E)** *Key Words:* premature rupture of the membranes
Premature rupture of the membranes and prematurity in general refer to any occurrence before 37–38 weeks of gestation. (**Ref. 3**, p. 438)

146. **(B)** *Key Words:* severe pre-eclampsia
The development of convulsions in the absence of neurological disease is pathognomonic for eclampsia. All the other statements apply to severe pre-eclampsia. (**Ref. 3**, pp. 428–429)

147. **(B)** *Key Words:* neonatal death
The leading cause of neonatal death is prematurity. (**Ref. 3**, p. 254)

148. **(C); 149. (B); 150. (A)** *Key Words:* true labor, false labor
Uterine contractions are palpable in both true and false labor. However, in false labor, the cervix does not dilate; in true labor, sedation is generally ineffective. (**Ref. 3**, p. 340)

References

1. Beckmann CRB, Ling FW, Barzansky BM et al. (eds): *Obstetrics and Gynecology for Medical Students.* Baltimore, MD, Williams & Wilkins, 1992.

2. DeCherney AH, Pernoll ML (eds): *Current Obstetric & Gynecologic Diagnosis and Treatment,* 18th ed. Norwalk, CT, Appleton & Lange, 1994.

3. Gant NF, Cunningham FG (eds): *Basic Gynecology and Obstetrics.* Norwalk, CT, Appleton & Lange, 1993.

4. Jacobs AJ, Gast MJ (eds): *Practical Gynecology.* Norwalk, CT, Appleton & Lange, 1994.

5. Cunningham GF et al. (eds): *Williams Obstetrics,* 19th ed. Norwalk, CT, Appleton & Lange, 1993.

7

Public Health and Preventive Medicine

Richard H. Hart, MD, DrPh

DIRECTIONS: Each of the questions or incomplete statements below is followed by a list of suggested answers or completions. Select the **one** that is best in each case.

---

1. A 2-year-old child is being seen for a well child check-up. Which of the following is a leading potential cause of death for this child, for which a preventive measure is available, and which should be addressed with the parents?
   A. Lead toxicity
   B. Motor vehicle accident
   C. Tuberculosis
   D. Pneumonia

2. For a 40- to 50-year-old male with no know medical problems, which of the following screening tests should routinely be performed?
   A. Urinalysis
   B. Sigmoidoscopy
   C. Cholesterol
   D. Prostate specific antigen

3. A slender 50-year-old caucasian female with fair skin is being seen for a routine Papanicolaou (Pap) smear. She is post-menopausal and in good health with no known medical problems. Her activity level is sedentary, and she spends most of her time indoors. Which of the following preventive measures would be **MOST APPROPRIATE?**
   A. Electrocardiogram
   B. Discussion of aspirin therapy
   C. Discussion of estrogen replacement surgery
   D. Instruction to use skin protection from UV light

4. Treatment of a person with AIDS using AZT is what level of prevention?
   A. Primary prevention
   B. Secondary prevention
   C. Tertiary prevention
   D. All of the above

5. Treatment of a person with AIDS using trimethoprim-sul-famethoxazole reflects which level of prevention?
   A. Primary prevention
   B. Secondary prevention
   C. Tertiary prevention
   D. All of the above

6. The crude birth rate (CBR), the most fundamental fertility measure, uses
   A. all births in the numerator and total population in the denominator
   B. all births in the numerator and women 15–44 years of age in the denominator
   C. the sum of all of the age-specific fertility rates by single years of age
   D. births to women in a specific age range in the numerator

7. *Fertility* refers to
   A. the capacity to bear children
   B. the probability of conceiving in a given month
   C. the actual birth of living offspring
   D. the probability of conceiving in a given year per 1000 women

8. The country with the highest life expectancy at birth for males, reaching 75.5 years in 1986, is
   A. Canada
   B. United States
   C. Japan
   D. Sweden

9. As we near the year 2000, what percentage of the world's population is found in urban areas?
   A. 22%
   B. 40%
   C. 60%
   D. 75%

10. The main reason that population growth rates in lesser developed countries have accelerated during the past several generations is
    A. birth rates have increased in rural areas
    B. death rates have decreased
    C. death rates have remained steady due to better living conditions
    D. high fertility rates

11. A country with a rapidly growing population has which of the following characteristics?
    A. 40–50% of the population is less than 15 years of age
    B. A crude birth rate of 20–30
    C. High doubling time
    D. A low migration rate

12. If a country had a crude birth rate of 35/1000 people/year and a crude death rate of 15/1000/year, what would its growth rate be?
    A. 20%
    B. 2%
    C. 2.3%
    D. 5%

13. A 33-year-old caucasian male traveled to South America for three days. Within hours of his return he had onset of watery diarrhea and abdominal cramping. What is the **MOST LIKELY** etiology?
    A. *Yersinia enterocolitica*
    B. *Escherichia coli*

C. *Giardia*
D. *Salmonella*

14. Prophylaxis of traveler's diarrhea can be accomplished by
    A. trimethoprim-sulfamethoxazole
    B. penicillin
    C. metronidazole
    D. iodochlorhydroxyquin (Entero-Vioform)

15. Effective preventive measures include which of the following?
    A. consumption of ice-chilled beverages
    B. consumption of washed raw vegetables
    C. use of water treated with 1–2 drops of 1% chlorine bleach per quart of water
    D. use of water treated with 5–10 drops of 2% tincture of iodine per quart of water

16. Which of the following vaccines are required for travel in endemic areas?
    A. Yellow fever vaccine
    B. Small pox vaccine
    C. Meningococcal vaccine
    D. Japanese encephalitis vaccine

17. Which of the following is a potential condition associated with *E. coli* infection?
    A. Hemorrhagic colitis
    B. Hemolytic uremic syndrome
    C. Meningitis
    D. Osteomyelitis

18. Which of the following vaccines for nonimmune travelers is recommended for pregnant females?
    A. Measles, mumps, rubella vaccine
    B. Yellow fever vaccine
    C. Oral typhoid vaccine
    D. Tetanus toxoid vaccine

19. In general, for nonimmune HIV- (human immunodeficiency virus)-positive travelers, all the following vaccinations are contraindicated **EXCEPT**
    A. oral polio vaccine
    B. measles, mumps, rubella vaccine
    C. oral typhoid vaccine
    D. yellow fever vaccine

20. For immunizations in a healthy infant in the United States whose immunization schedule is up to date, all the following vaccines are appropriate for the six-month visit **EXCEPT**
    A. oral polio vaccine
    B. diphtheria, pertussis, tetanus vaccine
    C. measles, mumps, rubella vaccine
    D. *Haemophilus influenza,* type B vaccine

21. The oral typhoid vaccine would be **MOST APPROPRIATE** for travelers in which of the following situations?
    A. Children under the age of 2 years
    B. Travelers visiting endemic areas
    C. Women in the first trimester of pregnancy
    D. HIV-positive travelers

22. Immune globulin should be withheld or given with caution in all the following situations **EXCEPT** for persons
    A. with sensitivity to mercury
    B. receiving MMR concurrently
    C. with severe thrombocytopenia
    D. receiving OPT concurrently

23. Which is the **MOST APPROPRIATE** situation for the administration of measles (rubeola) immunization?
    A. Travelers with HIV infection
    B. Americans born before 1957
    C. Pregnant females in endemic areas
    D. Persons with congenital immunodeficiency

24. A 21-year-old college student presented to student health services with complaints of cough and fever for a few days. On physical examination, an erythematous maculopapular rash is present, and

Koplik spots are present on the oral mucosa. Which of the following is **TRUE** concerning this illness?

A. This illness is more common and more severe in children

B. In the typical form, the rash appears first on the torso and then spreads to the extremities

C. Conjunctivitis, excessive lacrimation, and photophobia are common symptoms

D. Prompt administration of immune globulin soon after exposure does *not* alter the course of the illness

25. The single **MOST USEFUL** method to control measles (rubeola) in the United States has been

A. isolation of exposed individuals

B. good sanitation in crowded institutions

C. enactment and enforcement of school immunization laws

D. maintaining high levels of passive immunity

26. Which of the following is **TRUE** about current vaccinations for influenza?

A. The World Health Organization makes recommendations every two to three years to the Centers for Disease Control and Prevention and vaccine manufacturers on the formulation of the vaccines

B. An increased incidence of Guillain-Barré has been observed in association with the influenza vaccine in the past ten years

C. The most common current vaccines are trivalent with two A strains and one B strain

D. Vaccination of high-risk groups has only a modest effect on mortality rates

27. Efforts to control influenza in the United States has **BEST** been achieved by

A. isolation

B. prophylaxis

C. immunization

D. ultraviolet irradiation

28. Which of the following is the **LEAST LIKELY** mode of transmission for varicella?
    A. Airborne droplets
    B. Direct contact
    C. Fomites
    D. Blood exposure

29. Which of the following is **FALSE** about the prevention and treatment of *Haemophilus influenzae*?
    A. Chemoprophylaxis with rifampin for household contacts under 6 years of age has been recommended for patients with *Influenzae meningitis*
    B. For normal, healthy infants, immunization for *H. influenzae* begins at 2 months of age
    C. A three-stage vaccination is available for primary immunization and a booster
    D. Treatment for life-threatening illnesses from *H. influenzae* may include both chloramphenicol and ampicillin

30. Which of the following statements is **TRUE** concerning the epidemiology of *Haemophilus influenzae*?
    A. 95% of cases of *H. influenzae* meningitis occur in children over 5 years of age
    B. The incidence in Alaskan natives is 10 times the national average
    C. The incidence of *H. influenzae* infection is lowest in the spring
    D. The incidence of *H. influenzae* meningitis is higher in whites than in African-Americans

31. Concerning the epidemiology of Pneumococcus (*Streptococcus pneumonia*), which of the following statements is **FALSE**?
    A. The most common cause of community-acquired bacterial pneumonia
    B. Responsible for most cases of otitis media
    C. One of the three most common causes of bacterial meningitis
    D. A low case fatality rate in cases of meningitis because of its great susceptibility to penicillin

Questions 32–33: After a problem of fever and malaise, a 23-year-old pregnant female in her first trimester presents with a history of a nonspecific maculopapular rash that lasted 3 days; she also had cervical lymphadenopathy.

32. Her unborn child may be at increased risk for all the following congenital cardiac abnormalities **EXCEPT**
A. tetralogy of Fallot
B. patent ductus arteriosus
C. myocardial necrosis
D. pulmonary stenosis

33. The infant is also at increase risk for developing which of the following endocrinopathies?
A. Diabetes insipidus
B. Precocious puberty
C. Gout
D. Gigantism

34. Which of the following methods has been **MOST EFFECTIVE** in the control and prevention of pertussis in the United States?
A. Isolation
B. Conferment of passive immunity
C. Conferment of active immunity
D. Restriction of fomite transmission

35. The **MOST COMMON** cause of mortality associated with varicella infection in the adult population is
A. sepsis
B. pneumonia
C. encephalitis
D. meningitis

36. Immunizations that are **NOT APPROPRIATE** for the human immunodeficiency- (HIV)-positive traveler include
A. measles, mumps, rubella vaccine
B. inactivated polio vaccine
C. bacillus Calmette-Guerin vaccine
D. pneumococcal vaccine

37. Of the following immunizations, which one would be **MOST APPROPRIATE** for the HIV-positive traveler?
    A. Oral polio vaccine
    B. Bacillus Calmette-Guerin vaccine
    C. Yellow fever vaccine
    D. Immune globulin

38. Which of the following is the only virus that has been isolated from breast milk following a mother's immunization?
    A. Yellow fever
    B. Rubella
    C. Hepatitis B
    D. Polio

39. Precautions for the administration of oral polio vaccine include avoidance of vaccination in the presence of which of the following situations?
    A. An immunodeficient household contact
    B. Prematurity
    C. Diarrhea
    D. Breast feeding

40. In general, which of the following should be considered a precaution when administering the diphtheria, tetanus, pertussis vaccine?
    A. Family history of convulsions
    B. Family history of sudden infant death syndrome
    C. Temperature of 105° F (40.5° C)
    D. Prematurity

41. Current strategies recommended by the Centers for Disease Control and Prevention for epidemiologic control and prevention of sexually transmitted diseases in the U.S. population include all the following **EXCEPT**
    A. barrier methods
    B. contact tracing
    C. screening programs
    D. disease reporting

42. Syphilis remains an important sexually transmitted disease in the United States, despite declining after reaching a peak in the latter half of the 1980s, because of all the following **EXCEPT**
   A. its association with HIV transmission
   B. its escalating rate among male homosexuals
   C. its preventability and curability
   D. its effect on perinatal mortality and morbidity

43. All the following trends are reflective of gonorrhea infection in the United States during the 1980s **EXCEPT** a(n)
   A. increase in the incidence among white homosexual males
   B. increase in the incidence among African-American teenagers
   C. decrease in the incidence among the U.S. population
   D. decrease in the incidence among white Americans

44. Since the emergence of clinically significant penicillinase-producing *Neisseria* gonorrhea (PPNG), antibiotic resistance has been associated with all the following drugs **EXCEPT**
   A. tetracyclines
   B. aminoglycosides
   C. third-generation cephalosporins
   D. penicillins

Questions 45–47: Choose the organism that is **MOST CLOSELY** associated with the statements. Each answer may be used once, more than once, or not at all.

   A. *Neisseria gonorrhea*
   B. *Chlamydia trachomatis*
   C. *Yersinia enterocolitica*
   D. *Streptococcus fecalis*

45. The etiology of the most common sexually transmitted bacterial genital infection _____

46. Plasmid mediated resistance has hampered the progress in treatment _____

47. Chromosomally mediated resistance has hampered progress in treatment _____

Questions 48–52: A 30-year-old male comes into a community clinic with complaints of several lesions at the base of his penis. He is sexually active and has never had anything like this before. He complains that he has had these painful lesions for about seven days.

48. What is the **MOST LIKELY** causative organism?
    A. *Chlamydia trachomatis*
    B. Herpes simplex virus-2
    C. *Haemophilus ducreyi*
    D. *Treponemum pallidum*

49. What is the **BEST** method for definitive diagnosis for this acute infection?
    A. Serologic assay
    B. Viral isolation from tissue culture
    C. Tanck preparation
    D. Darkfield examination of tissue

50. Which of the following neoplasms has been strongly correlated with this sexually transmitted disease?
    A. Anal carcinoma
    B. Vulvar carcinoma
    C. Cervical carcinoma
    D. Vaginal carcinoma

51. Which of the following are possible associated syndromes?
    A. Epididymitis
    B. Aseptic meningitis
    C. Penile carcinoma
    D. Prostatitis

52. What is the **MOST APPROPRIATE** management?
    A. Erythromycin
    B. Acyclovir
    C. Ceftriaxone
    D. Tetracycline

53. Which of the following is **MOST TRUE** concerning herpes simplex virus-2 (HSV-2) infection and genital lesions?
   A. In patients with HSV-2 antibodies, the majority noticed symptoms associated with their HSV-2 infection
   B. In 75% of cases of confirmed HSV-2 transmission, no lesions were present at the time of transmission
   C. HSV-2 infection is *not* associated with increased HIV risk among homosexuals
   D. HSV-2 infection ranks third as a cause of genital ulcerations

54. Efforts to aid in the diagnosis and control of subclinical human papilloma virus (HPV) infection include detecting all the following **EXCEPT**
   A. koilocytes on cytological smears
   B. HPV viral cultures
   C. immunochemical strains for HPV antigen
   D. HPV nucleic acid sequences

55. Which of the following is **TRUE** regarding HPV and subclinical infection?
   A. HPV is not usually transmitted in the absence of lesions
   B. Cervical cancer can be a sequelae of HPV infection despite the absence of HPV lesions
   C. Subclinical HPV penile infections are thought to be uncommon
   D. Most of the 57 types of HPV are associated with genital infections

56. For the control of hepatitis B infection (HBV), which of the following groups would it be **MOST IMPORTANT** to vaccinate in terms of controlling transmission?
   A. Homosexual males
   B. Hemodialysis patients
   C. Institutionalized patients
   D. Health care workers

57. The long-term effects of HBV infection include an increased risk for all the following **EXCEPT**
   A. fulminant hepatitis
   B. hepatic thrombosis
   C. chronic active hepatitis
   D. hepatocellular carcinoma

58. A pregnant 23-year-old woman comes into a primary care clinic and receives a diagnosis of pelvic inflammatory disease. She is at **LEAST** risk for developing which of the following complications?

    A. Premature rupture of membranes

    B. Spontaneous abortion

    C. Chorioamnionitis

    D. Prematurity

59. To most effectively use available resources to prevent neonatal infection with herpes simplex virus (HSV), which of the following would be the **BEST** strategy?

    A. Caesarean delivery

    B. Screening prior to delivery for maternal HSV

    C. Reducing the duration of infectivity (decreasing viral transmission)

    D. Changing sexual practices of high-risk core groups

60. Human papilloma virus (HPV) infection has been strongly associated with all the following neoplasms **EXCEPT**

    A. vulvar

    B. testicular

    C. anal

    D. cervical

Questions 61–64: Select the virus **MOST STRONGLY** associated with the disease. The answers may be used once, more than once, or not at all.

    A. Human papilloma virus (HPV)

    B. Hepatitis B infection (HBV)

    C. Human immunodeficiency virus (HIV)

    D. Herpes simplex virus-2 (HSV-2)

61. Penile carcinoma _____

62. Hepatocellular carcinoma _____

63. Non-Hodgkins lymphoma _____

64. Anal carcinoma _____

Questions 65–66: A 21-year-old male, with signs of urethritis, conjunctivitis, and arthritis, has just received a presumptive diagnosis of an accompanying sexually transmitted disease (STD).

65. Which is the **MOST LIKELY** organism to cause the associated STD?
    A. *Neisseria gonorrhea*
    B. *Chlamydia trachomatis*
    C. *Treponemum pallidum*
    D. *Gardnerella vaginalis*

66. The treatment of choice for this STD includes
    A. doxycycline
    B. penicillin
    C. metronidazole
    D. trimethoprin-sulfamethoxazole

67. Treatment for Reiter's syndrome, with its triad of urethritis, conjunctivitis, and arthritis, consists of all the following **EXCEPT**
    A. systemic steroids
    B. nonsteroidal antiinflammatory drugs
    C. analgesics
    D. cytotoxic drugs

Questions 68–71: Select the syndrome characterized by the presence of the symptom or response. The answers may be used once, more than once, or not at all.

    A. Reiter's syndrome
    B. Gonoccocal arthritis
    C. Both of the above

68. Conjunctivitis _____

69. Balanitis _____

70. **MOST LIKELY** to affect the upper extremities _____

71. Responds to penicillin _____

72. Which of the following is the **MOST FREQUENTLY** reported AIDS-defining illness?
   A. Invasive cervical carcinoma
   B. Pneumocystic carinii pneumonia
   C. HIV wasting syndrome
   D. Candida infections

73. Choose the control method that is **MOST APPROPRIATE** to control the AIDS epidemic in the regional area of New York.
   A. Use of a needle exchange program
   B. Stressing condom usage and safer sexual practices
   C. Both
   D. Neither

74. Choose the control method that is **MOST APPROPRIATE** to control the AIDS epidemic in Southeast Asia.
   A. Use of a needle exchange program
   B. Stressing condom usage and safer sexual practices
   C. Both
   D. Neither

75. Of the following, which is the most rapidly increasing cause of years of potential life lost?
   A. Unintentional injuries
   B. HIV
   C. Prematurity
   D. Cancer

76. All the following are part of the new Center for Disease Control and Prevention 1993 AIDS Surveillance **EXCEPT**
   A. invasive cervical carcinoma
   B. CD4 positive T-lymphocyte percentage of total <14
   C. recurrent vaginal yeast infections
   D. pulmonary tuberculosis

77. HIV infection has been clearly associated with each of the following neoplastic conditions **EXCEPT**
   A. Kaposi's sarcoma
   B. non-Hodgkins lymphoma
   C. squamous cell carcinoma of the anus
   D. invasive cervical carcinoma

78. In 1993 the number of cases of AIDS attributed to heterosexual transmission to an uninfected partner was highest in which of the following groups?
    A. Intravenous drug users
    B. Transfusion recipients
    C. Persons with hemophilia
    D. Bisexual males

79. The following symptoms are common in *Salmonella typhimurium* infection **EXCEPT**
    A. fever
    B. chill
    C. malaise
    D. diarrhea

80. Effective treatment of *Salmonella typhimurium* include all the following **EXCEPT**
    A. chloramphenicol
    B. septra
    C. erthromycin
    D. ciprofloxacin

81. The following are **TRUE** concerning vibrio cholerae **EXCEPT**
    A. protein endotoxin
    B. water is primary vehicle of infection
    C. bloody diarrhea
    D. noninvasive

82. All the following are *bacterial* causes of gastrointestinal infection **EXCEPT**
    A. *Salmonella*
    B. *Shigella*
    C. *Yersinia entercolitica*
    D. *Giardia lambia*

83. Which of the following is **NOT TRUE** concerning *Legionella*?
    A. Transmitted by water droplets, especially from water coolers
    B. Drug of choice is erythromycin
    C. Transmissible from person to person
    D. Older persons at greater risk

84. Which of the following is **NOT TRUE** concerning *Giardia lambia*?
   A. Humans are the main reservoirs
   B. Day care centers are commonly affected
   C. Transmitted by fecal oral route
   D. Amphotericin is the drug of choice

85. Which of the following is **TRUE** about staphylococcal food poisoning?
   A. Toxin is heat labile
   B. Onset is gradual
   C. Staphylococci are found in high concentrations in contaminated food
   D. Foods rich in protein and handled often are primarily affected (custards, cream fillings, and sliced meats)

86. Which is **NOT TRUE** of salmonella food poisoning?
   A. Incubation is usually 48–96 hours
   B. Diarrhea is present
   C. Primary source is raw meat and meat products
   D. Poultry is affected more than beef

87. The following drugs are effective against *Salmonella typhimurium* **EXCEPT**
   A. chloramphenicol
   B. ampicillin
   C. trimethaprim/sulfamethoxazole
   D. erythromycin

88. Which of the following do **NOT** contribute to *Clostridium perfringens* food poisoning?
   A. Cooking meat in large quantities
   B. Prolonged storage at room temperature
   C. Rapid cooling of food
   D. Inadequate reheating of food

89. Which of the following is **TRUE** concerning botulism?
   A. *Clostridium botulinum* is a gram-positive, aerobic bacillus
   B. Symptoms are caused by a preformed toxin
   C. The toxin is heat stable
   D. Most outbreaks are due to commercial canning

90. Which of the following is **NOT TRUE** concerning food poisoning from *Vibrio parahaemolyticus*?
   A. It is the leading cause of food poisoning in Japan
   B. Primary source is crustaceans from warm coastal waters
   C. Incubation time is about 2–4 hours
   D. It causes salmonellosislike symptoms

91. Which of the following are associated with seafood poisoning?
   A. *Vibrio parahaemolyticus*
   B. Ciguatera
   C. Red tide
   D. All of the above

92. Appropriate treatment of *Shigella* infections include all the following **EXCEPT**
   A. TMP/SMZ
   B. ampicillin
   C. norfloxacin
   D. antidiarrheal agents

93. The proper order of incidence (highest to lowest) of nosocomial infections is
   A. lower respiratory tract, urinary tract, surgical wound, bloodstream
   B. urinary tract, lower respiratory tract, surgical wound, bloodstream
   C. lower respiratory tract, urinary tract, bloodstream, surgical wound
   D. urinary tract, surgical wound, lower respiratory tract, bloodstream

Questions 94–96: Select the organism that **BEST** suits the description in the question. The answers may be used once, more than once, or not at all.

   A. *Legionella pneumonia*
   B. *Streptococcus pneumonia*
   C. Candida
   D. Enterococci

94. One of the top three nosocomial bloodstream pathogens _____

95. Causes sporadic and occasionally epidemic lower respiratory tract infections in certain hospitals _____

96. An important cause of bloodstream infections in patients on chemotherapy _____

Questions 97–98: Select the infection that **BEST** suits the description in the question. The answers may be used once, more than once, or not at all.

    A. *Haemophilus influenzae*
    B. Hepatitis A virus
    C. Cytomegalovirus
    D. *Shigella*

97. A symptomatic infection that affects children, day care staff, and close family _____

98. Inapparent in children attending day care facilities but likely to be significant in their adult contacts _____

99. Regarding epidemic typhus, all the following are true **EXCEPT**
    A. it is usually confined to remote areas of Africa
    B. overcrowding, poverty, and infrequent bathing are social factors
    C. fever, chills, and faint macular rash over the trunk are common
    D. erthromycin is usually curative and is the treatment of choice

100. Regarding scrub typhus, all the following are true **EXCEPT**
    A. mostly self-limiting if untreated
    B. seen in hot, wet tropical climates
    C. life cycle involves larval mites (chiggers)
    D. doxycycline is particularly reliable

101. Rickettsial infections are associated with all the following **EXCEPT**
    A. obligate intracellular parasite
    B. severe headaches, fever, myalgia, and rash
    C. trench fever and Brill-Zinnsser disease
    D. transmission to man is primarily by direct inoculation through biting

102. Which of the following is **MOST CLOSELY** associated with Q fever?
    A. Maculopapular rash
    B. Limited to the Western Hemisphere
    C. Insecticide spraying of cattle, sheep, and goats may be effective control
    D. Formaldehyde vaccine is commercially available

Questions 103–106: Match the disease named in the question with one of the following. The answers may be used once, more than once, or not at all.

    A. Human body louse
    B. No rash
    C. Western Hemisphere

103. Q fever _____

104. Trench fever _____

105. Rocky Mountain spotted fever _____

106. Select the **BEST** answer regarding human plague.
    A. Penicillin is effective and is the treatment of choice
    B. Fever, chills, and lymph node pain occur within 7 days
    C. Diagnosis is best made with serology
    D. Mode of transmission is fecal oral

107. The infected female *Anopheles* mosquito inoculates malarial sporozoites into a human while feeding. Within 30 minutes, these sporozoites
    A. enter RBCs
    B. enter hepatocytes
    C. become schizonts
    D. release merocytes

108. Ideally, the diagnosis of malaria in a febrile patient is confirmed by
    A. serology testing
    B. liver biopsy
    C. identification of malaria parasites on a blood smear (Giemsa stain)
    D. fever, chills, and sweats in a person with no prior exposure to the parasite

109. Which of the following species of *Plasmodium* causes the **MOST** deaths?
    A. *P. falciparum*
    B. *P. vivax*
    C. *P. malariae*
    D. *P. ovale*

110. Placental malaria infection is commonly associated with each of the following **EXCEPT**
    A. severe anemia
    B. low birth weight
    C. premature birth
    D. toxemia

111. The most drug-resistant malarial parasites in the world are currently found in
    A. sub-Sahara Africa
    B. the region of Thailand and Burma
    C. the Amazon region of Brazil
    D. the Middle East

112. Successful treatment of *Pneumocystis carinii* pneumonia in an HIV-positive patient will
    A. increase the prevalence of AIDS by increasing the incidence of AIDS
    B. increase the prevalence of AIDS by increasing the duration of AIDS
    C. not alter the prevalence of HIV in the community
    D. represent a form of tertiary prevention of *Pneumocystis carinii* pneumonia
    E. increase the incidence of AIDS

113. The risk of acquiring hepatitis A is measured by the
   A. incidence times the average duration of hepatitis A
   B. number of existing cases divided by the duration of hepatitis A
   C. incidence of Hepatitis A
   D. number of new cases of hepatitis A
   E. number of existing cases divided by the population at risk

Questions 114–116: In a community of 100,000 persons, there were 1000 existing cases of disease X at the beginning of 1993. During 1993, 100 new cases of this disease were diagnosed, while 500 persons died of disease X during the year. Assume that disease X is a nonrepeating chronic illness.

114. The annual prevalence of disease X for this population during 1993 was
   A. 75/100,000
   B. 101/100,000
   C. 500/100,000
   D. 1000/100,000
   E. 1100/100,000

115. The risk for disease X for this population during 1993 was
   A. 75/100,000
   B. 101/100,000
   C. 500/100,000
   D. 1000/100,000
   E. 1100/100,000

116. The risk of death from disease X for this population during 1993 was
   A. 75/100,000
   B. 101/100,000
   C. 500/100,000
   D. 1000/100,000
   E. 1100/100,000

Questions 117–120: Match the following with the descriptions in the questions. Each choice may be used only once.

    A. Infectivity
    B. Pathogenicity
    C. Viability
    D. Virulence

117. The propensity for *Neisseria meningitides* to produce severe and fatal disease _____

118. The capacity of the HIV virus to survive in a defined environment outside the human body _____

119. The capacity of the *Influenza* virus to enter, survive, and multiply inside a host _____

120. The capacity of toxigenic *E. coli* to produce the functional, morphologic, and pathologic changes that cause symptomatic disease _____

121. An example of fomite transmission of a disease-producing agent would be transmission from
    A. clothing contaminated by body lice
    B. dust particles contaminated by rhinovirus
    C. mountain spring water contaminated by *Giardia*
    D. bite of mosquito infected by *Plasmodium vivax*
    E. food contaminated by *Staphylococcus*

Questions 122–125: Match the following choices with the descriptions in the questions. Each choice may be used only once.

    A. Cross-sectional
    B. Case control
    C. Ecologic
    D. Cohort

122. An investigation evaluated the association between the incidence of pancreatic cancer and the sale of beef among South American countries. _____

123. A research team follows 1200 HIV-positive patients at an outpatient clinic over three years to determine the incidence of cerebral toxoplasmosis. _____

124. Urine samples were collected from 29,000 pregnant women admitted for delivery to 202 hospitals throughout the state for determination of maternal alcohol and drug use at the time of the infants' delivery. _____

125. Medical records of 73 people with hepatitis B were reviewed to determine if there is an association between their previous vaccination status and their chances of contracting hepatitis B. _____

126. Specificity is the probability that a person
   A. with latent syphilis will have a reactive RPR
   B. without syphilis will have a reactive RPR
   C. without syphilis will have a nonreactive RPR
   D. with syphilis will have a false positive RPR
   E. with syphilis has a reactive RPR

Public Health and Preventive Medicine

Answer Key

1. B	25. C	49. B	73. A
2. C	26. C	50. C	74. B
3. C	27. C	51. B	75. B
4. B	28. D	52. B	76. C
5. A	29. A	53. B	77. C
6. A	30. B	54. B	78. A
7. C	31. D	55. B	79. D
8. C	32. A	56. A	80. C
9. B	33. B	57. B	81. C
10. B	34. C	58. B	82. D
11. A	35. B	59. D	83. C
12. B	36. C	60. B	84. D
13. B	37. D	61. A	85. D
14. A	38. B	62. B	86. A
15. D	39. A	63. C	87. D
16. A	40. C	64. A	88. C
17. A	41. C	65. B	89. B
18. D	42. B	66. A	90. C
19. B	43. A	67. A	91. D
20. C	44. C	68. C	92. D
21. A	45. B	69. A	93. D
22. D	46. A	70. B	94. D
23. A	47. A	71. B	95. A
24. C	48. B	72. B	96. C

97. D	105. C	113. C	121. A
98. B	106. B	114. E	122. C
99. D	107. B	115. B	123. D
100. A	108. C	116. C	124. A
101. D	109. A	117. D	125. B
102. C	110. D	118. C	126. C
103. B	111. B	119. A	
104. A	112. B	120. B	

Public Health and Preventive Medicine

Answers and Comments

1. **(B)** Motor vehicle accidents are a leading cause of death for children age 2 years and above. Most such fatalities would be preventable by the use of a car seat. Counseling parents regarding the use of a car seat as well as safety belts for older children, is an important preventive measure. (**Ref. 2,** pp. xxxix–xlv)

2. **(C)** A serum total cholesterol is indicated every five years, starting by age 35 years or earlier. The other preventive measures listed are recommended by some major authorities, starting after age 50, except for urinalysis, which is recommended to start after age 60. (**Ref. 8,** p. 163)

3. **(C)** For a slender caucasian female who is postmenstrual, there is an increased risk of osteoporosis. It is thus appropriate to discuss estrogen replacement therapy with her and ask about possible contraindications (e.g., history of breast cancer or active liver disease). Another important measure would be discussion of an exercise program. The other measures listed could be helpful in certain specific populations but are not needed in her case. (**Ref. 2,** pp. 239–242)

4. **(B)** Treatment of a disease that is already present, to reduce the severity of its consequences, is secondary prevention. Antiviral

therapy for AIDS is direct treatment of the disease and thus is secondary prevention. Tertiary prevention would be limitation of disability through rehabilitation. (**Ref. 5,** pp. 4–5, 119; **Ref. 10,** pp. 56–57)

5. **(A)** Treatment that prevents the development of a disease is primary prevention. Treating a person with AIDS using trimethoprim-sulfamethoxazole is intended to prevent *Pneumocystis carinii* pneumonia. Thus, it is a primary preventive measure for pneumonia and a tertiary prevention for AIDS. (**Ref. 5,** pp. 4–5; **Ref. 10,** pp. 56–57)

6. **(A)** The CBR uses all births as the numerator and the total population, regardless of gender or age, as the denominator. The general fertility rate (GFR) also uses all births as the numerator but is based on a denominator comprising all women of childbearing age, most often defined as women 15 to 44 years of age. The age-specific fertility rate (ASFR) is calculated using births to women in a specific age interval as the numerator and women in the same age interval as the denominator. The total fertility rate (TFR) is the sum of all the age-specific fertility rates by single years of age. (**Ref. 5,** p. 43)

7. **(C)** Fertility, in its most specific sense, refers to the actual birth of living offspring. Fecundity is the capacity to bear children, and fecundability is the probability of conceiving in a given month. (**Ref. 5,** p. 44)

8. **(C)** Life expectancy in the world is generally increasing. In recent years, Japan has become the country with the highest life expectancy at birth for males reaching 73.8 years in 1981 and 75.5 years in 1986, among 40 nations for which current information is available. (**Ref. 5,** p. 48)

9. **(B)** The movement of people to cities (urbanization) is one of the dominant characteristics of population change in the twentieth century. At the beginning of the century, fewer than one out of every seven persons in the world lived in a city. As we near the year 2000, more than 40% of the world's population is found in urban areas. (**Ref. 5,** p. 51)

10. **(B)** With birth rates having apparently held steady during most of human history, we must look to decreases in death rates to explain why growth rates have shot up the last 200 years. This is mainly due to improvements in public sanitation, advances in agriculture, and the control of infectious diseases, which have resulted in a decline in death rates, particularly with regard to infant and child mortality. (**Ref. 7**, p. 52)

11. **(A)** The highest percentage of people under 15 is indicative of the explosive growth potential of most developing nations. In most developing nations this percentage is 40 to 50%. By contrast, the percentage under 15 in most industrialized countries is 20 to 30%. (**Ref. 7**, p. 59)

12. **(B)** Since birth rates represent additions to a population and death rates represent subtractions, a change in population size is represented by the difference between the two, i.e., by the growth rate of that population. Growth rates can be calculated simply by subtracting the death rate from the birth rate, and they are normally expressed as a percent, not per 1000 as in birth and death rates. (**Ref. 7**, p. 48)

13. **(B)** Enterotoxigenic *Escherichia coli* (*E. coli*) is the most likely etiology. It is the most common cause of diarrhea in travelers. The diarrhea is usually characterized by watery consistency and abdominal cramping. Vomiting and high temperatures are unusual. Diarrhea usually lasts one to eight days and is usually self-limited. (**Ref. 3**, pp. 531–533; **Ref. 5**, p. 62)

14. **(A)** Prophylaxis with trimethoprim-sulfamethoxazole can prevent this diarrhea. However, usually this illness is self-limited and requires only hydration and rest. The problem associated with widespread use of antibiotic prophylaxis can lead to resistance. Pepto-Bismol has been shown to lessen the duration and severity of diarrhea associated with *Escherichia coli*. (**Ref. 5**, p. 162)

15. **(D)** When traveling to countries where the water is unsafe, it is necessary to carry one's own water or use only water that has been purified for drinking. Chlorine tablets can be taken on such trips to accomplish this purpose. Water can also be purified by adding 2–4 drops of 5% chlorine bleach or by adding 5–10 drops of 2%

tincture of iodine. Boiling water is an even better purifying method. (**Ref. 5,** pp. 62, 179)

16. **(A)** Yellow fever vaccination is required for travel to tropical Africa and to Central and South America. This vaccination provides protection for ten years. Vaccination for smallpox is no longer necessary since it has been eradicated, the last case being seen in October 1977. Meningococcal vaccination is recommended during the seasons it is most likely to be transmitted in those parts where transmission is possible (Saudi Arabia, Nepal, etc.). Japanese encephalitis is recommended for travel to high-risk areas in rural Asia. (**Ref. 5,** pp. 60–61)

17. **(A)** Hemorrhagic colitis has been associated with the *Escherichia coli* strain 0156:H7. Hemolytic uremic syndrome has also been associated with *Shigella dysenteriae* and *Salmonella typhimurium.* Disseminated *Yersinia* infection can be associated with meningitis and osteomyelitis. (**Ref. 1,** p. 76)

18. **(D)** In general, pregnant travelers should avoid live vaccines. Included among the live vaccines are measles, mumps, and rubella (MMR); yellow fever; oral polio vaccine (OPV); and oral typhoid. The MMR is an absolute contraindication during pregnancy. The injectable form of the polio vaccine (IPV) is the preferred vaccine against polio during pregnancy. However, if immediate protection is needed, the oral vaccine is permissible. Injectable typhoid is permitted if the risk justifies it. Vaccinating the mother against tetanus also affords protection to the unborn fetus. It is preferred to delay vaccination until the second or third trimester. As an aside, hepatitis B vaccine can also be administered to a pregnant patient. (**Ref. 1,** p. 76)

19. **(B)** In general for HIV patients and other immunocompromised patients, the live vaccines are to be avoided. However, in the case of measles, mumps, and rubella (MMR), it is thought that the risks outweigh the benefits as measles can be so devastating in these patient. (**Ref. 5,** p. 68)

20. **(C)** The measles, mumps, and rubella (MMR) vaccine would not be appropriate for the six-month visit but rather is given after 12 to 15 months. Prior to this time, the infant is protected by

maternal antibodies (passive immunity), and the vaccine would be inactivated. (**Ref. 12,** pp. 43, 44)

21. **(A)** Typhoid can be common among young children, but they usually have mild cases. The importance of vaccination increases as access to reasonable medical care decrease. The injectable form of the typhoid vaccine would be more beneficial for HIV-positive persons. (**Ref. 12,** pp. 105–111)

22. **(D)** Immune globulin can be given either two weeks after measles or MMR immunization, or six weeks (preferably three months) before MMR immunization. Immune globulin should be given with caution to persons with an allergy or sensitivity to mercury or thimerosal. Intramuscular injections should be avoided when possible in patients with coagulation disorders, platelet defects, or thrombocytopenia. Immune globulin can be given with yellow fever and oral polio vaccines. (**Ref. 12,** pp. 83–85)

23. **(A)** Measles is not contraindicated for HIV-positive persons. It is felt that the disease manifestations of measles in these persons far outweigh the risks. However, in people with congenital immunodeficiency, the MMR is contraindicated. Persons born prior to 1957 probably have a natural immunity from previous infection. The MMR is always contraindicated in pregnancy. (**Ref. 12,** pp. 42–47)

24. **(C)** Measles is more common in children but not more severe. The risk of complications is highest among the very young or the very old. The incubation period for measles is 10 to 12 days. Usually the first symptoms are fever and malaise, followed by cough, coryza, and conjunctivitis. (**Ref. 3,** pp. 825–826)

25. **(C)** All the mentioned strategies are useful; however, the most successful has been the enactment and enforcement of school immunization laws. Passive immunity is associated with the newborn period up to about 12 months and is conferred by maternal antibodies. (**Ref. 5,** p. 65)

26. **(C)** The World Health Organization makes yearly recommendations to the Centers for Disease Control and Prevention. It is necessary to do this often because of the changing strains.

Influenza A epidemics are more common than B epidemics, hence the 2 A strains and 1 B strain. Guillain-Barré has not been observed in association with influenza vaccines since 1976. (**Ref. 5,** p. 84)

27. **(C)** Efforts to control influenza in the United States have been most successful with two methods: vaccination and chemoprophylaxis with amantidine. (**Ref. 5,** p. 84)

28. **(D)** Varicella has been known to spread by all the routes mentioned; however, blood-borne is not one of the most common methods. (**Ref. 5,** p. 91)

29. **(A)** Chemoprophylaxis with rifampin is given to household contacts less than two years of age patients with *Haemophilus influenzae*. Both a three-stage and a two-stage vaccination with subsequent boosters are available. Immunization for *Haemophilus influenzae* usually begins at the two-month visit in a normal healthy infant. Aggressive treatment with chloramphenicol and ampicillin is preferable in the case of life-threatening illnesses (e.g., meningitis, epiglottitis). (**Ref. 5,** pp. 86, 87)

30. **(B)** Ninety-five percent of *Haemophilus influenzae* meningitis cases occur in children less than 5 years of age. Peak incidence is in children 6 to 7 months old. The incidence is lowest in the summer and peaks in the fall and spring. The incidence of *H. influenzae* is three times higher in the African-American population than the white population. (**Ref. 5,** p. 86)

31. **(D)** *Streptococcal pneumoniae* is the most common cause of community-acquired bacterial pneumonia. It is also responsible for most cases of otitis media. *Pneumococcus, Neisseria,* and *Haemophilus* are the most common causes of meningitis. The case fatality ratio for meningitis secondary to pneumococcus is high in persons over 40 years of age. (**Ref. 5,** p. 87)

32. **(A)** The "three-day measles," or rubella, is characterized by a relatively mild maculopapular rash that lasts three days or less. The rash begins on the face and spreads downward. Contraction of rubella during the first trimester is particularly dangerous and may result in numerous congenital abnormalities of the fetus. Possible

cardiac manifestations included are patent ductus arteriosus, pulmonary stenosis, and myocardial necrosis. (**Ref. 5,** pp. 70–71)

33. **(B)** Precocious puberty has been associated with congenital rubella infection, as has diabetes mellitus, growth retardation, and growth hormone deficiency. (**Ref. 5,** p. 71)

34. **(C)** The most effective strategy for the prevention and control of pertussis is active immunization. This highly contagious infection has a secondary attack rate of close to 90%. (**Ref. 5,** p. 75)

35. **(B)** Pneumonia is the most common cause of mortality in adults. Sepsis and encephalitis are also common causes of mortality in children. (**Ref. 5,** p. 90)

36. **(C)** Bacillus Calmette-Guerin vaccine is absolutely contraindicated for patients with HIV. Measles, mumps, rubella vaccine is preferred to risking measles infection. Pneumococcal and tetanus vaccines are also permissible. (**Ref. 9,** Vol. 40, No. RR-12, 1991, p. 59)

37. **(D)** Immune globulin is appropriate for HIV-positive travelers. The injectable form of the polio vaccine is preferable to the live, oral form. Yellow fever vaccination is also not recommended except in the case of substantial risk in an HIV-positive patient. The bacillus Calmette-Guerin vaccine is never indicated for HIV-positive patients. (**Ref. 12**)

38. **(B)** Rubella vaccine virus is the only one to be isolated from breast milk. However, this should not be considered a contraindication for immunization in the postnatal period. There has been no indication that babies receiving breast milk from mother immunized against rubella have been harmed. (**Ref. 9,** Vol. 38, No. 13, 1989)

39. **(A)** Breast feeding, diarrhea, and prematurity are not contraindications to receiving the oral polio vaccine. However, persons with household contacts who are immunocompromised should not receive the oral polio vaccine. (**Ref. 12**)

40. **(C)** A significantly elevated temperature should be considered a precaution when considering DPT vaccination. A family history of

convulsions, sudden infant death syndrome, or prematurity should not be considered a precaution to administering DPT vaccine. (**Ref. 12**)

41. **(C)** Barrier methods and total abstinence from sexual activity are the major modes of primary prevention. Contact tracing and subsequent treatment also contribute to primary prevention. Screening programs have their best efficacy in high-risk populations only. (**Ref. 5, pp. 108, 109**)

42. **(B)** Syphilis in all its stages is curable even today with penicillin. Treatment of syphilis may reduce possible concurrent transmission of other sexually transmitted diseases (e.g., HIV). During the last half of the 1980s, the incidence of primary and secondary syphilis increased dramatically. This was reflected most strongly in the low-income, minority, heterosexual populations. (**Ref. 5, pp. 102, 103**)

43. **(A)** There was an overall decrease in the incidence of gonorrhea in the U.S. population from 1975 to 1989 of approximately 30%. This decrease was thought to be secondary to a reduction in high-risk sexual practices of white Americans. Unfortunately, this message is not reaching the inner city, teenager/adolescent, minority population, since transmission rates in this group are increasing. (**Ref. 5, p. 104**)

44. **(C)** In 1976, clinically significant PPNG became evident. The three classes of drugs now less effective are tetracyclines, penicillins, and aminoglycosides (especially spectinomycin). The recommendations for treatment of gonococcal infections tend now towards third-generation cephalosporins. (**Ref. 5, p. 104**)

45. **(B)** *Chlamydia trachomonas* is the cause of the most common sexually transmitted bacterial genital infection. (**Ref. 5, p. 104**)

46. **(A)** Plasmid-mediated resistance has become an increasing problem with gonococcal therapy with tetracyclines. (**Ref. 5, p. 104**)

47. **(A)** Chromosomally mediated resistance has contributed to treatment failure of gonococcal infections with penicillins and tetracyclines. (**Ref. 5, p. 104**)

48. **(B)** The etiology of initial onset of multiple painful genital lesions of a sexually transmitted origin is herpes simplex virus-2. (**Ref. 5,** p. 105)

49. **(B)** Viral isolation of HSV-2 from tissue culture is the definitive method for identification of this viral infection. The yield is further increased if this is a primary infection and when the lesions are vesicular (as opposed to ulcerative). Presumptive diagnosis can be made from the tanck preparation in the office setting. Darkfield examination technique establishes the definitive diagnosis of *Treponema pallidum* infection. Fluorescent monoclonal antibody strain helps establish the diagnosis of *Chlamydia trachomatis*. (**Ref. 5,** p. 111)

50. **(C)** Squamous cell carcinoma of the cervix has been strongly associated with HSV-2 infection. Anal, vaginal, and vulvar carcinoma have been linked to papilloma virus. (**Ref. 5,** p. 108)

51. **(B)** Aseptic meningitis has been associated with HSV-2 infection. Epididymitis has been associated with *Neisseria gonorrheae* and *Chlamydia trachomatis*. Penile carcinoma has been linked to human papilloma virus. Prostatitis may be linked to *N. gonorrheae*. (**Ref. 5,** p. 100)

52. **(B)** Acyclovir is still the treatment of choice to lessen morbidity and possible recurrences of HSV-2 clinical manifestations. (**Ref. 5,** p. 112)

53. **(B)** In patients having HSV-2 antibodies, only one in three ever noticed having symptoms related to HSV-2 infection. And in patients with primary HSV-2, 75% of their sexual contacts never noticed any genital lesions. HSV-2 is the leading cause of genital ulceration in the United States. (**Ref. 5,** pp. 105, 106)

54. **(B)** We are not yet able to determine HPV by viral culture. Detection of coilocytes on cytological smears, immunochemical strains, or nucleic acid sequences are the methods most often used. A fourth method includes determination of HPV infection by using polymerase chain reactions (PCR) from cervical smears. With the aid of this technique, HPV is being detected despite an otherwise normal Papanicolaou smear. (**Ref. 5,** pp. 106, 107)

55. (B) HPV can be transmitted in the absence of genital lesions or symptoms and probably occurs mostly under these circumstances. If appropriate follow-up is not done after a suspicious Papanicolaou smear, there could be progression to cervical carcinoma and possible death. (**Ref. 5,** pp. 106, 107)

56. (A) The U.S. vaccination program for the hepatitis B virus has traditionally focused on the vaccination of health care workers, institutionalized patients, and hemodialysis patients. However, these persons are not responsible for the majority of known HBV infection transmission. Most cases are transmitted through sexual contact or IV drug use. (**Ref. 5,** p. 107)

57. (B) Possible long-term effects associated with hepatitis B infection include chronic carrier status, fulminant hepatitis, chronic active hepatitis, and hepatocellular carcinoma. (**Ref. 5,** p. 107)

58. (B) Gonococcal infection during pregnancy has been associated with an increased risk of premature rupture of membranes, chorioamnionitis, and prematurity. Spontaneous abortion is also a possible outcome; however, this is mostly associated with primary herpes infection. (**Ref. 5,** p. 108)

59. (D) Concentrating on promoting safer sexual practices for high-risk groups is currently the most cost-effective. Caesarean delivery and prenatal screening are not currently considered to be cost-effective. Reducing the duration of infectivity would not be considered to be reliable at this time. (**Ref. 5,** pp. 108, 109)

60. (B) Human papilloma virus has been associated with several neoplasms including vulvar, anal, and cervical. Testicular cancer is not associated with HPV infection. (**Ref. 5,** p. 101)

61. (A) Penile cancer has been strongly associated with human papilloma virus. (**Ref. 5,** p. 101)

62. (B) Hepatocellular carcinoma has been strongly associated with hepatitis B infection. (**Ref. 5,** p. 101)

63. (C) Non-Hodgkins lymphoma has been linked to human immunodeficiency virus infection. (**Ref. 5,** p. 101)

64. **(A)** Human papilloma virus has been strongly associated with anal carcinoma. (**Ref. 5,** p. 101)

65. **(B)** *Chlamydia trachomatis* is the most likely sexually transmitted disease associated with the triad of urethritis, conjunctivitis, and arthritis. This syndrome is called Reiter's syndrome. (**Ref. 5,** p. 100)

66. **(A)** The treatment of choice for *Chlamydia trachomatis* is doxycycline. Tetracycline is also an alternative. Metronidazole is the treatment of choice for *Gardnerella vaginalis*. Penicillin is still the treatment for syphilis. Cephalosporins are becoming significant therapy for gonococcal infections. (**Ref. 5,** p. 112)

67. **(A)** Treatment for Reiter's syndrome is directed toward relief of symptoms. Nonsteroidal antiinflammatories and analgesics are used as with rheumatoid arthritis for inflammation and pain relief. However, systemic steroids are not used with Reiter's syndrome because of the fear that this would aggravate the dermatologic manifestations of the syndrome (e.g., keratoderma, blenorrhagica, and mucosal lesions). (**Ref. 3,** pp. 764–765)

68. **(C)** Both gonococcal arthritis and Reiter's syndrome are likely to be characterized by the presence of conjunctivitis. (**Ref. 3,** p. 556)

69. **(A)** Reiter's syndrome is most likely to be associated with the presence of balanitis. (**Ref. 3,** p. 556)

70. **(B)** Gonococcal arthritis is most likely to affect the upper extremities, while Reiter's syndrome is most likely to affect the lower extremities. (**Ref. 3,** p. 1689)

71. **(B)** Gonococcal arthritis responds to treatment with penicillin, while Reiter's syndrome is unresponsive to penicillin. (**Ref. 3,** p. 1689)

72. **(B)** AIDS is most frequently reported following an opportunistic infection. The opportunistic infection that occurs earliest would be the AIDS-defining illness. The most frequently reported AIDS-defining illness is *Pneumocystis carinii* pneumonia. (**Ref. 5,** p. 117; **Ref. 9,** Vol. 41, No. RR-17, 1992)

73. **(A)** A survey of seroprevalence in the New York area in 1985 revealed a seropositive rate of approximately 57% in intravenous drug users. However, the seropositive rate in child-bearing females was 14%. This latter group is thought to represent heterosexual transmission. (**Ref. 5,** p. 119)

74. **(B)** In parts of Southeast Asia, the incidence of AIDS among prostitutes is high. Safer sexual practices would be the most advantageous method to try to control the spread of human immunodeficiency infection in that region. (**Ref. 5,** p. 119)

75. **(B)** Although unintentional injuries, prematurity, and cancer are very common causes of years of potential life lost, HIV infection is increasing the fastest as the cause of years of potential life lost. (**Ref. 5,** p. 121)

76. **(C)** Invasive cervical carcinoma, CD4-positive T-lymphocyte count <200/UL or CD4-positive T-lymphocyte percentage of total lymphocytes <14, pulmonary tuberculosis, and recurrent pneumonia are all part of the revised classification system for HIV infection and expanded case definition for AIDS surveillance. Recurrent yeast infections may be an indication of HIV seropositivity in females; however, this is not a part of the expanded case definition. (**Ref. 9,** Vol. 41, No. RR-17, 1992)

77. **(C)** Squamous cell carcinoma of the anus has been associated with male homosexuality but not necessarily HIV infection. Kaposi's sarcoma, non-Hodgkins lymphoma, and invasive cervical carcinoma are neoplastic conditions that have been associated with HIV infection. (**Ref. 5,** p. 108)

78. **(A)** In 1993 the greatest risk factor associated with heterosexual HIV transmission was, of course, having a partner who was HIV-positive. The second most common risk factor was being the sexual partner of an intravenous drug user. (**Ref. 9,** Vol. 43, No. 9, 1994)

79. **(D)** Common symptoms include fever, malaise, chills, vomiting, headaches, and joint pain. Diarrhea is uncommon. (**Ref. 6,** pp. 173, 174)

80. **(C)**   Chloramphenicol is the drug of choice, but ampicillin, septra, and ciprofloxacin are all acceptable alternatives. (**Ref. 6,** p. 175)

81. **(C)**   Vibrio cholera is caused by a gram-negative bacteria. Symptoms are caused by a protein endotoxin that turns on the adenylate cyclase and increases electrolyte secretion into the intestinal lumen. Symptoms include rice water stools and vomiting. It can be fatal in hours, and rehydration and electrolyte replacement are crucial. Water is the primary vehicle of infection. Bloody diarrhea is not usual for vibrio cholera. (**Ref. 6,** pp. 176–178)

82. **(D)**   *Giardia lambia* is a protozoan. (**Ref. 6,** pp. 186, 187)

83. **(C)**   There is no evidence that *Legionella* is transmissible from person to person. (**Ref. 6,** pp. 181–183)

84. **(D)**   The drug of choice for the treatment of *Giardia lambia* is Flagyl (metronidazole). (**Ref. 6,** pp. 186–188)

85. **(D)**   The cause of staphylococcal food poisoning is *Staphylococcus aureus,* which produces five heat-stable enterotoxins. Incubation period is two to four hours. Onset of nausea, vomiting, abdominal cramps, and salivation is abrupt. Staphylococci are found in low concentrations in contaminated food. (**Ref. 6,** pp. 194, 195)

86. **(A)**   *Salmonella* is a gram-negative bacillus. Common signs and symptoms include diarrhea, abdominal cramps, fever, headaches, nausea, vomiting. Incubation is usually 6 to 48 hours. The source of contamination is usually raw meat and meat products, dairy products, and eggs. Prevention is by proper food handling, storage of food, and hand washing. (**Ref. 6,** pp. 195, 196)

87. **(D)**   The drug of choice is chloramphenicol. Patients with cholelithiasis often need cholecystectomy to eliminate carriage of *S. typhimurium.* (**Ref. 6,** p. 195, **Ref. 13,** p. 263)

88. **(C)**   *Clostridium perfringens* is an anaerobic, gram-positive bacilli that is spore-forming. It produces both heat-stable and heat-labile spores. Of the five toxicological types, A and C cause

human gastroenteritis. Common symptoms include abdominal cramps and diarrhea with occasional nausea. Fever and vomiting are usually absent. The incubation period is 6 to 24 hours. (**Ref. 6,** pp. 195, 196)

89. **(B)** *Clostridium botulinum* is a gram-positive, anaerobic, spore-forming bacillus. The spores are ubiquitous and worldwide. Symptoms are caused by a preformed toxin. The toxin prevents the release of acetylcholine and interrupts the transmission of nerve impulses. The result is flaccid paralysis. The toxin is heat-labile, and 90% of outbreaks are due to home canning. (**Ref. 6,** pp. 196, 197)

90. **(C)** The incubation time is about 12 hours. (**Ref. 6,** p. 198)

91. **(D)** *Vibrio parahaemolyticus* is one of the leading causes of food-borne disease in Japan. Crustaceans from warm coastal marine waters are primarily affected. Ciguatera toxin is produced by dinoflagellates attached to algae on coral reefs. Fish eat the algae and concentrate the toxin. Paralytic shell fish poisoning is caused by ingestion of toxic dinoflagellates of the *Gonyaulax* species. Mollusks (mussels and clams) concentrate the neurotoxin saxitoxin. The toxic dinoflagellates bloom and cause "red tide." (**Ref. 6,** p. 198)

92. **(D)** Antidiarrheal agents are contraindicated, because they prolong symptoms and increase the chance of bacteremia. (**Ref. 13,** p. 263)

93. **(D)** Urinary tract infections (UTIs) are the most common hospital-acquired infections, accounting for about one-third of all nosocomial infections. Surgical wound infections are the second most common, then lower respiratory tract infections, and finally bloodstream infections. (**Ref. 5,** pp. 203–205)

94. **(D)** Gram-positive organisms including coagulase-negative staphylococci, *Staphylococcus aureus,* and the enterococci account for most nosocomial bloodstream infections. (**Ref. 5,** p. 205)

95. **(A)** *Legionella pneumophila* causes sporadic and occasionally epidemic lower respiratory tract infections in some hospitals. The organisms are spread through air conditioning units. (**Ref. 5,** p. 205)

96. (C) Chemotherapy, because of its immunosuppressive effects, predisposes individuals to a wide variety of infections. One of the most serious types is candidal bloodstream infections. These infections are associated with a significantly high mortality rate compared to other bloodstream infections. (**Ref. 5,** p. 205)

97. (D) Shigella is easily transmitted by close person-to-person contact among children and by environmental contamination caused by children who are not toilet-trained. (**Ref. 5,** p. 209)

98. (B) Hepatitis A is spread by the fecal oral route, with transmission occurring between household and sexual contacts. Hepatitis A can also be spread through contact with contaminated fomites. It can survive on environmental surfaces for at least one month. Hepatitis A is typically a mild illness in young children but can cause substantial morbidity in adults. (**Ref. 5,** p. 209)

99. (D) Epidemic typhus has disappeared from much of the world except remote areas of Africa, Asia, Central and South America. After an incubation period of two weeks, there is an abrupt onset of fever, chills, malaise, muscle aches, and severe headaches. Approximately five days later, a faint pink macular rash usually develops over the trunk. Tetracycline or chloramphenicol is usually curative if given early. Certain social factors that predispose to epidemic typhus, including overcrowding, poverty, and infrequent bathing or changing of clothes, are especially common during cold weather or periods of war. (**Ref. 5,** p. 233)

100. (A) Scrub typhus, also known as tsutsugamushi disease, Japanese river fever, or tropical typhus, was first described in sixteenth century China, and its ancient name means chigger fever. Most infections are mild to moderate in severity. Significant morbidity occurs regularly, however, and mortality rates range from 0 to 30% if untreated. Larval mites (chiggers) are the vectors and reservoirs. It is especially common in tropical and subtropical areas, including rain forests, riverbanks, and sea shores. Doxycycline appears to be particularly reliable, and relapses are rare following its use. (**Ref. 5,** p. 234)

101. (D) Transmission to man is through vector feces contaminating the bite wound or other skin breaks. Most of the rickettsioses are characterized by the syndrome of severe headache, fever, myalgia, and rash of a specific pattern. There is no rash with Q fever. The rickettsia are obligate intracellular parasites that can propagate only in living cells. Serology is the mainstay of laboratory diagnosis. Epidemic typhus, scrub and murine typhus, Brill-Zinnsser disease, Q fever, and trench fever are all included in the rickettsial diseases of man. Epidemic typhus is usually cured by tetracycline or chloramphenicol, and recovery is complete with immunity to reinfection. However, it may recur decades later as Brill-Zinnsser disease, which is usually milder with little or no rash. (**Ref. 5,** pp. 231–235)

102. (C) Q fever is essentially worldwide in distribution, although it is uncommon in the United States. After an incubation period of two to four weeks, fever, headache, malaise, weakness, and weight loss may last a few days or weeks, but no rash occurs. Domestic animals, including cattle, sheep, and goats, are the main source of human illness. Location of dairy and other livestock operations away from population centers, disinfection, and appropriate disposal of infected animal tissues and regular spraying of cattle, sheep, and goats for control of ectoparasites may be effective. A formaldehyde vaccine is available commercially for the epidemic typhus, but none is available for Q fever. (**Ref. 5,** p. 236)

103. (B) Q fever has no rash. (**Ref. 5,** pp. 235–236)

104. (A) The natural life cycle of *Rochalimaea quintana* (formerly *Rickettsia*) (trench fever) involves man and the human body louse. (**Ref. 5,** pp. 235–236)

105. (C) Rocky Mountain spotted fever and Q fever are important tick-borne typhus diseases. Rocky Mountain spotted fever has been recognized as a distinct entity in the United States and Canada since the late 1800s. (**Ref. 5,** pp. 235–236)

106. (B) The classic form of *Y. pestis* infection in humans is bubonic plague. Other clinical forms (septicemia, pneumonic, meningeal) usually occur as complications of bubonic plague. In addition to flea bites, entry sites can include mucus membranes of the eye and oropharynx as well as broken skin. Within two to seven days of exposure, the onset of illness is heralded by fever, chills, and pain in the area of lymph nodes, and eventually lymph node enlargement (bubo). It is best diagnosed by a culture of material aspirated from a fluctuant bubo. The penicillins are not effective against *Y. pestis*. The most effective antibiotic is streptomycin. (**Ref. 5,** pp. 238, 239)

107. (**B**)   Thirty minutes after malaria sporozoites are inoculated into a human, they enter hepatocytes, initiating the exoerythrocytic stage of development. Primary tissue schizogony of parasites takes 7 to 15 days in the liver. The schizonts then rupture, and the resulting merozoites enter RBCs. The RBC schizogenic cycle leads to maturation of the parasites, with ring stage parasites becoming schizonts; these rupture and release merozoites into the bloodstream. These invade RBCs, and the erythrocytic cycle is continued. (**Ref. 5,** p. 240)

108. (**C**)   The classic malaria illness occurs in a person with no prior exposure to the parasite, who experiences fever, chills, sweats, headaches, back pain, and malaise. Ideally the diagnosis of malaria in a febrile patient is confirmed by the identification of malaria parasites on a blood smear. (**Ref. 5,** p. 240)

109. (**A**)   *P. falciparum* causes the most severe form of the disease, often with neurologic manifestations, renal failure, hemolytic anemia, hypoglycemia, and acute pulmonary edema. (**Ref. 5,** p. 240)

110. (**D**)   Malaria in pregnancy is associated with low birth weight, anemia, acute pulmonary edema, still birth, premature labor, hypoglycemia, and fetal distress. (**Ref. 3,** p. 285)

111. (**B**)   On the borders of Thailand, mefloquine resistance in *P. falciparum* has increased rapidly over the past five years. These regions contain the most drug-resistant parasites in the world and in the past have acted as harbingers of resistance patterns elsewhere in the tropics. The management of multidrug resistant infections is difficult; quinine and tetracycline remain effective, but compliance with the seven-day regimen is poor. (**Ref. 4,** 1994, p. 170:971–7)

112. (**B**)   Successful secondary prevention measures have no direct effect on disease incidence. Instead, secondary prevention can

alter prevalence by changing the duration of disease. Secondary prevention measures for otherwise fatal diseases can increase prevalence by increasing duration when treatment prevents death but does not offer a cure. (**Ref. 10,** pp. 56–57)

113. **(C)** Incidence measures risk of a disease within a defined population and time period. The terms *risk* and *cumulative incidence* are frequently used synonymously in the health literature. (**Ref. 10,** pp. 22–23)

114. **(E); 115. (B); 116. (C)** The annual prevalence of X is computed using the number of existing cases of disease during 1993 (old and new cases = 1100) as the numerator and the entire population at the beginning of the year as the denominator. The risk of disease X is the annual incidence of disease X during 1993 and is equal to the number of new cases of disease X (100) divided by the population at risk at the beginning of the year (100,000 minus the 1000 existing cases); so it is 100 divided by 99,000, or 101. Risk of death, or mortality proportion, is deaths from a specific cause divided by the population at risk of death from that cause at the beginning of the time period. (**Ref. 10,** pp. 22, 42, 43, 51)

117. **(D); 118. (C); 119. (A); 120. (B)** *Viability* is the capacity of an agent to survive in a defined environment outside the host. *Virulence* is the propensity of an agent to produce severe and fatal disease. *Pathogenicity* is the property of an agent that determines the extent to which overt disease is produced in an infected population, i.e., the capacity of an agent to produce the functional, morphologic, and pathologic changes that cause symptomatic disease. *Infectivity* is the agent characteristic that embodies capability to enter, survive, and multiply in the host. (**Ref. 10,** p. 89)

121. **(A)** A fomite is an article that conveys infection to others because it has been contaminated by pathogenic organisms. Examples include a handkerchief, drinking glass, door handle, clothing, and toys. (**Ref. 10,** p. 89)

122. **(C); 123. (D); 124. (A); 125. (B)** Ecologic studies use groups as the unit of comparison, rather than individuals, when assessing relationships between two or more characteristics (e.g., cancer and sale of beef). The "ecologic fallacy" occurs when bias is intro-

duced by assuming than an inference that is observed at the group level also applies to the individual. Cross-sectional studies simultaneously evaluate exposure and outcome in a population. Observational studies can be categorized as cohort or case control. In a case control study, the risk of exposure to a cause by those with a health problem (cases) is compared with the risk of exposure of those who do not have the health problem (controls). It is a retrospective study, where outcomes that are rare or that have a long latency or incubation period are studied. Cohort studies begin with a case group made up of individuals exposed to the hypothesized cause of a health problem. The comparison group is one that is not exposed, but has similar demographic, behavioral, and biological characteristics. The groups are compared and characterized according to the rates at which the health problem occurs in each group. (**Ref. 5,** pp. 24–25)

126. (**C**) Specificity is the probability that a person not having a disease will test negative on a test for that disease. (**Ref. 10,** p. 238)

References

1. Centers for Disease Control and Prevention: *Health Information for International Travel,* HHS publication no. 93-8280. Atlanta, GA, Department of Health and Human Services—Public Health Service, August 1973.

2. Fisher M (ed): *Guide to Clinical Preventive Services* (Report of the U.S. Preventive Services Task Force). Baltimore, MD, Williams & Wilkins, 1989.

3. *Harrison's Principles of Internal Medicine,* 12th ed. New York, McGraw-Hill, 1990.

4. *Journal of Infectious Disease.* 1994.

5. Last JM, Wallace RB (eds): *Maxcy-Rosenau-Last Public Health and Preventive Medicine,* 3rd ed. Norwalk, CT, Appleton & Lange, 1992.

6. Last JM, Wallace RB: *Public Health and Preventive Medicine,* 3rd ed. Norwalk, CT, Appleton & Lange, 1992.

7. Nadakavukaren A: *Man and Environment,* 3rd ed. Prospect Heights, IL, Wadeland Press.

8. McGinnis MJ (ed): *The Clinician's Handbook of Preventive Services.* U.S. Department of Health and Human Services, Public Health Service, Office of Disease Prevention and Health Promotion, Washington, DC, 1994.

9. *MMWR,* Vol. 40, No. RR-12, 1991.

10. Morgan JW: *Concise Epidemiology,* 3rd ed. Bryn Mawr, CA, MDM Consulting, 1994.

11. Nadakavukaren A: *Our Global Environment, a Health Perspective,* 4th ed. Prospect Heights, IL, Waveland Press, Inc., 1995.

12. *Travel and Routine Immunizations: A Practical Guide for the Medical Office.* Shoreland Medical Marketing, Inc., 1994.

13. Woodley M, Whelan A: *The Washington Manual.* Boston, Little Brown and Co., 1992.

COMPREHENSIVE

Go, *First Aid for the USMLE Step 2*, 150 pp., paperback, A2591-4

Goldberg, *The Instant Exam Review for the USMLE Step 2, 2/e*, 250 pp., paperback, A4328-0

Catlin, *A&L Review for the USMLE Step 2, 2/e*, 287 pp., paperback, A0266-5

INTERNAL MEDICINE

Goldlist, *A&L Review of Internal Medicine*, 275 pp., paperback, A0251-7

OBSTETRICS & GYNECOLOGY

Julian, *A&L Review of Obstetrics and Gynecology, 5/e*, 416 pp., paperback, A0231-9

PEDIATRICS

Hansbarger, *MEPC: Pediatrics, 9/e*, 248 pp., paperback, A6223-0

Lorin, *A&L Review of Pediatrics, 5/e*, 222 pp., paperback, A0057-8

PUBLIC HEALTH

Hart, *MEPC: Preventive Medicine and Public Health*, 350 pp., paperback, A6319-6

Penalver, *Public Health and Preventive Medicine Review, 2/e*, 120 pp., paperback, E5936-9

SURGERY

Metzler, *MEPC: Surgery, 11/e*, 317 pp., paperback, A6195-0

Wapnick, *A&L Review of Surgery, 2/e*, 156 pp., paperback, A0220-2

See reverse side for more A&L review titles